Barbara Mertins / Renate Delucchi Danhier (eds.)

Diversity in Cognition

PETER LANG
Lausanne - Berlin - Bruxelles - Chennai - New York - Oxford

Library of Congress Cataloging-in-Publication Data
A CIP catalog record for this book has been applied for at the Library of Congress.

Bibliographic information published by the Deutsche Nationalbibliothek.
The German National Library lists this publication in the German National Bibliography; detailed bibliographic data is available on the Internet at http://dnb.d-nb.de.

ISSN 1434-6710
ISBN 978-3-631-90344-5 (Print)
E-ISBN 978-3-631-90345-2 (E-Book)
E-ISBN 978-3-631-90346-9 (E-PUB)
DOI 10.3726/b21118

Published by Peter Lang GmbH, Berlin, Deutschland

info@peterlang.com - www.peterlang.com

This publication has been peer reviewed.

Table of contents

Barbara Mertins

Introduction

The title of the book in your hands is *Diversity in Cognition*, a topic that has gained prominence in scientific, educational, and general discourse in the European and North American contexts. With the concept of inclusion replacing integration, diversity in thinking has become crucial in various settings of human life. While people differ in terms of appearance, gender, moral values, and other characteristics, it is worth examining from a cognitive point of view whether individuals from different cultures and linguistic backgrounds approach the external world from diverse perspectives. These ideas go back to Wilhelm von Humboldt who formulated in his book from 1836 (Humboldt 2009) that "language is the forming organ of thought" (German: *Sprache ist das bildende Organ des Gedanken*). Later on, at the beginning of the 20th century, Edward Sapir and Benjamin Lee Whorf as well as Franz Boas developed further the idea of language/grammar affecting human cognition and perception, and corroborated it with the first empirical data (Boas 1966; Sapir 1921; Whorf 1956). Dan Isaac Slobin's famous paper from 1996 (Slobin 1996) has shifted the focus of linguistic relativity research from a static description of language and thought to a dynamic view on language processes, and thus on thinking and speaking. Modern research on linguistic relativity has brought in experimental research methods such as eye-tracking or EEG (electroencephalogram) and added a language processing perspective. The effects of language on cognition and partially also on perception has been proven for a number of different cognitive domains, such as locomotion (von Stutterheim et al. 2012; Mertins 2018), space (Levinson et al. 2002), gender (Boroditsky et al. 2003) or color (Roberson et al. 2000, 2005) in native, non-native and bilingual/multilingual speakers of different ages. Linguistic relativity or *thinking-for-speaking* (Slobin 1996) or *seeing-for-speaking* (Mertins 2018) has developed into an established research field which is currently expanding to new cognitive domains (e.g., numerical cognition, Gordon 2004) and participant groups (e.g., infants and young children Loewenstein & Gentner 2005).

Diversity in cognition presents a central theme within psycholinguistics research, with individual differences in particular interpreted in the light of such diversity. These observations also hold true for different types of acquisition: whether in second or foreign language acquisition or in bilingual first language acquisition, the search for universals and universal features has largely been replaced by the focus on cross-linguistic, language-specific, group-specific and individual differences. Among other things, these entail differences in cognition, language use or relevant extra-linguistic variables (e.g., socio-economic status or whether someone is left- or right-handed).

Some of the research articles featured in this volume are written in English, while others are in German. The German articles include a long abstract in English, to enable non-German speakers to access the research findings. The decision to include both English and German papers in this book was driven by the idea of diversity in thinking and publishing. English has been the lingua franca of science for the past five decades, and the majority of research articles are published in English. However, only a small number of active academics in the relevant fields for this book are native English speakers. It is essential to note that non-nativeness in a language does not diminish the value or interest of research results and ideas. Therefore, this book is bilingual to ensure that valuable research findings and ideas from non-native English scholars are not overlooked, removing at least in part the hurdles for non-native English scholars.

The approach taken in the present book is interdisciplinary, including various theoretical frameworks and methodologies, as well as research fields. It utilizes a range of methods that span from experimental setups, including eye-tracking, to data elicitation and corpus analyzes. In terms of speaker groups investigated, the volume is also diverse, encompassing monolingual and bilingual children and (young) adults, as well as second language and native speakers.

This edited volume comprises eight articles that approach the topic of diversity in cognition from various perspectives. Leimbrink, Harwardt, Lowes and Mertins investigated the connection between language, music and cognition on the basis of a large corpus of folk songs in Czech, English, German, and French. The findings indicate that specific musical variables, such as the upbeat or the overall pitch range, are driven by language-specific differences related to the underlying prosodic systems of the investigated languages. The authors interpreted the results as an effect of linguistic relativity on music composition. The second study examining linguistic relativity is by Marklová and Mertins. Its focus was on the perception of goal-oriented locomotion in young monolingual and bilingual adults and the study employed eye-tracking. Although the authors stipulate differences between bilingual and monolingual speakers, no relevant differences were found. The third study by Hanna S. Andresen also examined goal-oriented motion in verbalizations of English, German, and Norwegian native speakers. Her study clearly shows support of language-specific perspectives on event construal and is thus in line with the linguistic relativity principle.

The book includes two meta-studies, both drawing from a large body of previous studies. The first study by Maryam Fatemi looks into the distribution of gender marking within the entire Indo-European language family. It shows that grammatical gender marking concerns only a small number of European languages and cannot be considered a common grammatical category in this language family. The other meta-study by Katrin Odermann critically reviews previous research on meta-linguistic awareness in monolingual and bilingual children. It concludes that this area has been seriously under-studied for bilingual children and that some of the conclusions from monolingual children have been wrongly transferred into the bilingual context. The paper by Christopher J. Hall employs a cognitive perspective on English as a *Lingua Franca* (ELF), as an expression of linguistic diversity. Within this approach, it is shown how the phenomenon of ELF obliges all speakers to reconfigure traditional ontologies of English in terms of the individual resources that diverse language users deploy in usage events. The study by Hendrik Trescher discusses critically the so-called "easy language" actively used in German-speaking countries, for example, for people with special linguistic or cognitive needs. The volume concludes with a novel article by Renate Delucchi Danhier that attempts to visualize the diversity of academics involved in diversity research by using authentic personal information from these academics.

Although the articles in this book are diverse and differ in many aspects, they share several commonalities. Firstly, all papers present empirical evidence that contradicts the notion of universal cognition or a universal view of the world. This suggests that speakers with different linguistic backgrounds and/or cultures view and approach external reality differently. Some contributions ground their findings within the linguistic relativity principle, other emphasize individual factors and cross-linguistic variation. Secondly, all papers assume implicitly or explicitly the immense role of linguistic input in language learning, as well as general learning. This aspect is particularly important and visible in studies on child or adult learners. Overall, input is relevant not only in terms of its quantity, but also in terms of its quality and complexity.

Finally, the immense relevance of diversity in cognition and in thinking has explicit consequences for other fields of research and other aspects of human life. Making the assumption that people come from very different points of departure diminishes the idea of shared common ground. In other words, one could say that successful communication of any kind is rather a matter of good luck than a rule. Taking the findings of the studies in this volume and the general findings on diversity in language and cognition seriously, several consequences must follow, for example in pedagogy, didactics, language learning or even human justice. Also, given that most of the research presented here is biased, due to the European origin of the authors, one must assume that other views and data on the presented topics must exist. To conclude, diversity in cognition definitely leads to the liberating thought that there is no ultimate truth.

Literaturverzeichnis

Boas, F. (1966) [1911]. Introduction. In F. Boas (ed.), *Handbook of American Indian languages* (pp. 1–79). Lincoln, NE: University of Nebraska Press.

Boroditsky, L., Schmidt, L. A., & Phillips, W. (2003). Sex, syntax, and semantics. In D. Gentner & S. Goldin-Meadow (eds.), *Language in mind: Advances in the study of language and thought* (pp. 61–79). Cambridge, MA: MIT Press.

Gordon, P. (2004). Numerical cognition without words: Evidence from Amazonia. *Science, 306*(5695), 496–499. https://doi.org/10.1126/science.1094492

Humboldt, W. von. (2009) [1836]. *Über die Verschiedenheit des menschlichen Sprachbaues und ihren Einfluß auf die geistige Entwickelung des Menschengeschlechts*. Cambridge: Cambridge University Press.

Levinson, S. C., Kita, S., Haun, D. B. M., & Rasch, B. H. (2002). Returning the tables: Language affects spatial reasoning. *Cognition, 84*(2), 155–188. https://doi.org/10.1016/S0010-0277(02)00045-8

Loewenstein, J., & Gentner, D. (2005). Relational language and the development of relational mapping. *Cognitive Psychology, 50*(4), 315–353. https://doi.org/10.1016/j.cogpsych.2004.09.004

Mertins, B. (2018). *Sprache und Kognition: Ereigniskonzeptualisierung im Deutschen und Tschechischen*. Berlin, New York: De Gruyter.

Roberson, D., Davidoff, J., Davies, I. R. L., & Shapiro, L. R. (2005). Color categories: Evidence for the cultural relativity hypothesis. *Cognitive Psychology, 50*(4), 378–411. https://doi.org/10.1016/j.cogpsych.2004.10.001

Roberson, D., Davies, I., & Davidoff, J. (2000). Color categories are not universal: Replications and new evidence from a stone-age culture. *Journal of Experimental Psychology: General, 129*(3), 369–398. https://doi.org/10.1037/0096-3445.129.3.369

Sapir, E. (1921). *Language: An introduction to the study of speech*. Harcourt.

Slobin, D. (1996). From "thought to language" to "thinking for speaking". In J. J. Gumperz & S. C. Levinson (eds.), *Rethinking linguistic relativity* (pp. 70–96). Cambridge: Cambridge University Press.

von Stutterheim, C., Andermann, M., Carroll, M., Flecken, M., & Schmiedtová, B. (2012). How grammaticized concepts shape event conceptualization in language production: Insights from linguistic analysis, eye tracking data, and memory performance. *Linguistics, 50*(4). https://doi.org/10.1515/ling-2012-0026

Whorf, B. L. (1956). *Language, thought, and reality: Selected writings.* Cambridge, MA.

Maryam Fatemi

Synchronic overview of grammatical gender marking in Indo-European languages

Abstract: In line with the theories of *linguistic relativity* (Whorf 1956), *thinking for speaking* (Slobin 1996), and *seeing for speaking* (Mertins 2018), which all argue that the grammatical feature of the language we speak influences the way we see the world and conceptualize it, grammatical gender makes a relevant category to explore such effect on our thoughts. The morphosyntactic feature of gender is linguistically marked in high number of languages in diverse forms. These diverse forms of representing gender of animate and inanimate entities in languages are based on semantic, morphological, and phonological principles. Different from the languages which express gender according to the aforementioned principles, the instance of a language like Farsi, with no grammatical gender-marking system, has depicted that gender information of the nouns can also be optionally represented by lexical description in postnominal positions. Such diverse forms of representing gender in various languages have made this grammatical feature a valid and relevant category for studying diversity in cognition. Looking at the literature on the influence of grammatical gender on thought, the issues of the WEIRD bias as well as Eurocentric bias have been observed. The results of such biased studies on only European languages can explain neither the linguistic variation nor can be taken as the basis for showing the possible cognitive diversity triggered through such variations. The goal of this article is to explicitly address the issues of the WEIRD bias as well as the Eurocentric bias by initially critically reviewing 43 empirical studies on grammatical gender in linguistic relativity and secondly exploring the current state of 413 Indo-European languages concerning +/- grammatical gender features, including the many languages without any expression of grammatical gender. The results of the critical review on 43 studies proves additional evidence for Eurocentric and WEIRD bias in the linguistic relativity framework, since in these studies only 20 languages were considered, among which fifteen Indo-European languages mainly spoken in Europe. The findings of this study on the state of 413 Indo-European languages concerning +/ - grammatical gender feature firstly convey that 72 % of the Indo-European languages are spoken outside Europe. Secondly, it was found that only 198 languages have linguistic proof for the absence or presence of gender-marking systems. Furthermore, the results have revealed that most of these languages, 96 in number, express gender in a twofold system of masculine and feminine. Finally, out of all Indo-European languages, 215 languages have not been linguistically studied regarding their expression of grammatical gender.

Keywords: linguistic relativity, thinking for speaking, seeing for speaking, grammatical gender, Indo-European languages, WEIRD bias, Eurocentric bias

1. Introduction

Eurocentrism, which is the tendency to view the European ideas and social standards as the basis for evaluative judgments of other practices, has been widely criticized (Joseph et al. 1990). Eurocentric bias can be observed not only in social relations and politics, but also in research, specifically including linguistic research.

Following Eurocentrism, the term "WEIRD" societies was coined (Henrich, Heine & Norenzayan 2010; Henrich 2020), which refers to the *Western Educated Industrialized Rich Democratic* societies. Most scientific studies in various fields are concentrated on WEIRD people. In linguistics, psycholinguistics, and corpus linguistics, the majority of studies have looked merely into the languages spoken in Europe, which make up approximately 1 % of the 7,099 existing languages spoken in the world. These facts lead to the question of how linguistic variations can be explained, when the existing research body has only taken 1 % of all languages into consideration. This article addresses explicitly the issue of the WEIRD bias as well as the Eurocentric bias by exploring the category of grammatical gender in 413 Indo-European languages, including the many languages without any expression of grammatical gender.

In a high number of languages, the morphosyntactic feature of gender is linguistically marked. Alvanoudi (2000, 2015) defines this feature as a grammaticized agreement system, which correlates with specific semantic characteristics of the noun such as sex, animacy or humanness. These features are realized outside the noun itself. That is, the agreement is applied through morphosyntactic marking of the words that the gendered noun is morphosyntactically related to (Boroditsky et al. 2003a; Corbett 1991). The term *gender* has been interchangeably used with the term *noun class* in literature. Alvanoudi (2000) has proposed that the term *noun class* should be used as the cover term for both *gender* and *noun class* and the term *gender* should be utilized for the systems including two or three genders which always have at least feminine and masculine. Alvanoudi (2000) argues in his typological approach that nouns are assigned to specific classes not only based on *semantic* but also on *morphological* and *phonological* principles.

Semantic principles refer to the systems in which the meaning of a noun determines its gender. For instance, in Dravidian languages such as Kolami, Parji and Ollari nouns denoting male humans belong to one class and nouns denoting female humans and any other non-male entities belong to a different class (Corbett 1991). An opposite pattern can be observed in Diyari, an Australian Indigenous language. Diyari differentiates between nouns denoting female human/animates and the rest, which comprise male human/animates and all inanimates (Dixon 1972). Dyirbal, which is another Australian Indigenous language spoken in North Queensland, categorizes the nouns yet differently. There are four different classes: (i) *bayi* referring to males and non-human animates, (ii) *balan* referring to females, fire, water, battle, and most birds, (iii) *balam* referring to non-protein food, and (iv) *bala* for the rest (Dixon 1972).

A completely different take on the classification of nouns can be seen in Manambu, a language belonging to the Ndu family spoken in Papua New Guinea. The nouns are categorized into feminine and masculine based on their size and shape. For example, adult humans are categorized based on their sex, however, bigger or older children are classified as masculine, and smaller or younger children are referred to as feminine. Furthermore, longer, and larger inanimate objects are categorized as masculine, while smaller and/or rounder objects are categorized as feminine (Aikhenvald 2012).

In the Indo-European languages such as Danish, Icelandic, Spanish, Polish, German, Italian, Serbian/Croatian/Bosnian, Portuguese, Swedish, and Greek, the gender assignment is mainly motivated semantically when it refers to a human and some animals. That is, nouns in these languages denoting female humans and some animals are usually grammatically feminine, and nouns denoting male humans and some animals are usually grammatically masculine (Hellinger & Bussmann 2001, 2002, 2003). Therefore, there is a grammatical congruency between the gender of the nouns and the articles and/or the adjectives which precede the nouns (the same agreement rules exist in animate and inanimate). For instance, the German nouns in Example 1 show the sex of the person both lexically and grammatically:

Example 1:

Masculine-Definite
(a) Deutsch

Der	*groß-e*	*Mann*
The (M.D.A.)	tall-NOM.SG.	man
'The	tall	man'

Feminine-Definite
Deutsch

Die	*groß-e*	*Frau*
The (F.D.A.)	tall-NOM.SG.	woman
'The	tall	woman'

Masculine-Indefinite
(b) Deutsch

Ein	*groß-er*	*Mann*
A (M.ND.A.)	tall-NOM.SG.	man
'A	tall	man'

Feminine-Indefinite
Deutsch

Eine	*groß-e*	*Frau*
A (F.ND.A.)	tall-NOM.SG.	woman
'A	tall	woman'

Masculine-animate
(c) Deutsch

Der	*schnell-e*	*Tiger*
The (M.D.A.)	fast-NOM.SG.	(male) tiger
'The	fast	tiger'

Feminine-animate
Deutsch

Die	*schnell-e*	*Tigerin*
A (F.D.A.)	fast-NOM.SG.	(female) tiger
'The	fast	tiger'

At the same time, in the Indo-European languages, gender assignment in inanimate nouns such as in food (e.g., egg, bread) or furniture (e.g., chair, table) is generally considered to be semantically arbitrary. The peculiarity of gender assignment does not end with assigning a feminine, masculine and/or neutral gender to inanimate objects. But rather, in some of the languages of this family, speakers are required to not only mark objects as gendered through modifying articles, pronouns, and adjectives according to the gender of the noun, but also to add affixes to verbs to agree with the gender of the noun in specific tenses. For instance, in Czech, which belongs to the Slavonic group of languages in the Indo-European family, the verbal suffix *-y* is used in the past tense only when the referred noun is plural feminine animate, children, and/or all inanimate. On the other hand, the verbal suffix *-i* marks the past tense for the plural masculine animate. Moreover, this distinctive assignment of grammatical gender on verbs is observable only in written language and as mentioned in the past tense.

Knowing this grammatical information in Czech, which is a pro-drop language, is important in order to be able to infer the nature of the subject in the sentence, especially the gender of the subject.

Example 2:

(a) Czech

Včera	*šl-i*	*do*	*kina.*
Yesterday	went-he	to	cinema
'Yesterday	he went	to	the cinema'

(b) Czech

Včera	*šl-y*	*do*	*kina.*
Yesterday	went-they	to	cinema
'Yesterday	they went	to	the cinema'

In (2a), the verbal suffix *-i* marks that the subject of this sentence must be masculine, whereas in (2b) the verbal suffix *-y* can only refer to the animate feminine referent, and/or to children based on the context. However, from the pragmatic point of view, the inanimate referent is not conveyed here, as the inanimate referent cannot go to the cinema. A lack of this grammatical information in Czech leads to false interpretation of the meaning of sentences.

Furthermore, morphological, and phonological principles play an important role in gender assignment. For instance, in Russian not only does the semantic distinction of sex specify the gender of the noun (e.g., *mat* "mother" is gendered as feminine and *otec* "father" is gendered as masculine), but also in other cases nominative, accusative, genitive, dative, instrumental and prepositional nouns are classified as masculine, feminine and neuter according to morphological principles. Nouns of declension 1, which usually end in a consonant are masculine (e.g., zakon "law"), nouns in declension 2 and 3 which end in -a and- я are feminine (e.g., škola "school"), and nouns of declension 4, which end in -o, -e, or -ë are neuter (e.g., vino "wine") (Corbett 1991). In Katcha, a Kordofanian language spoken in Sudan, nouns beginning with m- are feminine, except for the nouns which have a male referent (Heine 1982).

Different from the languages which express gender semantically, morphologically or phonologically, which has consequences for the syntactic structure, Farsi, another Indo-European language mainly written and spoken in Iran, is a genderless language. In this language, nouns are not classified into gendered classes. Consequently, there is no gender marking related to case marking. Furthermore, pronouns in third person singular are not gendered either. Example 3 gives the translations of the above Examples 1. It should be mentioned that Farsi is written from right to left.

Example 3:

Masculine
(3a) Farsi

-	بزرگ /bozorg/	مرد /Mærd/
-	tall	man
'The	tall	man'

Feminine
Farsi

	بزرگ /bozorg/	زن /zæn/
	tall	woman
'The	tall	woman'

Masculine/Feminine-animate
(3b) Farsi

	بزرگ /bozorg/	ببر /bæbr/
	big	tiger
'the	big	tiger'

As shown in Example 3, in Farsi, nouns (whether animate and/or inanimate) can be directly used to refer to definiteness. In other words, nouns are definite by default. Indefiniteness is expressed through adding either the suffix ی *(-i)* to the noun, or the article یک */Yek/*, similar to the English *a/an* used before the singular nouns, which doesn't attribute any gendered meaning to the noun. However, referring to the gender of an animal or an inanimate object is possible but optional through descriptively adding the translations of the lexemes (feminine and masculine) only in the postnominal position. It is important to stress that the sequence of adjective and noun in Farsi is "nouns + adjective". Due to the lack of grammatical gender marking, personal pronouns in Farsi only provide information about person and number. Example 4 gives the translation of the English sentence "He came" in Farsi.

Example 4:

Farsi

است. **/ast/**	مرد/mard/	یک /yek/	او/u/	آمد . /amad/	او /u/
Is	man	M.ND.A.	he/she	came	he/she
'He	came.'				

Conforming to the above explained facts about the grammatically genderless system of nouns in Farsi, including all animate/inanimate nouns (e.g., *cat, dog, door, window, desk*), nouns referring to jobs (e.g., *teacher, engineer*) are genderless as well. However, in accordance with the Farsi syntax, it is possible to add gender information to the noun. As described above, such information can be further added to the noun phrase in the postnominal position. For instance, the genderless word *teacher* /ʔɑmuzeˈgɑɹ̊/ can refer both to a feminine teacher or a masculine teacher. If a Farsi speaker would like to give information about the gender of a teacher, they can do so by adding a gendered lexeme in the postnominal position.

Grammatical gender has been studied in different linguistic fields such as psycholinguistics (Levelt, Roelofs & Meyer 1999; Friedmann & Biran 2003), cognitive linguistics (Evans & Green 2006; Lakoff 1987) or linguistic relativity (Lucy 1997). The framework of the present article is the field of linguistic relativity. Linguistic relativity is a theory which can be traced back to the linguistic-philosophical work of Wilhelm von Humboldt in the beginning of 19th century, where he described language as the "formative organ of thought". The principles of his theory could be equated with the later Sapir-Whorf hypothesis, which was proposed and supported with first empirical evidence in the 20th century. According to the Sapir-Whorf hypothesis[1] the grammatical features of the language we speak influences the way we see the world, conceptualize, categorize, and speak about it. In other words, speakers of different languages apply different language-specific perspectives on one and the same event existing in the external world (Boroditsky et al. 2003a; Lucy 1992; Mertins 2018; Slobin 1996; Whorf 1956, 2012). Studies focusing on linguistic relativity and grammatical gender have experimentally tested the effects of grammatical gender on the conceptualization and interpretation of nouns by speakers of different languages (Dilkina, McClelland & Boroditsky 2007; Schiefke & Stefanowitsch 2004; Landor 2014; Haertlé 2017). These studies have shown that grammatical gender can

1 This principle is later called *thinking for speaking* by Slobin (1996), and *seeing for speaking* by Mertins (2018).

lead to different kinds of conceptualizations. In other words, it affects cognitive processes and speakers' categorizations of the external world. However, most of these studies have concentrated on languages spoken in Europe, in which gender is grammatically marked. As a consequence of the WEIRD bias, this view on grammatical gender must be skewed.

In order to get a more impartial view of how gender influences thought, a detailed, systematic study is necessary that focuses on all alive languages from the Indo-European family, including languages without grammatical gender marking. Additionally, the strong focus of the research so far on preferences from English or German speakers cannot be taken as a basis for other, especially less studied languages. To broaden the focus in this way will help to identify possible differences in the conceptualization of objects in gendered compared with non-gendered languages.

The present study raises the following question: What is the current state of Indo-European languages concerning the presence or absence of grammatical gender features? Based on the existing linguistic and psycholinguistic research, one could hypothesize that most of the Indo-European languages are gendered. This is not the case, but rather a false impression given that the majority of the existing studies have investigated languages marking grammatical gender. The goal of this study is to show the linguistic bias of the current research in the field of linguistic relativity on the one hand, and to provide an overview of the expression of grammatical gender in all spoken L1 Indo-European languages on the other. In line with John Lucy (1997), only the study of languages in cross-linguistic contexts enables us to gain a full insight into the features, which would show support for the linguistic relativity hypothesis.

The structure of this paper is as follows: Section 2 encompasses a meta-analysis of existing studies on grammatical gender within the frame of linguistic relativity by critically reviewing a large-scale study. In Section 3 follows the overview of how Indo-European languages depict grammatical gender in their systems. Section 4 contains a presentation of the findings from the previous section. In Section 5 the overall results from Sections 2 and 3 are discussed. The article closes with a summary and a conclusion.

2. Criticism of a review on 43 empirical studies on grammatical gender in linguistic relativity

Many studies have examined the influence of grammatical gender on thought (Boroditsky et al. 2003b; Chen & Su 2011; Flaherty 2001; Konishi 1993; Sera, Berge & Pintado 1994; Vigliocco et al. 2005). A systematic and large-scale review of 43 empirical studies (from 1993 to 2018) was carried out by Samuel, Cole and Eacott (2019), in which all studies investigated the topic of the influence of grammatical gender on thought, testing 5,895 participants in total. The authors of this review classified these 43 articles based on the methods each study implemented and their findings in terms of +/- support for the hypothesis. In addition, six other parameters were part of the review:

1. The first parameter is *saliency of gender or sex* referring to the task of *voice assignment*. In this task the participants are instructed to explicitly assign a biological sex to the objects by assigning/attributing a female or male voice, when seeing a word or a picture.
2. The second parameter is *language*. This parameter controls the extent to which the tasks use language for finding evidence of the effect of language on thought as opposed to a non-verbal or a non-linguistic task such as application of eye-tracking methods. Therefore, the tasks were classified into two groups: Studies with high recruitment of language in their tasks and studies with low recruitment of language in their tasks.
3. The third parameter is *gendered language*. The underlying hypothesis here is that if someone's language creates a gender-bias conceptualization of the objects, such a conceptualization and gender-bias world view should be observed not only in the context of that particular gendered language, but also in the context of a non-gendered language. Accordingly, the studies were classified in terms of whether the participants were tested in a gendered or in a non-gendered language.
4. The next, and for this paper most relevant parameter, is the *number of genders*. It is important to pay attention that all of the 43 studies investigated only gendered languages, and excluded non-gendered languages. Consequently, the authors of this systematic review classified the studies in terms of whether the participants spoke a two- or three-gendered language and considered English as a non-gendered language.

5. The fifth parameter is *the effect with animate and inanimate targets,* which deals with the question of whether the studies reviewed only showed the influence of grammatical gender on the conceptualization of animate targets.
6. The final parameter is the *age* of the participants, i.e., stronger effects in support of linguistic relativity have been found among adults than children. Based on the results of these studies, weaker effects at younger ages are possibly consistent with less experience of younger children with grammatical gender. Furthermore, formal and institutional instructions play an important role in the formation of meta-linguistic knowledge about grammatical gender.

The methods implemented across the different articles for testing the effect of grammatical gender on the conceptualization of objects were as heterogeneous as *property judgment*, *voice choice*, *sex assignment*, *extrinsic affective Simon task*, *priming*, *similarity judgment*, *association*, and *object-name memory association*.

Along with the applied methods and the parameters listed above, the results of these 43 articles have been classified into three groups: *support* (studies showing consistent effects of grammatical gender on conceptualization), *mixed support* (studies showing partial confirmation of the influence of grammatical gender on thought, e.g., an effect of one particular gender only), and *no support* (studies showing no evidence for any effect of grammatical gender on thought).

Table 1 lists these 43 studies structured in separate columns according to the information about the *languages* being tested, the applied *method*, the percentage of the *overall studies applying a specific method*, and the results of the overall meta-analysis.

Table 1: Summary of 43 empirical studies on grammatical gender and linguistic relativity

Studies	Flaherty 2001; Imai et al. 2014; Saalbach et al. 2012; Haertlé 2017; Konishi 1993; Sedlmeier,Tipandaj, & Jänchen 2016; Semenuks et al. 2017; Landor 2014; Mickan, Schiefke & Stefanowitsch 2014; Montefinese et al. 2019	Almutrafi 2015; Athanasopoulos & Boutonnet 2016; Beller et al. 2015; Bender er al. 2016a; Bender et al. 2018; Haertlé 2017; Kurniski et al. 2016; Lambelet 2016: Ramos & Roberson 2011; Sera et al. 1994; Sera et al. 2002; Vernich 2017; Vernich, Argus, & Kamandulyte-Merfeldiene 2017; Bassetti 2007; Kurinski & Sera 2011; Forbes et al. 2008;	Pavlidou & Alvanoudi 2013; Pavlidou & Alvanoudi 2018; Belacchi & Cubelli 2012; Bender et al. 2016b; Flaherty 2001; Nicoladis 2019; Nicoladis et al. 2016; Nicoladis & Foursha Stevenson 2012; Sera et al. 1994;	Bender et al. 2016a, 2016b, 2018	Bender et al. 2011; Sato & Athanasopoulos 2018; Bender et al. 2011; Degani 2007; Mickan et al. 2014; Samuel et al. 2016
Languages	Spanish, English, German, Japanese, Polish, French, Tamil, Romanian, Finno-Ugric (the traditional name of Ulric Languages), Semitic, Italian	Arabic, English, French, Spanish, Norwegian, German, Polish, Hungarian, Portuguese, Estonian, Italian, Lithuanian, Italian, Russian	Greek, German, Italian, English, Spanish, Russian, French	German	German, French, English, Spanish, Romanian, Lithuanian, Italian, Bulgarian, Latvian, Ukrainian
Task type	Property judgment	Voice choice	Sex assignment	EAST	Priming
Percentage of the overall studies	37 %	28 %	12 %	9 %	8 %
support	3 %	64 %	66 %	11 %	34 %
Mixed support	23 %	22 %	26 %	56 %	-
No support	74 %	14 %	8 %	33 %	66 %

Based on the data presented in Table 1, it can be concluded that the absence/presence of a grammatical gender effect on conceptualization is highly related to the task/method used in a study. More specifically, when the tasks *voice choice* or *sex assignment* were used, in which the participants were explicitly asked to assign a biological gendered voice or a name when naming objects, the influence of grammatical gender was stronger. Following the argumentation of Samuel et al. (2019), these two tasks form the cornerstone for proving the linguistic relativity theory (in terms of *support*: voice choice 64 %; sex assignment 66 %). By contrast, the tasks *association*, and *property judgement* stand at the other end of the continuum, providing evidence for the absence (no support) of such effects.

In conclusion, it is important to consider the fact that all of the 43 empirical studies mentioned above investigated only fifteen Indo-European languages, all spoken in Europe, and five non-Indo-European languages. These fifteen languages cover merely 3.5 % of the 413 languages spoken within the Indo-European family. Such linguistic focus confirms yet again the Eurocentric bias often found in linguistic studies. In order to reduce this bias and to gain a more comprehensive as well as evidence-based view on the cross-linguistic occurrence of grammatical gender, the inclusion of other Indo-European languages into the analysis is a must. In line with this argumentation, in the following a detailed scrutiny of 413 Indo-European languages will be presented and analyzed in terms of +/- grammatical gender.

3. Indo-European languages

The backbone for the analyzes in the present paper was the language database *Glottolog* version 4.6 (Hammarström et al. 2022), which is a comprehensive reference information for the world's languages, with focus on the lesser-known languages. According to this database, the Indo-European language family represents one of the overall existing 427 language families. The Indo-European family consists of 581 languages, from which only 413 of the languages are alive and spoken, with the rest being extinct. In line with *Glottolog*, these 413 languages, including languages which are moribund,[2] threatened,[3] or endangered,[4] were considered for the purpose of the current study.[5] Following Hammarström et al. (2022), the Indo-European language family was classified as following:

2 This term refers to languages which are severely endangered and are near to death.

3 This term refers languages which are still spoken, but threatened to language change or lost.

4 This term refers the languages which are massively endangered but not yet extinct.

5 The classification does not include any extinct languages, such as the Anatolian group.

Classical Indo-European

- Albanian
- Armenic
- Balto-Slavic
- Celtic
- Germanic
- Graeco-Phrygian
- Indo-Iranian
- Italic

Figure 1 presents a map of the geographical distribution of all Indo-European languages, including the extinct groups.

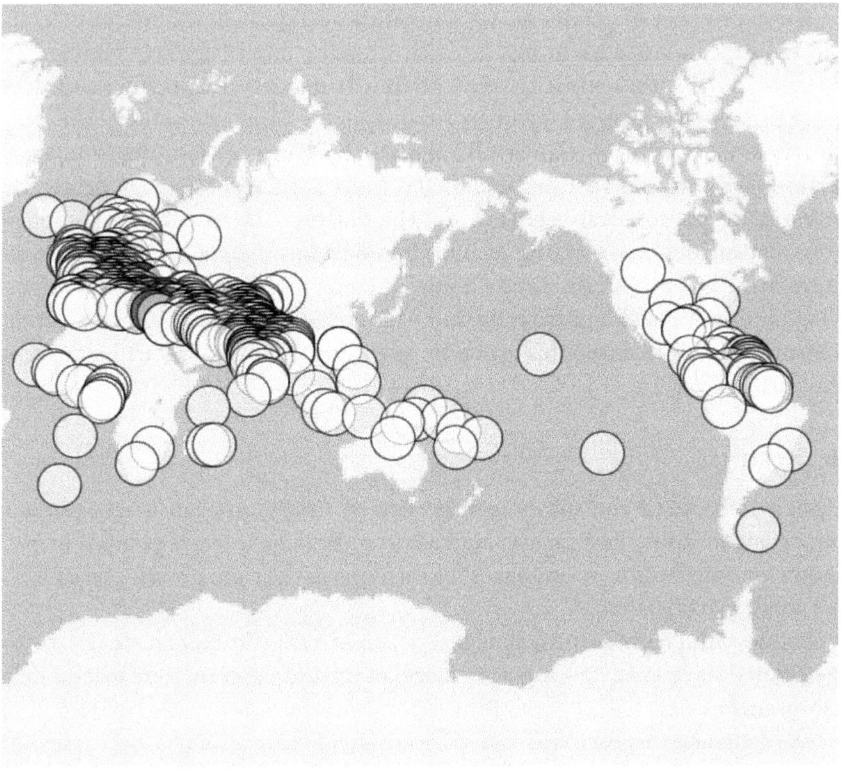

Figure 1: A map of the main Indo-European languages

As shown in Figure 1, contrary to what the name of this family of languages might imply, the languages of this group are not merely spoken in Europe and Asia but are rather spoken in a broader scope of continents such as in Africa, Australia, and even Central America. However, the fact that the density of the geographical location of these languages is mostly in the Middle East and Europe cannot be neglected.

All language groups listed above divide into subgroups called *sub-branch languages*. Each of these *sub-branch languages* also includes various dialects. For instance, Swedish is a sub-branch language belonging to the *Germanic* group and it branches further into four different dialects: *Götamal*, *old Swedish*, *Standard Swedish* and *Sveamal*. In this article, dialects in any sub-branch language are not part of the analysis.

The expression of gender as a grammatical feature is found not only in the Indo-European language group, but also in many other language families, for instance in the Afroasiatic languages, Atlantic Languages, Australian Languages, Austroasiatic Languages, Dravidian Languages, or Languages of the Americas. Despite this diversity, grammatical gender is far from constituting a universal feature (Ibrahim 2014). Even within the Indo-European language group, the marking of grammatical gender is not the default: "The inner distribution of grammatical gender marking is not homogenous within the entire Indo-European family" (Allassonnière-Tang & Dunn 2020). In order to find out whether or not a language from the Indo-European family belongs to +/- gender systems, we will examine this group by analyzing each sub-branch language in the next section.

4. Results

Having introduced the sub-branch groups of Indo-European languages, it is important to know how many languages are spoken in each group. Figure 1 shows the distribution of languages for each one of the eight groups presented in the above classification.

In line with Figure 2, the languages spoken in each sub-branch are not evenly distributed since most languages are found in the Indo-Aryan, Iranian, and Italic sub-branches.

The languages in each sub-branch were divided in terms of +/- expression of grammatical gender into five categories: (1) NGG – languages without grammatical gender; (2) 1GG- languages with one grammatical gender; (3) 2GG – languages with two grammatical genders; (4) 3GG – languages with three grammatical genders; and (5) No Info – no information found. It is important to stress that in this paper the 1GG group includes languages with pronominal genders, such as English. There are other linguistic approaches, in which English is considered a non-gendered language (Sabourin, Stowe & de Haan 2006). The summary of the analyzes carried out for the purpose of this article are presented in Figure 3.

In Figure 3, the different sub-branch groups are plotted on the x-axis whereas the y-axis shows the number of languages belonging to each category, marked with a different color.[6]

Overall, only seven languages of all the analyzed Indo-European languages belong to the 1GG category. There are three languages in the Iranian, one in the Indo-Aryan, one in the Graeco-Phrygian, and two in the Germanic sub-branch group. As for the category 2GG, there are 96 languages in total, from which 39 languages were identified for the Indo-Aryan, 33 in the Italic, 13 in the Iranian, five in the Celtic, four in the Germanic, and two languages in the Balto-Slavic sub-branches. Regarding the 3GG systems, a total of 34 languages were identified belonging to this category. The majority, eleven languages, were found in the Balto-Slavic sub-branch, followed by seven languages in the Indo Aryan, four languages in the Germanic as well as in the Italic sub-branch. In the Graeco-Phrygian group there were four languages, and finally Albanian with three languages. The last category No GG was found in 61 languages in total, with 44 languages in the Iranian group, followed by the Indo-Aryan with 10 languages and the Italic sub-branch with two languages. The sub-branch Armenic with a total of two languages also belongs to No GG. Finally, there was one language in the Germanic, and one language in the Graeco-Phrygian sub-branch, which belong to the No GG category.

6 As for 215 languages no linguistic information regarding their grammatical gender marking system is available, the category of No Info has not been presented in Figure 3.

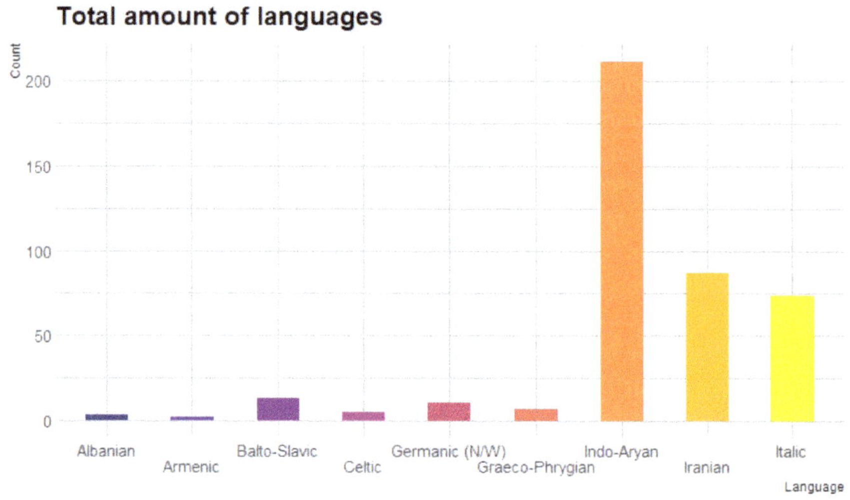

Figure 2: The number of languages in each sub-branch of Indo-European family

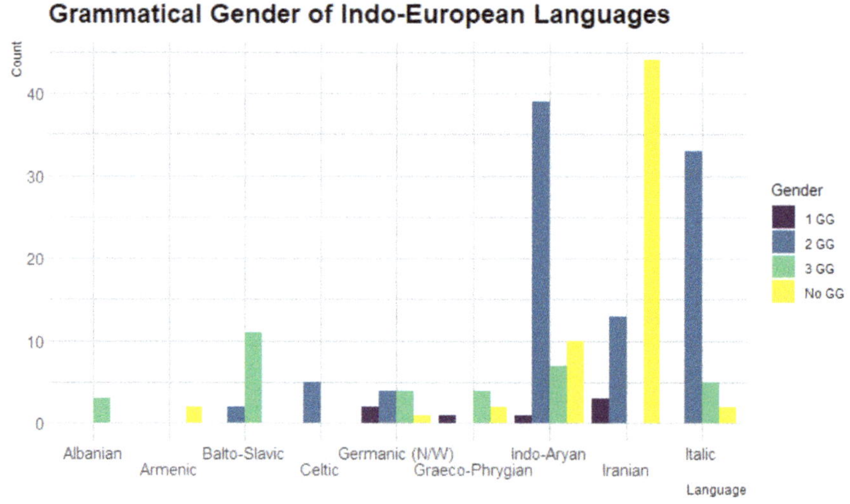

Figure 3: Grammatical gender of each sub-branch in Indo-European family

Looking at the results, it can be further observed that the sub-branches of Germanic and Indo-Aryan include more diverse grammatical gender systems, since both sub-branches have languages belonging to all four categories. Although Germanic languages are considered as languages with gender systems, it is important to highlight that the only Germanic language without a grammatical gender marking system is Afrikaans. This language is indeed the youngest fully standardized member of the West Germanic branch, spoken in South Africa. It is also considered as a daughter of Dutch and is characterized by extreme simplifications of Dutch morpho-syntax, including missing Dutch's gender system (Brown & Ogilvie 2009).

On the other hand, Armenic, Albanian, and Celtic sub-branches show the least diversity in terms of grammatical gender, since the two languages in the Armenic sub-branch only include No GG systems and all three languages from the Albanian sub-branch express grammatical gender in a threefold system, i.e., in the 3GG category. Finally, the alive languages belonging to the Celtic sub-branch assign gender solely in a twofold system of feminine and masculine.

It is also important to note that languages categorized as 1GG, 2GG, 3GG, and NGG made up only 47.9 % (198 languages) of the total number of languages spoken in the Indo-European family. This means that for more than half of the spoken languages in the Indo-European family, no linguistic research is available. Out of all 413 languages spoken in this family, only seven of them express gender as one category, mostly expressed as a pronominal feature; 96 languages have a twofold gender system, 34 express the category gender in a threefold system, and 61 languages have no grammatical genders at all.

In addition, taking the gendered Indo-European languages, it can be observed that most of them, 96 in total, have a twofold gender system. This means that among the Indo-European languages, most of the languages show a strong correlation between biological sex and grammatical gender for all animates (humans and animals), when compared to the three-gendered languages such as German.

Taking the three principles of semantic, morphological and phonological gender assignment into consideration, the results of the present study further confirm the fact mentioned in section 1 of the current article, that gender assignment in the Indo-European languages is mainly motivated semantically when referring to humans and some animals.

Given the high number of languages considered for this analysis, the detailed results for every sub-branch language are presented in appendices A1, A2, A3 and A4.

5. Discussion

Taken the Eurocentric and WEIRD biases in research in general and specifically in linguistic and psycholinguistic studies, this article has found additional evidence for these biases in the linguistic relativity framework, specifically in research on grammatical gender. In the systematic review of Samuel et.al. (2019), 43 empirical studies with the focus on grammatical gender marking on different languages were reviewed. Having critically re-assessed these 43 articles, it was found that only twenty languages were taken into account, among which fifteen Indo-European and five non-Indo-European languages. These fifteen Indo-European are mainly spoken in Europe.

These results inspired me to study all languages alive in the Indo-European family, with the focus on their underlying grammatical gender marking systems. The findings of the present study firstly convey that 72 % of the Indo-European languages are spoken outside Europe. These languages belong to the sub-branch languages of Indo-Aryan and Iranian languages, which all together comprise 298 languages of the total of 413 alive languages in this language family. Secondly, it was found that only 198 languages have linguistic proof for the absence or presence of a gender-marking systems. These languages belong to the sub-branches of Indo-Aryan, Italic, Iranian, Celtic, Germanic, Balto-Slavic, Albanian, Armenic, and Graeco-Phrygian groups. Furthermore, the results have revealed that most of these languages express gender in a twofold system of masculine and feminine. Therefore, it can be claimed that most of the grammatical gender of nouns referring to animals and humans in these twofold gendered languages are congruent with their biological sex. This confirms that the majority of the gendered Indo-European languages classify nouns based on the semantic principle. However, it should not be overlooked that the classification of inanimate nouns among these twofold gendered languages are semantically arbitrary. The reason is that these nouns are, by definition, inanimate and have therefore no biological sex, i.e., gender is not an intrinsic characteristic of those nouns (Bender et al. 2018). Finally, out of all Indo-European languages, 215 languages have not been linguistically studied regarding their expression of grammatical gender.

Moreover, having presented the categories of grammatical gender marking systems among Indo-European languages, it is also important to include the precise nature of grammatical gender marking systems. The categories of No GG, 1GG, 2GG and 3GG can be explained as forming a continuum, on each of their extreme ends including the categories of No GG and 3 GG. It is important to mention that *sex* and *gender* are distinguished from the sociological perspective.

Sex is a biological term, which refers to the chromosomes, hormonal profiles, and internal and external sex organs, since *gender* is a cultural term and denotes the characteristics that societies or cultures delineate along the spectrum of masculinity and femininity (Butler 2002). Taking German as an example for a 3 GG language, some nouns referring to human/animals can be claimed to carry a grammatical gender inconsistent with their social gender, due to the existence of the third neuter gender. For instance, the lexeme *girl* in German is expressed with neutral gender *das Mädchen*, although by virtue of being probably socially feminine, the neutral grammatical gender would not accord with the social gender. No GG languages, on the other hand, do not in any way mark gender grammatically. However, it can be argued that despite the absence of this grammatical feature, nouns can be associated with specific genders culturally. As mentioned above, 1GG languages refer to the languages with pronominal genders. Such languages pronominally refer to humans and animals consistent with their social gender. 2GG languages in the Indo-European family form two groups. One group divides the nouns into feminine and masculine such as Spanish, French, and Italian. This group forms the most frequent type of twofold gender marking systems among the Indo-European languages. The second group, which is less common, take a different approach in their classification of the nouns: They classify nouns into *gendered* and *neuter* categories. Dutch and Swedish are two instances of such Indo-European languages with a different take on the classifications of nouns. Looking at Samuel et al. (2019), it should also be emphasized that such languages have also been excluded in their review.

In this discussion, the focus is also on the areas which need addressing in future research on grammatical gender in linguistic relativity. Although the systematic review by Samuel et al. (2019) provided evidence for the effect of grammatical gender on conceptualization and thought, testing only fifteen languages of the 413 Indo-European languages does not provide comprehensive results. The generalization of these findings based on only fifteen languages to the complete family can be considered as debatable. Following John Lucy (1997), it is only through cross-linguistic studying of languages that we can gain full insights into the features, which show support for linguistic relativity. Thus, more languages need to be studied to have a better understanding of language-specific effects of grammar on the conceptualizations of the world. As the results of the current data on the Indo-European languages have proven, there exists a diversity in the marking of grammatical gender within the Indo-European family. Consequently, studies must be carried out including languages which mark gender semantically, morphologically and phonologically, but also including languages which do not express gender grammatically at all. An example of a language with no gender marking system is Farsi, in which gender information can be presented through a lexical description and/or by context. As mentioned above, although nouns in Farsi do not mark gender, conveying such information through the lexical insertion of the words *masculine* and *feminine* in postnominal positions is possible and does not violate the underlying structural rules. Therefore, the concept of gender/sex does exist in Farsi, albeit not grammatically marked. Comparing the results of empirical studies on such non-gendered languages with gendered languages is therefore essential to fill the gap in study of the effects of linguistic diversity on cognition.

Another potential point of relevance of taking more non-gendered languages into consideration, besides finding further support for linguistic relativity, is the acquisitional perspective, especially in migration contexts. In line with the main topic of the current study, it is also relevant to pose the following questions: How do native speakers of non-gendered languages acquire and master gendered languages, such as German, French, or English? How do second language speakers of these languages adjust to the extreme gendered classifications of every noun? Having briefly introduced Farsi as one example of a non-gendered language, one could relate the above raised questions with the consistent increase in migration among Iranians. According to a study at Stanford University in 2020, the total number of Iranian migrants grew from about 130,000 in 1970 to 3.1 million in 2020 (Azadi et al. 2020). Among the countries which host the largest number of Iranian migrants are the United States (32 %), Canada (14 %), Germany (11 %), United Kingdom (6 %) and Sweden (5 %). In accordance with this diaspora of Iranian speakers to countries in which gendered languages are the dominant language of the society in every aspect, it is relevant to study the linguistic behavior of Farsi speakers in acquiring such languages.

This study is not free of limitations. The biggest limitation is that there is no comprehensive resource for all spoken languages in the Indo-European family that could serve as a basis for the analysis. Although there exists reliable linguistic works such as *Encyclopaedia of Languages of the World* (Brown & Ogilvie 2009), they are not up to date because they do not include information on language change and are therefore inaccurate. As pointed out before, the list of languages in the appendix display a large number of languages belonging to the category of *No Info*. This means it is difficult to draw conclusions on the results. Nonetheless, the results prove the fact that further research is necessary to fill in the gaps considering many other understudied languages.

6. Conclusions

Based on the analyzes of the current article, diverse forms of representing gender of animate and inanimate entities (semantically, morphologically, phonologically, and by lexical description) in various languages have made this grammatical feature a valid and relevant category for studying diversity in cognition. In line with the linguistic relativity theory, grammatical gender is a relevant feature for finding evidence for the effects of language on conceptualization. Nevertheless, the findings of this study clearly manifest the existence of the Eurocentric and the WEIRD bias in studies on grammatical gender within the linguistic relativity principle. The current study showed that the review by Samuel et al. (2019) is clearly affected by both biases. On the basis of the present study, it can be concluded that among all Indo-European languages a long list of understudied languages exists. Therefore, a more comprehensive and evidence-based research on all, especially understudied Indo-European languages is necessary in order to corroborate the findings on the effects of grammatical gender on thought. This article has further paved the way for future studies by providing the existing linguistic information about all sufficiently documented alive languages from the Indo-European family on the +/- expression of grammatical gender.

References

Adib, D. (1972). *Further data on khuniite from the Tschah Khuni Mine, Anarak, Iran.*

Aikhenvald, A. Y. (2000). *Classifiers: A typology of noun categorization devices.* Oxford: Oxford University Press.

Aikhenvald, A. Y. (2012). Round women and long men: Shape and size in gender choice in Papua New Guinea and beyond. *Anthropological Linguistics, 54*(1), 33–86.

Alam, S. (2011). Word formation in Surjapuri. *Language in India, 11*(3), 487–497.

Alimova, K. (2020). Dari word-forming transposotion phenomenon. *International Journal of Pharmaceutical Research, 12*, 516–521.

Allassonnière-Tang, M. & Dunn, M. (2020). The evolutionary trends of grammatical gender in Indo-Aryan languages. *Language Dynamics and Change, 11*(2), 211–240.

Almutrafi, F. (2015). *Language and cognition: Effects of grammatical gender on the categorisation of objects* (Unpublished doctoral thesis). Newcastle University, Newcastle upon Tyne, UK.

Alvanoudi, A. (2015). *Grammatical gender in interaction: Cultural and cognitive aspects. Brill's studies in language, cognition and culture: v. 9*. Brill, Leiden, The Netherland.

Andonova, E., D'amico, S., & Decescovi, A. (2004). Gender and lexical access in Bulgarian. *Perception & Psychophysics, 66*(3), 496–507.

Anonby, E. J. (2003). Update on Luri: How many languages? *Journal of the Royal Asiatic Society of Great Britain & Ireland, 13*(2), 171–197. Retrieved (03/2023) from https://doi.org/10.1017/S1356186303003067

Arora, A. (2020, December 6). *Historical phonology and other observations on historical phonology and other observations on Kholosi.* Georgetown University, Washington, United States.

As-Sultan, Ab. H. J. (2010). Causative in Shabaki. *Acta Linguistica, 4* (2), 79–88.

Athanasopoulus, P. (2009). Cognitive representation of colour in bilinguals: The case of Greek blues. *Bilingualism: Language and Cognition, 12*(1), 83–95.

Athanasopoulos, P. & Boutonnet, B. (2016). Learning grammatical gender in a second language changes categorization of inanimate objects: Replications and new evidence from English learners of L2 French. In R. Alonso (Ed.), *Cross-linguistic influence in second language acquisition* (pp. 173–192). Bristol, UK: Multilingual Matters.

Audring, J. (2008). Gender assignment and gender agreement: Evidence from pronominal gender languages. *Morphology, 18*(2), 93–116. Retrieved (03/2023) from https://doi.org/10.1007/s11525-009-9124-y

Azadi, P., Mirramezani, M., & Mesgaran, M. B. (2020). Migration and brain drain from Iran. *Stanford Iran, 2040*, 1–30.

Baart, J. (1999). *Sketch of Kalam Kohistani grammar: Studies in languages of Northern Pakistan*. Quaid-i-Azam University and Summer Institute of Linguistics, Islamabad, Pakistan.

Bano, S., Deo, A., & Butt, M. (2019). Achievement predicates and tense paradigms in Hazaragi. *Proceedings of the LFG'19 Conference*, 394–414.

Barber, H. & Carreiras, M. (2005). Grammatical gender and number agreement in Spanish: An ERP comparison. *Journal of Cognitive Neuroscience, 17*(1), 137–153.

Barker, M. S., Nelson, N. L., & Robinson, G. A. (2020). Idea formulation for spoken language production: The interface of cognition and language. *Journal of the International Neuropsychological Society: JINS, 26*(2), 226–240.

Bartens, A. & Sandström, N. (2008). Explaining Kabuverdianu nominal plural formation. *Language Complexity: Typology, Contact and Change*, 94, 305–320, John Benjamins, Amsterdam, The Netherlands.

Bashir, E., Conners, T. J., & Hefright, B. (2019). *A descriptive grammar of Hindko, Panjabi, and Saraiki. Mouton-CASL Grammar Series: volume 4*. De Gruyter Mouton.

Bassetti, B. (2007). Bilingualism and thought: Grammatical gender and concepts of objects in Italian–German bilingual children. *International Journal of Bilingualism, 11*, 251–273.

Batzarov, Z. (2000). *Orbis Latinus: Descriptive grammar of the Occitan language.* https://www.orbilat.com/Languages/Occitan/Grammar/index.html

Bavanpouri, M., Mirzaei Al-Husseini, S. M., & Fathi Iranshahi, T. (2021). Investigation of meaning and phonological processes of Arabic words involved in Laki language [In Persian]. *Journal of Language Teaching, Literature & Linguistics, 4*(1), 29–48.

Baxter, A. N. (1988). *A grammar of kristang (malacca creole portuguese).* The Australian National University.

Belacchi, C. & Cubelli, R. (2012). Implicit knowledge of grammatical gender in preschool children. *Journal of Psycholinguistic Research, 41*, 295–310.

Beller, S., Brattebø, K. F., Lavik, K. O., Reigstad, R. D., & Bender, A. (2015). Culture or language: What drives effects of grammatical gender? *Cognitive Linguistics, 26*, 331–359.

Bender, A., Beller, S., & Klauer, K. C. (2011). Grammatical gender in German: A case for linguistic relativity? *Quarterly Journal of Experimental Psychology, 64*, 1821–1835.

Bender, A., Beller, S., & Klauer, K. C. (2016a). Crossing grammar and biology for gender categorisations: Investigating the gender congruency effect in generic nouns for animates. *Journal of Cognitive Psychology, 28*, 530–558.

Bender, A., Beller, S., & Klauer, K. C. (2016b). Lady Liberty and Godfather Death as candidates for linguistic relativity? Scrutinizing the gender congruency effect on personified allegories with explicit and implicit measures. *Quarterly Journal of Experimental Psychology, 69*, 48–64.

Bender, A., Beller, S., & Klauer, K. C. (2018). Gender congruency from a neutral point of view: The roles of gender classes and conceptual connotations. *Journal of Experimental Psychology: Learning, Memory, and Cognition, 44*, 1580–1608.

Benkato, A. (2015). Recent work in Yaghnobi studies. *Iran and the Caucasus, 19*(3), 283–294.

Bernstein, J. (1991). DPs in French and Walloon: Evidence for parametric variation in nominal head movement. *Probus, 3*(2). Retrieved (03/2023) from https://doi.org/10.1515/prbs.1991.3.2.101

Bhattacharya, S., Choudhury, M., Sarkar, S., & Basu, A. (2005). Inflectional morphology synthesis for Bengali noun, pronoun and verb systems.

Proceedings of the National Conference on Computer Processing of Bangla (NCCPB 05), 34–43.

Borijan, H. (2004). Review: Northern Talysh by Wolfgang Schulze. *Iran & the Caucasus, 8*(1), 165–168.

Borjian, H. (2008). *The Komisenian dialect of aftar. Advance online publication.* Retrieved (03/2023) from https://doi.org/10.7916/D8N02H9X

Borjian, H. (2014). What is Judeo-Median – and how does it differ from Judeo-Persian? *Journal of Jewish Languages, 2*(2), 117–142.

Borjian, H (2019). *The Caspian language of Šahmirzād. Journal of the American Oriental Society, 2*(139), 361–380.

Borjian, H. [Habib] (2019). The Mazandarani dialect of Kalijān Rostāq. *Iranian Studies, 52*(3–4), 551–573. Retrieved (03/2023) from https://doi.org/10.1080/00210862.2019.1611371

Borjian, H. (2021). *Essays on three Iranian language groups: Taleqani, Biabanaki, Komisenian*. Bristol, CT (USA), ISD LLC.

Boroditsky, L. (2012). How the languages we speak shape the ways we think. In M. Spivey, K. McRae, & M. Joanisse (Eds.), *The Cambridge handbook of psycholinguistics* (pp. 615–632). Cambridge University Press, Cambridge, United Kingdom. Retrieved from https://doi.org/10.1017/CBO9781139029377.042.

Boroditsky, L. & Schmidt, L. A. (2000). Sex, syntax, and semantics. In L. R. Gleitman & A. K. Joshi (Eds.), *Proceedings of the twenty second annual conference of the cognitive science society* (pp. 42–46). Mahwah, NJ: Erlbaum.

Boroditsky, L., Schmidt, L. A., & Phillips, W. (2003a). Sex, syntax, and semantics. *Language in Mind: Advances in the Study of Language and Thought* (22), 61–79.

Boroditsky, L., Schmidt, L. A., & Phillips, W. (2003b). Can quirks of grammar affect the way you think? Grammatical gender and object concepts. *Proceedings of the Annual Meeting of the Cognitive Science Society* (25), 928–933.

Braine, M. D. (2014). What is learned in acquiring word classes – A step toward an acquisition theory. In Mechanisms of Language Acquisition, *The 20th annual Carnegie Mellon symposium on cognition.*

Brown, K. & Ogilvie, S. (2009). *Concise encyclopedia of languages of the world.* Elsevier Ltd, Oxford, United Kingdom.

Bussmann, H. & Hellinger, M. (Eds.). (2001, 2002, 2003). *Gender across languages: The linguistic representation of women and men.* J. Benjamins, Amsterdam, The Netherlands.

Butler, J. (2002). *Gender trouble*. Routledge, New York, United States.

Chambers, F. M. (1985). *An introduction to old Provençal versification* (Vol. 167). American Philosophical Society, Philadelphia, United States.

Chen, J.-Y. & Su, J.-J. (2011). Differential sensitivity to the gender of a person by English and Chinese speakers. *Journal of Psycholinguistic Research*, *40*(3), 195–203. Retrieved (03/2023) from https://doi.org/10.1007/s10936-010-9164-9

Chockalingam, K. (2016). *Languages of Tamil Nadu Lambadi an Indo-Aryan dialect*. Messrs Alamu Printing, Part XII, Vol-IX, India.

Comrie, B. (Ed.). (1987). *The world's major languages*. Croom Helm, New York, United States.

Corbett, G. (1991). *Gender: Textbooks in linguistics*. Cambridge University Press, Cambridge.

Dash, B. (2014). Kurmali noun inflection: Aspectual inquiry into gender and number. *International Journal of Linguistics* (3), 1–14. Retrieved (03/2023) from https://doi.org/10.13140/RG.2.1.4993.8004.

David, A. B. (2013). Descriptive grammar of Pashto and its dialects. *Descriptive Grammar of Pashto and Its Dialects (Vol.1)*. Walter de Gruyter, Berlin, Germany.

Degani, T. (2007). *The semantic role of gender: Grammatical and biological gender match effects in English and Spanish* (Unpublished master's thesis). University of Pittsburgh, Pittsburgh, PA.

Dhakal, D. N. (2011). *The Darai language*. UGS Press, Tribhuvan, Kirtipur, Kathmandu.

Dhanunjay, B. (2010). *Pangwali grammar write-up*. Retrieved (03/2023) from https://www.pangi.in/en/Pangwali-Linguistic-papers

Dilkina, K., McClelland, J. L., & Boroditsky, L. (2007). How language affects thought in a connectionist model. *Proceedings of the Annual Meeting of the Cognitive Science Society, 29,* 215–220.

Dixon, R. M. W. (1972). *The Dyirbal language of North Queensland*. London: CambridgeUniversity Press.

Dovudov, G., Pomikálek, J., Suchomel, V., & Smerk, P. (2011). Building a 50M Corpus of Tajik Language (RASLAN), 89–95.

Dryer, M. S. & Haspelmath, M. (2013). *The world atlas of language structures online*. Max Planck Institute for Evolutionary Anthropology. Retrieved (03/2023) from https://wals.info/feature/30A#2/26.7/148.9

Dwivedi, A. V. (2013). *A grammar of Bhadarwahi. Languages of the world. Materials: Vol. 495*. LINCOM Europa, Munich, Germany.

Enguita-Utrilla, J. M. (2008). Spanish and historical dialect in Aragon. *International Journal of the Sociology of Language*, *2008*(193/194). Retrieved (03/2023) from https://doi.org/10.1515/IJSL.2008.048

Evans, V. & Green, M. (2006). *Cognitive linguistics: An introduction*. Edinburgh University Press, Edinburgh, Scotland.

Everett, C. (2013). *Linguistic relativity*. De Gruyter Mouton, Berlin, Germany.

Fareed, N. (2016). Morphology of Mewati language. *Proceedings of the Conference on Language and Technology*, 25–32.

Firestone, C. & Scholl, B. J. (2016). Cognition does not affect perception: Evaluating the evidence for "top-down" effects. *The Behavioral and Brain Sciences*, *39*, e229.

Flaherty, M. (2001). How a language gender system creeps into perception. *Journal of Cross-Cultural Psychology*, *32*(1), 18–31.

Forbes, J. N., Poulin-Dubois, D., Rivero, M. R., & Sera, M. D. (2008). Grammatical gender affects bilinguals' conceptual gender: Implications for linguistic relativity and decision making. *Open Applied Linguistics Journal*, *1*, 68–76.

Friedmann, N. & Biran, M. (2003). When is gender accessed? A study of paraphasias in Hebrew anomia. *Cortex*, *39*(3), 441–463. Retrieved (03/2023) from https://doi.org/10.1016/S0010-9452(08)70258-2

Gambhir, S. K. & Moag, R. F. (1981). Fiji Hindi. A basic course and reference grammar. *Journal of the American Oriental Society*, *101*(4), 506. Retrieved (03/2023) from https://doi.org/10.2307/601362

Gnanadesikan, A. E. (2017). *Dhivehi: The language of the Maldives. Mouton-CASL grammar series: Vol. 3*. De Gruyter Mouton, Berlin, Germany.

Greenbaum, S. (1996). *English grammar*. Oxford University, Oxford, United Kingdom.

Gusain, L. (1999). *A discriptive grammar of Bagri* [PhD Dissertation]. New Delhi: Jawaharlal Nehru University.

Gusain, L., Ph.D. (2002). *Language in India: Eendangered language: A case study of Sansiboli*. Retrieved (03/2023) from http://www.languageinindia.com/dec2002/sansi.html

Haertlé, I. (2017). Does grammatical gender influence perception? A study of Polish and French speakers. *Psychology of Language and Communication*, *21*(1), 386–407.

Haig, G. & Khan, G. (Eds.). (2018). *The languages and linguistics of Western Asia: An areal perspective: (Vol. 6)*. Walter de Gruyter GmbH & Co KG, Berlin/ Boston.

Hammarström, H., Forkel, R., Haspelmath, M., & Bank, S. (2022). *glottolog/glottolog: Glottolog database 4.6.* Retrieved (03/2023) from https://doi.org/10.5281/zenodo.6578297

Heine, B. (1982). African noun class systems. In H. Seiler & C. Lehmann (Eds.), *Apprehension: Das sprachliche Erfassen von Gegenständen, i: Bereich und Ordnung der Phänomene* (pp. 189–216). Tübingen: Narr.

Henrich, J., Heine, S. J., & Norenzayan, A. (2010). Most people are not WEIRD. *Nature, 466*(7302), 29. Retrieved (03/2023) from https://doi.org/10.1038/466029a

Hickmann, M. (2000). Linguistic relativity and linguistic determinism: Some new directions. *Linguistics,* 38(2). Retrieved (03/2023) from https://doi.org/10.1515/ling.38.2.409

Hirvonen, M. & Igareda, P. (2017). Imaginary places–Verbalization of setting in the English, German and Spanish audio descriptions of Slumdog Millionaire. Minor *t*ranslating *m*ajor-*m*ajor *t*ranslating *m*inor-*m*inor *t*ranslating *m*inor, *341*, Diavlos Publications, Athens, Greece.

Ibrahim, M. H. (2014). *Grammatical gender.* De Gruyter Mouton, The Hague, Netherlands. Imai, M., Schalk, L., Saalbach, H., & Okada, H. (2014). All giraffes have female-specific properties: Influence of grammatical gender on deductive reasoning about sex-specific properties in German speakers. *Cognitive Science, 38*, 514–536.

Ivanovska, B. (2015). *The category of definiteness in language pair German-Macedonian.* Anchor Academic Publishing, Hamburg, Germany.

Ivanow, W. (1926). Two dialects spoken in the Central Persian desert. *Journal of the Royal Asiatic Society, 58*(3), 405–431.

Jenner, H. (1904). *A handbook of the Cornish language: Chiefly in its latest stages, with some account of its history and literature.* D. Nutt.

Joseph, G. G., Reddy, V., & Searle-Chatterjee, M. (1990). Eurocentrism in the social sciences. *Race & Class, 31*(4), 1–26. Retrieved (03/2023) from https://doi.org/10.1177/030639689003100401

Kalnaca, A. (2014). *A typological perspective on Latvian grammar.* DE GRUYTER OPEN. Retrieved (03/2023) from https://doi.org/10.2478/9783110411317

Karacan, H. & Khalid, H. S. (2016). Adjectives in Kurdish language: Comparison between dialects. *International Journal of Kurdish Studies, 2*(2), 15–23.

Karatsareas, P. (2011). *A study of Cappadocian Greek nominal morphology from a diachronic and dialectological perspective* [PhD Dissertation]. Wolfson College, Cambridge.

Karim, S. O. (2021). *The synchrony and diachrony of New Western Iranian nominal morphosyntax* [Doctoral dissertation, The Ohio State University)].

RIS. Retrieved (03/2023) from https://search.proquest.com/openview/92c24f6c9f4944f07333190c95228fe8/1?pq-origsite=gscholar&cbl=18750&diss=y

Karimi Doostan, G. H. & Tajalli, T. (2015). Definite and indefinite articles in Ardekani dialect of fars within the minimalist framework. *Journal of Researchers in Linguistics, 7*(2), 85–100.

Katz, J. & Pitzanti, G. (2019). The phonetics and phonology of lenition: A Campidanese Sardinian case study. *Laboratory Phonology: Journal of the Association for Laboratory Phonology, 10*(1), 16. Retrieved (03/2023) from https://doi.org/10.5334/labphon.18

Kaushanskaya, M. & Smith, S. (2016). Do grammatical-gender distinctions learned in the second language influence native-language lexical processing? *International Journal of Bilingualism, 20,* 30–39.

Kiran, S. & Peterson, J. (Preprint 2021). *Sadani/Sadri: Новые индоарийские языки.(New Indo-Aryan languages)* [Redcall. LEE Kulikov, I Oranskaya, A Yu Rusakov, 367–379].

Konishi, T. (1993). The semantics of grammatical gender: A cross-cultural study. *Journal of Psycholinguistic Research, 22*(5), 519–534. Retrieved (03/2023) from https://doi.org/10.1007/BF01068252

Korangy, A. & Mahmoodi-Bakhtiari, B. (2019). *Essays on typology of Iranian languages.* De Gruyter Mouton, Berlin/ Boston.

Korn, A. (2017). Notes on the nominal system of Bashkardi. *Transactions of the Philological Society, 115*(1), 79–97.

Koul, O. N. & Wali, K. (2006). *Modern Kashmiri grammar.* Dunwoody Press, Springfield, United States.

Kumar, P. & Grace, G. V. (2017). *A write-up of Bhariati grammar.* ILL, Dehradun, India.

Kurinski, E., Jambor, E., & Sera, M. D. (2016). Spanish grammatical gender: Its effects on categorization in native Hungarian speakers. *International Journal of Bilingualism, 20,* 76–93.

Kurinski, E. & Sera, M. D. (2011). Does learning Spanish grammatical gender change English-speaking adults' categorization of inanimate objects? *Bilingualism: Language and Cognition, 14,* 203–220.

Kushal, G. & Padra, B. (2021). Agreement in Sambalpuri: A lesser-known language. *Online International Interdisciplinary Research Journal* (11), 49–61.

Lakoff, G. (1987). *Women, fire and dangerous things: What categories reveal about the mind.* The University of Chicago Press.

Lambelet, A. (2016). Second grammatical gender system and grammatical gender-linked connotations in adult emergent bilinguals with French as a second language. *International Journal of Bilingualism, 20*, 62–75.

Lamm, W. (2001). *Scottish Gaelic*. LINCOM Europa, Munich, Germany.

Landor, R. V. (2014). *Grammatical categories and cognition across five languages: The case of grammatical gender and its potential effects on the conceptualisation of objects*. DataCite, Griffith University, Brisbane, Australia.

Lautin, J. (2016). *Grammatical gender in Hindukush languages: An aerial-typological study* [Bachelor's thesis]. Stockholm University, Stokholm, Sweden, a research project supported by the Swedish Research Council.

Learn Haitian: Haitian Gender. (n.d.). Retrieved (03/2023) from http://learn101.org/haitian_gender.php

Levelt, W. J., Roelofs, A., & Meyer, A. S. (1999). A theory of lexical access in speech production. *The Behavioral and Brain Sciences, 22*(1), 1–38; discussion 38–75. Retrieved (03/2023) from https://doi.org/10.1017/S0140525X99001776

Liljegren, H. (2008). *Towards a grammatical description of Palula: An Indo-Aryan language of the Hindu Kush*, Arkitektkopia AB, Stockholm, Sweden.

Liljegren, H. (2019). Gender typology and gender (in) stability in Hindu Kush Indo-Aryan languages. *Grammatical Gender and Linguistic Complexity* (1), 279–328.

Lipski, J. M. (2001). Chabacano/Spanish and the Philippine linguistic identity: Shedding light on the Chabacano language: Learning from general linguistic and similar cases (= *Estudios de Sociolingüística 2.2*), 119–164.

Lucy, J. A. (1992). *Language diversity and thought: A reformulation of the linguistic relativity hypothesis. Studies in social and cultural foundations of language: Vol. 0012*. Cambridge University Press, New York, United States.

Lucy, J. A. (1997). Linguistic relativity. *Annual Review of Anthropology, Vol. 0012*, 291–312.

Lucy, J. A. (2020, September 18). *Influence of language on thought: Relativity, acquisition, and standardization*. Department of Anthropology. University of New Mexico, Albuquerque, NM, via Zoom. Retrieved (03/2023) from https://www.youtube.com/watch?v=cMGwu396N50&t=267s

Maciuszek, J., Polak, M., & Świa Tkowska, N. (2019). Grammatical gender influences semantic categorization and implicit cognition in Polish. *Frontiers in Psychology, 10*, 2208.

MacKinnon, C. R. (1974). *The phonology and morphology of Dezfuli-Shushtari: A study in West Persian dialectology*. University of California: Los Angeles.

Maffei, A. F. X. (1882). *A Konkani grammar*. Basel Mission & Tract Depository.

Martinez, I. M. & Shatz, M. (1996). Linguistic influences on categorization in preschool children: A crosslinguistic study. *Journal of Child Language, 23*(3), 529–545. Retrieved (03/2023) from https://doi.org/10.1017/s030500090000893x

Martins, C. & Santos, I. (2015). Standardising mirandese: Processes and challenges. *Sociolinguistica, 29*(1), 141–156.

Matras, Y. (2005, cop. 2002). *Romani: A linguistic introduction* (1st ed.). Cambridge University Press. Retrieved (03/2023) from https://doi.org/10.1017/cbo9780511486791

Matras, Y. (2012). *A grammar of Domari. Mouton Grammar Library [MGL]: Vol. 59*. De Gruyter Mouton: De Gruyter. Retrieved (03/2023) from https://doi.org/10.1515/9783110291421

Maurer, P. (2008). A first step towards the analysis of tone in Santomense. *Roots of Creole Structures*, Vol. xvii, 253–261.

Maurer-Cecchini, P. (2021). *A grammar of Tuatschin: A Sursilvan Romansh dialect*. Language Science Press, Berlin, Germany.

Mehta, J. (2018, November 2). *Here's everything you need to know about Mewari language*. Retrieved (03/2023) from https://www.udaipurblog.com/mewari-language.html

Melissaropoulou, D. (2019). Morphological innovations in Propontis Tsakonian. *He Morphology of Asia Minor Greek*, Vol.13, 284–314.

Mertins, B. (2018). *Sprache und Kognition*. DE GRUYTER, Berlin, Deutschland.

Michaelis, S. M., Maurer, P., Haspelmath, M., & Huber, M. (Ed.). *The survey of pidgin and creole language structures*. Oxford University Press, USA.

Mickan, A., Schiefke, M., & Stefanowitsch, A. (2014). Key is a llave is a Schlussel: A failure to replicate an experiment from Boroditsky et al. 2003. *Yearbook of the German Cognitive Linguistics Association, 2*, 39–50.

Mirdehghan, M. & Yusefi, S. (2013). Case and case marking in Vafsi. *Language Studies, 3*(5), 85–105.

Montefinese, M., Ambrosini, E., & Roivainen, E. (2019). No grammatical gender effect on affective ratings: Evidence from Italian and German languages. *Cognition and Emotion, 33*, 848–854. Retrieved (03/2023) from https://doi.org/10.1080/02699931.2018.1483322

Moreton, R. L. (2001). *Mississippi Gulf Coast French: Phonology and morphology*. Tulane University, Language, Linguistics.

Newmark, L., Hubbard, P., & Prifti, P. (1982). *Standard Albanian: A reference grammar for students*. Stanford University Press.

Nicoladis, E. (2019). [Unpublished data].

Nicoladis, E., Da Costa, N., & Foursha-Stevenson, C. (2016). Discourse relativity in Russian-English bilingual preschoolers' classification of objects by gender. *International Journal of Bilingualism, 20*, 17–29.

Nicoladis, E. & Foursha-Stevenson, C. (2012). Language and culture effects on gender classification of objects. *Journal of Cross-Cultural Psychology, 43*, 1095–1109.

Nourzaei, M., Jahani, C., Anonby, E., & Ahangar, A. A. (2015). *Koroshi: A corpus-based grammatical description*. Acta Universitatis Upsaliensis, Uppsala, Sweden.

Oberlies, T. (2011). *Pali: A grammar of the language of the Theravada Tipitaka. With a concordance to Pischel's Grammatik der Prakrit-Sprachen*. Walter de Gruyter, Berlin/ New York.

O'Donovan, J. (1845). *A grammar of the Irish language*.

Ojha, A. K., Behera, P., Singh, S., & Jha, G. N. (2015). Training & evaluation of POS taggers in Indo-Aryan languages: A case of Hindi, Odia and Bhojpuri. *The proceedings of 7th language & technology conference: Human language technologies as a challenge for computer science and linguistics*, 524–529.

Palmer, T. (2016). *Verbal morphology and grammatical aspect in Sarikoli* [Master Thesis]. University of North Dakota.

Parsieva, L. K. & Gatsalova, L. B. (2014). Linguistic and cultural specificity of the derivational category of grammatical persons' nominations in Ossetian language. *Journal of Language and Literature*, 5(4), 217–219.

Pavlidou, T.-S. & Alvanoudi, A. (2013). Grammatical gender and cognition. In N. Lavidas, T. Alexio, & A. Sougari (Eds.), *Major trends in theoretical and applied linguistics* (Vol. 2, pp. 109–124). London, UK: Versita.

Pavlidou, T.-S. & Alvanoudi, A. (2018). Conceptualizing the world as "female" or "male": Further remarks on grammatical gender and speakers' cognition. In N. Topintzi, N. Lavidas, & M. Moumtzi (Eds.), *Selected papers on theoretical and applied linguistics from ISTAL23*. Thessaloniki, Greece: School of English, Aristotle University of Thessaloniki.

Phillips, M. P. (2012). *Dialect continuum in the Bhil tribal belt grammatical aspects* [PhD Thesis]. University of London, London, England.

Phillips, W. & Boroditsky, L. (2003, August). *Can quirks of grammar affect the way you think? Grammatical gender and object concepts*. Paper presented at the 25th annual meeting of the Cognitive Science Society, Boston, MA.

Press, I. (1986). *A grammar of modern Breton. Mouton grammar library: Vol. 2*. Mouton de Gruyter

Pylyshyn, Z. W. (1984). *Computation and cognition*. MIT Press.

Rahimian, G. (1978). *Spoken Bakhtiari*. SIT Study abroad, SIT Graduate Institute, Brattleboro, Vermont.

Rajapurohit, B. B. (2012). *Grammar of Shina language and vocabulary: (Based on the dialect spoken around Dras)*. Central Institute of Indian Languages, Mysore, India.

Ramos, S. & Roberson, D. (2011). What constrains grammatical gender effects on semantic judgements? Evidence from Portuguese. *Journal of Cognitive Psychology, 23*(1), 102–111.

Rani Das, A. (October 2017). *A comparative study of Bangla and Sylheti grammar* [PhD Dissertation]. University of Naples Federico II, Napoli.

Rojavin, M. (2010,). The semantic category of gender in Russian and Ukrainian. *The Slavic and East European Journal, 54*(3), 503–526.

Saalbach, H., Imai, M., & Schalk, L. (2012). Grammatical gender and inferences about biological properties in German-speaking children. *Cognitive Science, 36*, 1251–1267.

Sabourin, L., Stowe, L. A., & de Haan, G. J. (2006). Transfer effects in learning a second language grammatical gender system. *Second Language Research, 22*(1), 1–29. Retrieved (03/2023) from https://doi.org/10.1191/0267658306sr259oa

Saksenā, B. (1971). *Evolution of Awadhi: (a branch of Hindi)* (2nd ed.). Motilal Banarsidass.

Samuel, S., Cole, G., & Eacott, M. J. (2019). Grammatical gender and linguistic relativity: A systematic review. *Psychonomic Bulletin & Review, 26*(6), 1767–1786. Retrieved (03/2023) from https://doi.org/10.3758/s13423-019-01652-3

Sande, H. (2013). Nouchi as a distinct language: The morphological evidence. *Annual Conference on African Linguistics* (44), 7–10.

Sato, S. & Athanasopoulos, P. (2018). Grammatical gender affects gender perception: Evidence for the structural-feedback hypothesis. *Cognition, 176*, 220–231.

Sedlmeier, P., Tipandjan, A., & Jänchen, A. (2016). How persistent are grammatical gender effects? The case of German and Tamil. *Journal of Psycholinguistic Research, 45*, 317–336.

Semenuks, A., Phillips, W., Dalca, I., Kim, C., & Boroditsky, L. (2017). Effects of grammatical gender on object description. In G. Gunzelmann, A. Howes, T. Tenbrink, & E. Davelaar (Eds.), *Proceedings of the 39th annual meeting of the Cognitive Science Society* (pp. 1060–1065). Austin, TX: Cognitive Science Society.

Sera, M. D., Berge, C. A., & Del Pintado, J. C. (1994). Grammatical and conceptual forces in the attribution of gender by English and Spanish speakers. *Cognitive Development*, *9*(3), 261–292. Retrieved (03/2023) from https://doi.org/10.1016/0885-2014(94)90007-8

Sera, M. D., Elieff, C., Forbes, J., Burch, M. C., Rodríguez, W., & Dubois, D. P. (2002). When language affects cognition and when it does not: An analysis of grammatical gender and classification. *Journal of Experimental Psychology: General, 131*, 377–397.

Siddique, K. (2006, June). *Memoni language project.* The Truth (As-Sidq). Retrieved (03/2023) from http://www.as-sidq.org/memoni/

Slobin, D. I. (1996). From "thought and language" to "thinking for speaking". In D. I. Slobin (Ed.), *Rethinking linguistic relativity* (pp. 70–96). Cambridge University Press, Cambridge, United Kingdom.

Slobin, D. I. (Ed.). (1996). *Rethinking linguistic relativity.* Cambridge University Press, Cambridge, United Kingdom.

Smith, I. R. (1977). *Sri Lanke Creole Portuguese phonology.* Cornell University.

Southworth, S. C. (1970). Review: A grammar of old Marathi by Alfred Master. *Linguistic Society of America, 46*(2, Part 1), 507–513.

Stemberger, J. P. (2006). Proper names in Slovene: Implications for defaults in inflectional morphology. *Proceedings of the Annual Meeting of the Cognitive Science Society, 28* (8), 2186–2191.

Taherkhani, N. & Ourang, M. (2013). A study of derivational morphemes in Lari & Tati as two endangered Iranian languages: An analytical-contrastive examination with Persian. *Journal of American Science, 9*(11s), 38–45.

Toker, H. (2014). *A practical guide to Hindko grammar.* Trafford Publishing, Mounton & Co.B.V, Hungary.

Trofimov, A. (2019). On the place of Parachi and Ormuri among the Iranian languages according to the data of annotated Swadesh lists. *Journal of Language Relationship, 16*(3–4), 277–292.

Trumpp, E. (1872). *Grammar of the Sindhi language: Compared with the Sanskrit-Prakrit and the cognate Indian vernaculars.* Trübner.

Truppi, C. (2019). Copulas in contact: Kriyol, Upper Guinea Creoles, and their substrate. *Journal of Ibero-Romance Creoles, 9*(1), 85–114.

Tucker, G. R., Lambert, W. E., & Rigault, A. A. (2019). The French speaker's skill with grammatical gender. *The French Speaker's Skill with Grammatical Gender.* Mounton & Co.B.V, Hungary.

Turner, R. L. (1932). The language of the Ashkun Kafirs. By G. Morgenstierne.: Extract from Norsk Tidsshrift for Sprogvidenskap, Bindii, 1929. pp. 192–289. *Journal of the Royal Asiatic Society, 6a4*(1), 173–175.

Uddin, N. & Uddin, J. (2019). A step towards Torwali machine translation: an analysis of morphosyntactic challenges in a low-resource language. *Proceedings of the 2nd Workshop on Technologies for MT of Low Resource Languages*, 6–10.

Vahman, F., Vahman, F., & Asatrian, G. (2002). *Notes on the language and ethnography of the Zoroastrians of Yazd* (Vol. 85). Kgl. Danske Videnskabernes Selskab.

van der Wal Anonby, C. A. (2015). *A grammar of Kumzari: A mixed Perso-Arabian language of Oman*. Leiden University, Doctoral dissertation.

Vernich, L. (2017). Does learning a foreign language affect object categorization in native speakers of a language with grammatical gender? The case of Lithuanian speakers learning three languages with different types of gender systems (Italian, Russian and German). *International Journal of Bilingualism, 23*, 417–436.

Vernich, L., Argus, R., & Kamandulytė-Merfeldienė, L. (2017). Extending research on the influence of grammatical gender on object classification: A cross-linguistic study comparing Estonian, Italian and Lithuanian native speakers. *Eesti Rakenduslingvistika Ühingu Aastaraamat, 13*, 223–240.

Vigliocco, G., Vinson, D. P., Paganelli, F., & Dworzynski, K. (2005). Grammatical gender effects on cognition: Implications for language learning and language use. *Journal of Experimental Psychology. General, 134*(4), 501–520. Retrieved (03/2023) from https://doi.org/10.1037/0096-3445.134.4.501

Villeneuve, A. J. (2011). *A sociolinguistic study of Vimeu French* [PhD Dissertation]. Indiana University, Indiana.

Visser, W. (2011). Historical gender change in West Frisian. *Morphology, 21*(1), 31–56.

Wam, C. (2019). *Grammatical gender in Afrikaans–simplification in action*. North-West University, Potchefstroom South Africa. Retrieved (03/2023) from https://www.ds.uzh.ch/dam/jcr:499d7d96-d307-410f-a924-ca927ecc3d6f/afrikaans_wanniecarstens.pdf

Wheeler, M., Yates, A., & Dols, N. (2002). *Catalan: A comprehensive grammar*. Routledge, England.

Whorf, B. (1956). *Language thought and reality*. MIT Press.

Whorf, B. L. (Ed.). (2012). *Language, thought, and reality, second edition: Selected writings of Benjamin Lee Whorf* (2nd ed.). The MIT Press.

Williams, S. J. (1986). *A Welsh grammar* (Repr). University of Wales Press.

Windfuhr, G. (2009). *The Iranian languages* (1st ed.). *Routledge language family Sseries*. Routledge, England.

Yadav, S. P. (July 2016). *A sociolinguistic survey of Chitoniya*. Linguistic Survey of Nepal, Department of linguisitcs, Tribhuvan University, Kathmandu, Nepal.

Appendix A.1

Name of the main branch	Name of L1 spoken languages	Number of grammatical gender
Albanian	Gheg and Tosk	Three genders: masculine, feminine, rare neutral
	Arvanitika	
	Arbëresh	
Armenic	Standard Armenic	No grammatical Gender
	East Armenic	
Baltic	Latvian/Lettish	Two genders: masculine and feminine
	Lithuanian	
Slavonic	Bulgarian	Three genders: masculine, feminine, rare neutral
	Macedonian	
	Serbo-Croat	
	Slovene	
	Czech	
	Slovak	
	Polish	
	Upper and lower Sorbian (Lusatian)	
	Russian	
	Ukrainian	
	Belorussian	

Name of the main branch	Name of L1 spoken languages	Number of grammatical gender
Celtic	Breton	Two genders: masculine and feminine
	Cornish	
	Welsh	

Name of the main branch	**Name of L1 spoken languages**	**Number of grammatical gender**
	Scotts Gaelic	
	Irish	
Northern Germanic	Norwegian	Three genders: masc., fem., neut.
	Modern Icelandic	Three genders: masc., fem., neut.
	Modern Danish	Two genders: common and neuter
	Modern Swedish	Two genders: common and neuter
Western Germanic	Modern German	Three genders: masc., fem., neut.
	Yiddish	Three genders: masc., fem., neut.
	Modern Dutch	Two genders: common and neuter
	Afrikaans	No grammatical Gender
	English	Pronominal gender
	Scots	Pronominal gender
	Frisian	Two genders: common (non-neuter) and neuter
Graeco-Phrygian	Apulia-Calabrian Greek/ Griko	No grammatical gender
	Cypriot Greek	No information found
	Romano-Greek	Three genders: masc., fem., neut.
	Cappadocian Greek	One gender: neutral
	Pontic	Three genders: masc., fem., neut.
	Modern Greek	Three genders: masc., fem., neut.
	Taskonian	Three genders: masc., fem., neut.

Appendix A.2

Name of the main branch	Name of L1 spoken languages	Number of grammatical gender
Indo-Aryan	Angika	No information found
	Bhojpuri	One gender: fem.
	Caribbean Hindustani	No information found
	Magahi	Two genders: masc., fem.
	Maithili	Two genders: masc., fem.
	Kudmali/Kurmali	Two genders: masc., fem.
	Oraon Sadri	No grammatical gender
	Sadri	No grammatical gender
	Panchpargania	No information found
	Pali	Three genders: masc., fem., neut
	Chitwania Tharu/ Chitoniya Tharu	No grammatical gender
	Dangaura Tharu	No information found
	Sonha	No information found
	Kathoriya Tharu	No information found
	Kochila Tharu	No information found
	Rana Tharu	Two genders: masc., fem.
	Buksa	No information found
	Majhi	No information found
	Musasa	No information found
	Kumhali	No information found
	Bote	No information found
	Darai	Two genders: masc., fem.
	Dewas-Done Danuwar	No information found
	Kochariya-East Danuwar	No information found
	Dhivehi	No grammatical gender
	Sinhala	Two genders: masc., fem.
	Veddah	No information found
	Domaaki	Two genders: masc., fem.
	Domari	Two genders: masc., fem.
	Archaic Angloromani	No information found
	Welsh Romani	No information found
	Kalo Finnish Romani	No information found
	Sinte-Manus Romani	No information found
	Balkan Romani	No information found

Name of the main branch	Name of L1 spoken languages	Number of grammatical gender
	Baltic Romani	No information found
	Caló	No information found
	Central Romani	Two genders: masc., fem.
	Vlax Romani	No information found
	Sauraseni Prakrit	No information found
	Bauria	No information found
	Bhili	No information found
	Chodri	No information found

Name of the main branch	Name of L1 spoken languages	Number of grammatical gender
Indo-Aryan	Dhodia-Kukna	No information found
	Dungra Bhil	No information found
	Gamit	No information found
	Adiwasi Garasia	No information found
	Rajput Garasia	No information found
	Malvi	No information found
	Mawchi	No information found
	Nimadi	No information found
	Pardhi	No information found
	Bhilali	No information found
	Nahali-Baglani	No information found
	Pauri Bareli	No information found
	Rathwi Bareli	No information found
	Palya Bareli	No information found
	Rathawi	No information found
	Vaagri Booli	No information found
	Noiri	No information found
	Vasavi	No information found
	Wagdi	Three genders: masc., fem., neut.
	Awadhi	Two genders: masc., fem.
	Bagheli	No information found
	Chhattisgarhi	Two genders: masc., fem.
	Powari	No information found
	Dubli	No information found
	Gujarati	Three genders: masc., fem., neut.
	Saurashtra	No information found
	Aer	No information found
	Kachi Koli	No information found

Name of the main branch	Name of L1 spoken languages	Number of grammatical gender
	Vaghri	No information found
	Wadiyara Koli	No information found
	Bagri	Two genders: masc., fem.
	Jandavra	No information found
	Dhatki	No information found
	Dhundari	No information found
	Hadothi	No information found
	Kabutra	No information found
	Kanjari	No information found
	Lambadi	No grammatical gender
	Merwari	No information found
	Gade Lohar	No information found
	Mewari	Two genders: masc., fem.
	Godwari	No information found
	Gujari	No information found
	Marwari	No information found

Name of the main branch	Name of L1 spoken languages	Number of grammatical gender
Indo-Aryan	Mewati	Two genders: masc., fem.
	Od	No information found
	Parya	No information found
	Shekhawati	No information found
	Bhaya	No information found
	Goaria	No information found
	Parkari Koli	No information found
	Dhanki	No information found
	Khandesi	No information found
	Middle Indo-Aryan	No information found
	Braj	Two genders: masc., fem.
	Bharia/Bhariati	Two genders: masc., fem.
	Bundeli	Two genders: masc., fem.
	Haryanvi	No information found
	Andaman Creole Hindi	No information found
	Fiji Hindi	No grammatical gender
	Hindi	Two genders: masc., fem.
	Urdu	Two genders: masc., fem.
	Kanauji	No information found
	Ghera	No information found

Name of the main branch	Name of L1 spoken languages	Number of grammatical gender
	Gurgula	No information found
	Bhatri	No information found
	Bhunjia	No information found
	Halbi	No information found
	Kamar	No information found
	Nahari	No information found
	Bengali	No grammatical gender
	Bishnupriya Manipuri	No information found
	Hajong	No information found
	Sylheti	Two genders: masc., fem.
	Kharia Thar	No information found
	Lodhi	No information found
	Mar Paharia of Dumka	No information found
	Rohingya	No information found
	Chakma	No information found
	Chittagonian	No information found
	Tangchangya	No information found
	Kurmukar	No information found
	Assamese	No grammatical gender
	Naga Pidgin	No information found
	Central-Eastern Kamta	No information found
	Rajbanshi	No information found
	Surjapuri	Two genders: masc., fem.
	Bodo Parja	No information found

Name of the main branch	Name of L1 spoken languages	Number of grammatical gender
Indo-Aryan	Kotia-Adivasi Oriya-Desiya	No information found
	Kupia	No information found
	Odia	No grammatical gender
	Reli	No information found
	Sambalpuri	No grammatical gender
	Garhwali	No information found
	Kumaoni	No information found
	Dotyali	No information found
	Jumli	No information found
	Nepali	Two genders: masc., fem.
	Jaunsari	No information found
	Bhadrawahi	Two genders: masc., fem.

Name of the main branch	**Name of L1 spoken languages**	**Number of grammatical gender**
	Churahi	No information found
	Bhattiyali	No information found
	Bilaspuri	No information found
	Chambeali	No information found
	Gaddi	No information found
	Pangwali	Three genders: masc., fem., neut
	Dogri	No information found
	Kangri	No information found
	Mandeali	No information found
	Hinduri	No information found
	Indo-Aryan Kinnauri	No information found
	Kullu Pahari	No information found
	Mahasu Pahari	No information found
	Chitral Kalasha	No information found
	Khowar	No information found
	Kashmiri	Two genders: masc., fem.
	Khah	No information found
	Gawri	Two genders: masc., fem.
	Torwali	Two genders: masc., fem.
	Indus Kohistani	No information found
	Bateri	No information found
	Mankiyali	No information found
	Chilisso	No information found
	Gowro	No information found
	Dameli	Two genders: masc., fem.
	Gawar-Bati	No information found
	Grangali	No information found
	Shumashti	No information found
	Northeast Pashayi	No information found
	Southeast Pashayi	No information found
	Northwest Pashayi	No information found
	Southwest Pashayi	No information found

Name of the main branch	**Name of L1 spoken languages**	**Number of grammatical gender**
Indo-Aryan	Brokskat	No information found
	Kohistani Shina	Two genders: masc., fem.
	Ushojo	No information found
	Kundal Shahi	Two genders: masc., fem.

Name of the main branch	Name of L1 spoken languages	Number of grammatical gender
	Shina	Two genders: masc., fem.
	Kalkoti	No information found
	Palula	Two genders: masc., fem.
	Savi	No information found
	Eastern Panjabi	No information found
	Sansi/Sansiboli	Two genders: masc., fem.
	Northern Hindko	Two genders: masc., fem.
	Southern Hindko	Two genders: masc., fem.
	Pahari Potwari	No information found
	Sirajic	No information found
	Saraiki	Two genders: masc., fem.
	Western Panjabi	No information found
	Kachchi	No information found
	Khetrani	No information found
	Jadgali	No information found
	Lasi	No information found
	Luwati	No information found
	Memoni	Two genders: masc., fem.
	Sindhi	Two genders: masc., fem.
	Sindhi Bhil	No information found
	Kholosi	Two genders: masc., fem.
	Katkari	No information found
	Goan Konkani/Konkani	Three genders: masc., fem., neut.
	Dungar Varli	No information found
	Marathi	Three genders: masc., fem., neut.
	Samvedi	No information found
	Varhadi-Nagpuri	No information found
	Konkan Marathi	No information found
	Phudagi	No information found
	Old Marathi	Three genders: masc., fem., neut.
	Chinali	No information found
	Lahul Lohar	No information found

Appendix A.3

Name of the main branch	Name of L1 spoken languages	Number of grammatical gender
Iranian	Gurani	No grammatical gender
	Bajelnai	No grammatical gender
	Shabaki	No grammatical gender
	Alamuti	No grammatical gender
	Kajali	No grammatical gender
	Karanic	No information found
	Shahrudi-Southern Talysh	No grammatical gender
	Kho´ni	moribund/pronominal gender (two genders: masculine, feminine)
	Maraghei	One gender, feminie
	North-Central Talysh	No grammatical gender
	Kabatei	Two genders: masc., fem.,
	Upper Taromi	No information found
	Harzani-Kilit	No information found
	Karingani-Kalasuri-Khoynarudi	No information found
	Alviri-Vidari	moribund/No grammatical gender
	Eshtehardi	No information found
	Rezajedri	No information found
	Takestani	No information found
	Ashtiani	No information found
	Vafsi	Two genders: masc., fem.
	Dimli	Two genders: masc., fem.
	Kirmanjki/Kurmanji	Two genders: masc., fem.
	Eastern-Baluchi	No grammatical gender
	Koroshi	No grammatical gender
	southern Baluchi	No grammatical gender
	Western Baluchi	No grammatical gender
	Gilaki	No grammatical gender
	Rudbari	No information found
	Mazandarani	No grammatical gender
	Shahmirzadi	No grammatical gender
	Kavir	No information found

Name of the main branch	Name of L1 spoken languages	Number of grammatical gender
	Gazic	No grammatical gender
	Judeo-Hamadani-Borujerdi	No grammatical gender
	Natanzic	No information found
	Soic	No information found
	Khunsaric	No information found
	Nayinic	No grammatical gender
	Zoroastrian Yazdi	No grammatical gender
	Sivandi	No information found
	Lasgerdi	No information found

Name of the main branch	Name of L1 spoken languages	Number of grammatical gender
Iranian	Sangisari	No information found
	Sorkhei-Aftari	No grammatical gender
	Central Kurdish	No grammatical gender
	Northern Kurdish	Two genders: masc., fem.
	Southern Kurdish	No grammatical gender
	Laki	No grammatical gender
	Semnani-Biyabuneki	No information found
	Digor Ossetian	No grammatical gender
	Iron Ossetian	No grammatical gender
	Yagnobi	No grammatical gender
	Ormuri	No grammatical gender
	Parachi	No grammatical gender
	Central Pashto	Two genders: masc., fem.
	Northern Pashto	Two genders: masc., fem.
	Southern Pashto	Two genders: masc., fem.
	Waneci	No information found
	Ishkashimi	No information found
	Sanglechi	No information found
	Sarikoli	No grammatical gender
	Shughni	No information found
	Yazgulyam	pronominal gender
	Bashkardi	No grammatical gender
	Fars Dialects	No grammatical gender
	Judeo-Tat	No grammatical gender

Name of the main branch	Name of L1 spoken languages	Number of grammatical gender
	Muslim Tat	No grammatical gender
	Aimaq	No information found
	Dari	No grammatical gender
	Dehwari	No information found
	Hazaragi	No grammatical gender
	Bukharic	No information found
	Tajik	No grammatical gender
	Judeo-Persian	No grammatical gender
	Western Farsi	No grammatical gender
	Kumzari	No grammatical gender
	Larestani	No grammatical gender
	Dezfuli-Shushtari	No grammatical gender/nearly extinct
	Bakhtiari	No grammatical gender
	Southern Luri	No grammatical gender
	Northern Luri	No grammatical gender
	Wakhi	No information found
	Munji	No information found
	Yidgha	No information found
	Ashkun	Two genders: masc., fem.

Name of the main branch	Name of L1 spoken languages	Number of grammatical gender
Iranian	Katë	Two genders: masc., fem.
	Nuristani Kalasha	Two genders: masc., fem.
	Tregami	Two genders: masc., fem.
	Prasun	Two genders: masc., fem.

Appendix A.4

Name of the main branch	Name of L1 spoken languages	Number of grammatical gender
Italic	Aromanian	Three genders: masc., fem., neut.
	Megleno Romanian	Three genders: masc., fem., neut.
	Romanian	Three genders: masc., fem., neut.
	Istro Romanian	Three genders: masc., fem., neut.
	Istriot	Two genders: masc., fem.
	Continental Southern Italian	Two genders: masc., fem.
	Italian	Two genders: masc., fem.
	Sicilian	Two genders: masc., fem.
	Emiliano	No information found
	Romagnol	No information found
	Judeo-Italian	Two genders: masc., fem.
	Ligurian	Two genders: masc., fem.
	Lombard	Two genders: masc., fem.
	Piemontese	Two genders: masc., fem.
	Sassarese Sardinian	Two genders: masc., fem.
	Venetian	Two genders: masc., fem.
	Friulian	Two genders: masc., fem.
	Ladin	Two genders: masc., fem.
	Cajun French	Two genders: masc., fem.
	Gulf Coast French	No information found
	Guianese Creole French	No information found
	Uaçá Creole French	No information found
	Haitian	Two genders: masc., fem.
	Guadeloupe-Martinique Creole French	Two genders: masc., fem.
	Saint Lucian Creole French	Two genders: masc., fem.
	Louisiana Creole French	Two genders: masc., fem.
	French	Two genders: masc., fem.
	Nouchi	Two genders: masc., fem.
	Morisyen	No information found
	Seselwa Creole French	No information found
	Réunion Creole French	No information found
	Tayo	No information found
	Picard	Two genders: masc., fem.,

Name of the main branch	Name of L1 spoken languages	Number of grammatical gender
	Arpitan	No information found
	Faeto and Celle San Vito Francoprovencal	No information found
	Walloon	Two genders: masc., fem.
	Romansh	Two genders: masc., fem.
	Catalan	Two genders: masc., fem.
	Gardiol	No information found
	Occitan	Two genders: masc., fem.

Name of the main branch	Name of L1 spoken languages	Number of grammatical gender
Italic	Old Provençal	Two genders: masc., fem.
	Asturian-Leonese-Cantabrian	No information found
	Mirandese	Two genders: masc., fem.
	Extremaduran	No information found
	Ladino	No information found
	Palenquero	No information found
	Peruvian Amazonian Spanish	No information found
	Chavacano	Two genders: masc., fem.
	Spanish	Two genders: masc., fem., three genders in pronouns masc., fem., neut.
	Fala	No information found
	Galician	No information found
	Cafundo	No information found
	Portuguese	Two genders: masc., fem.
	Malabar-Sri Lanka Portuguese	Two genders: masc., fem.
	Daman-Diu Portuguese	No information found
	Korlai Portuguese	No information found
	Angolar	No information found
	Annobonese	No information found
	Principense	No information found
	Sãotomense	Two genders: masc., fem.
	Macanese	No information found

Name of the main branch	**Name of L1 spoken languages**	**Number of grammatical gender**
	Malacca-Batavia Portuguese Creole	No grammatical gender
	Kabuverdianu	Two genders: masc., fem.
	Papiamento	No information found
	Upper Guinea Crioulo	No grammatical gender
	Minderico	No information found
	Aragonese	Three genders: masc., fem., neut
	Corsican	No information found
	Gallurese Sardinian	No information found
	Campidanese Sardinian	Two genders: masc., fem.
	Logudorese Sardinian	No information found
	South Lucanian	No information found

Kerstin Leimbrink, Janina Harwardt, Ian Lowes and Barbara Mertins

Zusammenhänge von Sprache, Musik und Kognition: Eine explorative Studie zu sprachspezifischen Merkmalen in deutschen, tschechischen, französischen und englischen Volksliedern

Abstract: In linguistic and musicological research, music and language are regarded as universal human forms of expression and means of communication that are temporally-organized and culturally-specific acoustic events. In the case of music, the emphasis is on the acoustic-emotional level of sounds. In language, on the other hand, the meaning-bearing side of lexical words is central. Phonological units are arbitrarily interpreted as lexical words and subordinated to a propositional world-structuring syntactic system. Psycholinguistic research shows that linguistic structures shape individual thinking, resulting in language- and culture-specific conceptualizations. However, only very few studies exist dealing with linguistic relativity in relation to composition and especially reception of music. The article presents a study on language-specific features in German, Czech, French, and English folk songs, showing specific linguistic structural features in the form of different rhythmic-melodic structures. On the basis of 400 folk songs, musical features such as pitch and pitch intervals, rhythm and meter, are compared statistically with the help of a multinomial logistic regression model. The findings display language-specific differences reflected in the presence of an upbeat, the preference for one meter over another, and the overall pitch range. Accordingly, it can be assumed that linguistic structures could also exert an influence on the auditory perception and processing as well as reception of music.

Keywords: Multilingualism research, language comparison, linguistic relativity, language-specific perception, cognition, language and music, music reception, thinking-for-speaking theory

1. Einführung

Musik und Sprache sind universelle menschliche Ausdrucksformen und Kommunikationsmittel, die als akustische Ereignisse zeitlich organisiert und kulturspezifisch geprägt sind. Beide sind voneinander unabhängig existierende syntaktische Systeme, die komplexe, hierarchisch strukturierte Sequenzen verwenden. Diese beruhen auf impliziten Strukturnormen. Bei beiden beinhaltet die syntaktische Verarbeitung die Integration diskreter Elemente in Strukturen höherer Ordnung – z. B. Wörter in der Sprache und Töne bzw. Akkorde in der Musik in Sätze und harmonische Sequenzen – die nach einer Reihe von kombinatorischen Prinzipien und auf der Folie eines spezifischen Hintergrundsystems erfolgt (vgl. Patel 2008).

Bei der Musik liegt die Betonung dabei auf der akustisch-emotionalen Ebene des lautlichen Ausdrucks – dem Klang. Durch die enge Beziehung zwischen musikalischen Elementen und Emotionen können Gefühle wie Spannung, Entspannung, Trauer, Freude etc. ausgedrückt werden. In der Sprache ist dagegen die bedeutungstragende Seite des lautlichen Ausdrucks (lexikalische Wörter) zentral. Phonologische Einheiten werden arbiträr als lexikalische Wörter interpretiert und einem propositional weltgliedernden syntaktischen System untergeordnet.

Die Zusammenhänge von Sprache, Musik und Kognition stellen ein weites interdisziplinäres Forschungsfeld bereit. Ein starkes Forschungsinteresse der Musikwissenschaft und zu einem geringeren Teil auch der Sprachwissenschaft gilt dem Ursprung von Musik und dessen Beziehung zur Sprachentwicklung in der Phylo- und Ontogenese (u.a. Papoušek & Papoušek 1981; Brown et al. 2001; Trehub 2000; Mithen 2005; Parncutt 2009; Wermke & Mende 2009; Leimbrink 2016). Einen Kurzüberblick dazu liefern die Kapitel 2 und 3.

Die Zusammenhänge von Sprache, Kultur und Kognition werden in verschiedenen wissenschaftlichen Disziplinen erforscht. In der Psycholinguistik wurden in den letzten Jahren vielfältige Einflüsse von sprachlicher, kultureller und individueller Vielfalt auf kognitive Prozesse untersucht (vgl. Mertins 2018). Dabei wurde herausgestellt, dass sprachliche Strukturen das individuelle Denken prägen, wodurch eine sprach- und kulturspezifische Prägung und damit auch soziokulturelle Vielfalt entstehen. Der Einfluss von Sprache(n) auf die Wahrnehmung und kognitive Verarbeitung, zusammengefasst im Konzept der Linguistischen Relativität, wird in Kapitel 3 näher beschrieben.

Ein bislang kaum erforschtes Feld stellen sprachspezifische Zusammenhänge von Sprache, Musik und Kognition dar. Nicht nachgewiesen ist, ob verschiedene Sprachen auch einen Einfluss auf die individuelle auditive Wahrnehmung und Verarbeitung von anderen auditiven Phänomenen wie z. B. Musik haben können.[1] Bisher gibt es keine Untersuchungen, die einen konkreten Anhaltspunkt für empirische Erhebungen des sprachspezifischen Musikhörens bereitstellen

---

1 Einflüsse auf andere Wahrnehmungen wie z.B. auf die visuell-räumliche sind bereits bestätigt worden. Es wurde gezeigt, dass die intraindividuelle Repräsentation von Musik räumlich wahrgenommen wird (z.B. hohe vs. tiefe Töne, ein naher vs. ferner

und beispielsweise der Frage nachgehen, ob melodisch-rhythmische Strukturen verschiedener Erstsprachen einen Einfluss auf die Strukturen der Wahrnehmung von musikalischen Stimuli haben. Die Autor*innen dieses Beitrags möchten sich dieser Fragestellung annähern und dafür erste empirische Grundlagen schaffen. Wir nehmen an, dass musikalische Errungenschaften wie Volkslieder aus verschiedenen Kulturkreisen und Epochen neben individuellen Merkmalen der Komponisti*nnen auch spezifische sprachstrukturelle Merkmale in Form unterschiedlicher rhythmisch-melodischer Strukturen aufweisen, die sich wie sprachstrukturelle Merkmale verschiedener Sprachen voneinander unterscheiden lassen. Dazu wurde eine Stichprobe von 400 Volksliedern der deutschen, tschechischen, französischen und englischen Sprache analysiert. Damit fokussiert dieser Beitrag den Zusammenhang von Sprache, Kognition und Musikwahrnehmung an der Schnittstelle von linguistischer Relativität und auditiver Wahrnehmung bzw. Verarbeitung von Musik und schafft erste empirische Voraussetzungen. Die Untersuchung und erste Ergebnisse werden in Kapitel 5 beschrieben. Es schließen sich eine Diskussion und ein Forschungsausblick in Kapitel 6 an.

2. Zusammenhänge von Sprache und Musik in der Phylogenese

> „.. the study of language evolution has much to gain from a joint consideration of music. This includes such important issues as evolution of the human vocal tract, the hominid brain expansion, human brain asymmetry, lateralization of cognitive function, the evolution of syntax, evolution of symbolic gesturing, and the many parallel neural and cognitive mechanisms that appear to underlie music and language processing." (Brown, Merker & Wallin 2001, 4)

Einschlägige Sprachhistoriker*innen gehen davon aus, dass unserer Sprache in der Evolution eine wenig artikulierte gesangsartige Protosprache vorausgegangen ist (Jespersen 1922; Wray 1998; Mithen 2005). Demnach waren die musikalischen Elemente in der frühen Sprachgeschichte reichhaltiger als heute. Nach Meinung vieler Forschender konnten unsere Vorfahren bereits singen, bevor sie sprechen lernten. Dies brachte ihnen einen entscheidenden Selektionsvorteil

---

Klang) (vgl. Griffiths 2003:168) und die kognitive Leitung vor allem bei musikalisch Trainierten beeinflusst (vgl. Altenmüller 2018). Das kognitive System bildet das prosodische Merkmal Tonhöhe als mentale Repräsentation des Raumes ab, wie Rusconi et al. (2006) zeigten.

bei der Paarung ein und diente der gegenseitigen Verständigung (Cross 2001; Mithen 2005).

Brown (2017) geht von einem gemeinsamen evolutionären Vorläufer, einer sogenannten „Musilanguage" aus – eine Art Mischung aus ‚*music*' und ‚*language*', die ihren Ursprung in emotionsgeladenen prosodisch modulierten vokalen Äußerungen hat. Dieser Vorläufer hatte zunächst eine gemeinschaftsstiftende Funktion und brachte dadurch einen evolutionären Vorteil mit sich. In dieser primären Ausdrucksweise waren Ausdruck und Gestaltung in der Kommunikation noch nicht voneinander getrennt. Bedeutung entstand durch die Variation von Tonhöhe und Rhythmus. Später entwickelten sich durch Gruppenbindung Formen der Urmusik, bei der mit einfachen Mitteln und Werkzeugen Klänge erzeugt wurden, wie es z. B. beim Didgeridoospiel, Urgesang oder Trommeln noch heute praktiziert wird.

Sprache und Musik sind somit wahrscheinlich evolutionär gemeinsam verankert, sie sind genetisch angelegt und werden von Generation zu Generation tradiert. Die Systeme verfügen über ähnliche strukturelle Merkmale. Dazu zählen Akzent, Rhythmus, Tonhöhe und Tonhöhenverlauf, Lautstärke, Sprechgeschwindigkeit und Stimmfärbung in der Sprache und Metrik, Rhythmik, Takt, Melodik, Dynamik, Tempo und Klangfarbe in der Musik. Einige akustische Merkmale verschiedener Emotionen wie Angst, Traurigkeit und Ärger stimmen in Sprache und Musik überein (vgl. Patel 2008). Weitergegeben werden die sprachlichen bzw. musikalischen Komponenten extragenetisch durch Lernen und Lehren, sie leben in der Veränderung und sind an menschliche Praxisfelder geknüpft. So ist die kindgerichtete Sprache der Bezugspersonen mit musikalischen Elementen angereichert, eine Kombination, die die frühen Vorläufer von Musik und Sprache bildet (Wallin, Merker & Brown 2001; Wermke & Mende 2009, 2011, 2013; Honing, Cate, Peretz, & Trehub 2015). Für den engen evolutionsbedingten Zusammenhang von Sprache und Musik spricht auch die Tatsache, dass das Wahrnehmen und Produzieren von Musik komplexe Vorgänge sind, die nahezu alle Bereiche des Gehirns involvieren, mehr als beim Sprechen. Zudem sind viele kognitive Verarbeitungsprozesse sowohl an der Wahrnehmung von Musik als auch an der von Sprache beteiligt (neuronale Korrelate dieser Verarbeitungsprozesse überlappen sich stark). Teile der prosodischen Merkmale wie die Tonhöhe werden ähnlich verarbeitet. Auch scheint der Einsatz von Musik Prozesse auf verschiedenen Ebenen der Sprachverarbeitung positiv zu beeinflussen und zu unterstützen wie z. B. die Wahrnehmung von Rhythmen. Verarbeitungsprozesse in einer Domäne profitieren von Training in der anderen Domäne (vgl. Besson et al. 2017).

Dennoch kann die Frage nach der Entstehung von Musik und Sprache bis heute (noch) nicht abschließend geklärt werden, da empirische Daten fehlen und auch das *Musilanguage – Modell* eher spekulativ und schwer zu überprüfen bleibt.

3. Sprache und Musik als sprach- und kulturspezifisch geprägte Ausdrucksformen in der Ontogenese

„... infants' first steps into language are based on prosodic information (that is, on the musical aspects of speech). Moreover, musical communication in early childhood (such as parental singing) appears to play an important role in the emotional, cognitive, and social development of children." (Kölsch 2013)

Bei dem hier skizzierten Forschungsvorhaben spielt die sprachspezifische Wahrnehmung und Verarbeitung prosodischer Merkmale in Sprache und Musik eine zentrale Rolle. Die Prosodie bezeichnet die melodische Gliederung gesprochener Sprache. Dazu gehören der Sprachrhythmus und die Sprachmelodie, Akzente, Klangfarbe, Pausen und die Variation der Lautstärke. Prosodische bzw. suprasegmentale Merkmale werden auch als „musikalische Aspekte des Sprachsignals" bezeichnet (Sallat & Jentschke 2015). Einige prosodische Tonmuster werden in verschiedenen Sprachen kommunikativ weitgehend universell verwendet (vgl. Patel 2008). So wird beispielsweise zur Beruhigung ein enger Tonraum und eine fallende Tonhöhenbewegungen eingesetzt – ähnlich wie bei Wiegen- und Schlafliedern.[2]

In der Spracherwerbsforschung besteht Konsens darüber, dass Sprache und Musik in der Ontogenese über diese gemeinsamen prosodischen Elemente erworben werden (vgl. Patel 2014). Föten erlernen nicht nur prosodische Elemente einer Sprache (z. B. DeCasper & Spence 1986), sondern auch die Merkmale der Musik, denen sie im Mutterleib ausgesetzt waren (z. B. Kisilevsky, Hains, Jacquet, Granier-Deferre & Lecanuet 2004). In der frühen Phase der Ontogenese werden sprachliche und musikalische Reize über verschiedene Tonhöhen und Rhythmen wahrgenommen. Föten sind einer Kombination aus körperlichen Phänomenen wie Herzschlag, Atemrhythmus und biochemischen

2 Die Prosodie hat darüber hinaus viele weitere Funktionen, wie z.B. die Angabe des emotionalen Zustands eines Sprechers, die Angabe der syntaktischen Struktur oder die Angabe von Hinweisen zur Gesprächsführung. Während des Spracherwerbs helfen prosodische Merkmale dem Säugling, Wort- und Phrasengrenzen zu erkennen. Dies ermöglicht es, Regelmäßigkeiten über die Anordnung von sprachlichen Mustern wie Phonemen, Wörtern und Phrasen zu erwerben (Sallat und Jentschke 2015).

Reaktionen wie z. B. Hormonausschüttung bei Freude, Wohlbefinden oder Angst ausgesetzt. Sie verfügen bereits im Uterus über die Fähigkeit zum auditiven Lernen und zur Gedächtnisbildung. Aufgrund der Erkenntnisse zum pränatalen Hören ist es wahrscheinlich, dass die intrauterin auditiv wahrgenommenen sprachspezifischen Intonationsverläufe und -muster der mütterlichen Sprechweise bereits die ersten Lautäußerungen Neugeborener und junger Säuglinge beeinflussen und dass hier bereits eine sprachspezifische Prägung stattfindet.

Über die Stimme der Mutter werden Wahrnehmungsschemata auf den Fötus übertragen, die die nachgeburtliche Wahrnehmung z. B. von angenehm empfundenen Stimmen und von Musik beeinflussen. Unmittelbar nach der Geburt äußert sich die stimmliche Prägung dadurch, dass die Stimme der Mutter anderen Stimmen vorgezogen wird. Studien zeigen dabei eine Aktivierung in hinteren Schläfenregionen, vorwiegend auf der linken Seite, sowie in Hirnarealen, die an der emotionalen Verarbeitung beteiligt sind (Amygdala, orbito-frontaler Kortex) (Beauchemin et al. 2011). Es gibt Hinweise darauf, dass sich der primäre auditorische Kortex vor der vollständigen Reifung an die mütterliche Stimme und den Herzschlag angepasst hat (Webb, Heller, Benson, & Lahav, 2015). Partanen et al. (2013) postulierten, dass die pränatale Hörerfahrung zur Entwicklung eines effektiveren neuronalen Netzes für die Tonverarbeitung führt. Die periodische Wahrnehmung des niederfrequenten mütterlichen Herzschlags ist für den Fötus eine wichtige rhythmische Erfahrung, die wahrscheinlich die neuronale Basis für das spätere auditorische Synchronisieren (Anpassung von Tonhöhen) schafft (vgl. Partanen et al. 2013).

Die pränatalen Hörerfahrungen haben einen starken Einfluss auf die Genauigkeit der Tonhöhenunterscheidung von Neugeborenen und auf die Struktur ihrer eigenen Lautäußerungen. Pränatal häufig erlebte und signifikante Melodietypen, die prosodisch typisch für die Erstsprache sind, z. B. eine steigende oder fallende Konturpräferenz, werden von Neugeborenen in ihren Lautäußerungen reproduziert (Dahlem 2008; Mampe et al. 2009; Wermke et al. 2016). Weitere Studien zeigen, dass ihre Gurr- und Babbellaute ebenfalls durch sprachspezifische Eigenschaften modifiziert sind (Vihman 1985, Fletcher & Garman 1986; Whalen et al. 1991; Fikkert 1994; Jusczyk 1997; Oller 2000). Somit zeigen sich anhand von einigen Studien, vor allem aus der Spracherwerbsforschung, viele Anhaltspunkte für die Prosodie als gemeinsamen Ursprung von Sprache und Musik in der Ontogenese, welche auch als kognitive Schnittstelle für die Forschung an linguistischer Relativität in Bezug auf Musik von Belang ist.

4. Linguistische Relativität und auditive Wahrnehmung und Verarbeitung von Musik

Bereits Wilhelm von Humboldt (2015/1820) war der Ansicht, dass Sprache und Denken untrennbar miteinander verbunden sind und dass mit jeder Sprache eine andere Weltsicht einhergeht. Damit stellte er die Grundlage für die Theorie der Linguistischen Relativität bereit. In diesem Kontext weisen Ergebnisse empirischer Studien der Psycholinguistik auf „eine wechselseitige Abhängigkeit zwischen den in der Grammatik einer Sprache vorhandenen sprachstrukturellen Merkmalen (z. B. Aspekt) und der Konzeptualisierung eines Ereignisses (z. B. Verlauf vs. Abgeschlossenheit)" hin (Mertins 2018: 16). Die Konzeptualisierung äußert sich u.a. in Bewegungen sowie in Gedächtnisleistungen, die man mit empirischen Verfahren der Psycholinguistik (z. B. Eye-Tracking) nachverfolgen kann. Die Basis für solche Studien ist der Umstand, dass unterschiedliche Konzeptualisierungsschemata die sprachspezifischen Unterschiede in der sprachlichen Enkodierung hervorrufen. Als theoretische Grundlage dient hierbei die sogenannte „Thinking-for-Speaking" – Hypothese (Slobin 1996), wonach Sprachen als Perspektiven bzw. Denkarten tituliert werden. Demnach beeinflussen grammatische Eigenheiten einer Einzelsprache die Konzeptualisierung von Situationen und Ereignissen.

Es stellt sich nun die Frage, ob es auch sprachspezifisch unterschiedliche Konzeptualisierungsschemata gibt, die sich in auditiven Prozessen wie bei der Rezeption von Musik äußern. Gibt es in Abhängigkeit von der erworbenen Erstsprache Präferenzen bei der auditiven Wahrnehmung von Melodien, Rhythmen und Klängen? Einige wenige Studien zeigen mithilfe von psychophysischen nonverbalen Tests, dass sich mentale Repräsentationen von musikalischer Tonhöhe bei Muttersprachlern des Niederländischen und des Farsi unterscheiden (Dolscheid et al. 2013). Während Niederländer Tonhöhen als *hoch* oder *tief* beschreiben, charakterisieren Farsi-Sprecher diese als *dünn* oder *dick*. Um zu testen, ob die Erfahrung im Umgang mit einer neuen Sprache die mentale Repräsentation der Tonhöhe beeinflussen kann, schulten Dolscheid et al. niederländische Muttersprachler darin, die Tonhöhe in Form der Dichte zu beschreiben, wie es Farsi-Sprecher tun. Nach dem Training ähnelte die Leistung der niederländischen Sprecher der Leistung von Farsi-Muttersprachlern. Dolscheid et al. kamen zu dem Schluss, dass Menschen, die unterschiedliche sprachliche Raum-Tonhöhen-Metaphern verwenden, auch Tonhöhen anders wahrnehmen. Folglich spielt die spezifische Sprache eine kausale Rolle bei der kognitiven Repräsentation von musikalischer Tonhöhe (Dolscheid et al. 2013: 613).[3]

Mannion et al. (2012) begründen die Übertragung des Konzeptes der linguistischen Relativität auf den Bereich Musik aus einer kulturellen Perspektive: Sprache und Musik als wesentliche Facetten der menschlichen Erfahrung und Kommunikation sind einzigartig. Sie sind in allen Kulturen allgegenwärtig. Sprache und Kultur reflektieren und erzeugen sich gegenseitig, genauso verhält es sich auch mit Musik und Kultur. Nach Meinung der Forschenden sollten Menschen danach streben, die vielen Erscheinungsformen der menschlichen Kultur zu verstehen und Maßnahmen ergreifen, um sie für künftige Generationen zu bewahren. Gerade in einer Welt, in der Intelligenz zunehmend künstlich nachgeahmt werden kann, Sprachenlernen durch immer stärkere Übersetzungsalgorithmen teilweise überflüssig wird und in der das kulturelle Handwerk stetig mechanisiert wird, erscheint es bedeutsam, an einem Wissen darüber festhalten zu können, woher der Mensch kommt und was seine Kognition ausmacht. Das Studium von sprachlichen und musikalischen Traditionen sowie damit verbundenen kognitiven Prozessen wirft Licht auf diese Zusammenhänge (vgl. Mannion et al. 2012).

So zeigt sich, dass zwar nur wenige Studien, die die Forschung bereits zum Thema der linguistischen Relativität in Bezug auf das Hören von Musik bereithält, auf Relativitätsphänomene im Sinne des Thinking-for-Speaking hinweisen, dass die Frage nach solchen kognitiven Präferenzen jedoch gerade mit den gegenwärtig vielfältigen experimentellen Forschungsmöglichkeiten einige tiefergehende Einblicke in das Feld offenlässt. Zum Zwecke der Vertiefung haben die Autor*innen daher anhand von Volksliedern aus vier europäischen Sprachen eine explorative Untersuchung zu sprachspezifischen Merkmalen in der Musik vorgenommen, die im folgenden Kapitel dargestellt wird.

5. Eine Untersuchung zu sprachspezifischen Merkmalen in deutschen, tschechischen, französischen und englischen Volksliedern

In diesem Kapitel werden erste Ergebnisse einer Untersuchung zu sprachspezifischen Merkmalen in deutschen, tschechischen, französischen und englischen Volksliedern präsentiert. Zunächst wird die Stichprobe vorgestellt und

3 Diese Ergebnisse konnten bei Konfliktbedingungen von Höhe und Dichte mit niederländischen und türkischen Sprechern reproduziert werden (Dolscheid et al. 2020).

das Vorgehen der Auswertung skizziert. Die Ergebnisse werden unter Zuhilfenahme des multinominalen logistischen Regressionsmodells vorgestellt und diskutiert.

5.1 Stichprobe und Auswertung

Das Untersuchungskorpus setzt sich aus 400 Volksliedern der vier europäischen Sprachen Deutsch, Tschechisch, Französisch und Englisch zusammen. Das Genre der Volkslieder eignet sich als alltagsnahe, wenig künstlerisch überformte[4] musikalische Produkte. Die Stichprobe umfasst in jeder Sprache 100 Lieder aus verschiedenen historischen Epochen vom 13. bis zum 20. Jahrhunderts und aus verschiedenen geographischen Herkunftsregionen. Sie beinhaltet unterschiedliche musikalische Formen wie Tanz- und Jagdlieder sowie Kinder- und Schlaflieder, in denen für alle Kulturen gemeinsame und lebensnahe Themen (Liebe, Beruf, Natur, Bewegungen u.a.) aufgegriffen werden.

Das Korpus wurde aus musikwissenschaftlich anerkannten Volksliedersammlungen zusammengestellt und mit Hilfe historisch-kritischer Quellen und Archiven überprüft (s. Tabelle 1). Alle 400 Volkslieder wurden in einem weiteren Schritt nach ausgewählten musikwissenschaftlichen Kriterien kodiert. Die einzelnen Analysekategorien sind am Beispiel des englischen Volksliedes „Banks Of Sweet Primroses“ in der Abbildung 1 dargestellt.

4 Auch Volklieder kommen nicht vollständig ohne künstlerische Formgebung aus, da sie vor allem schriftlich in Liedersammlungen tradiert wurden und somit meist nur eine, von einem Herausgeber ausgewählte, melodisch geformte Fassung von vielen verschiedenen mündlich tradierten Fassungen darstellen.

Tabelle 1: Sprachen und Quellen der ausgewählten Volkslieder

Sprache	Quellen
Deutsch	Carus-Verlag: Liederprojekt (Online): https://www.liederprojekt.org Die Liederkiste (Online): https://www.liederkiste.com Historisch-kritisches Liederlexikon der Albert-Ludwigs-Universität Freiburg. Online: https://www.liederlexikon.de Kiepenheuer & Witsch Verlag: Das Volksliederbuch. Köln: 1993 Liederarchiv (Online): https://www. lieder-archiv.de Reclam Verlag: Deutsche Volkslieder. Texte und Melodien. Stuttgart: 2006 Wikipedia (Online): https://www.wikipedia.de
Tschechisch	Školní Nakladatelstvi pro čechy a moravu: Naše Písně. Horák – Hutter. 1940
Englisch	The Penguin Book of English Folk Songs. Selected and edited by Ralph Vaughan Williams and A.L. Lloyd. London: 1959
Französisch	Clouzot: Chansons Populaires des Provinces de l'Ouest. Jérome Bujeaud. 1895 Heugel & Cie: Chansons populaires [Vincent d'Indy collection]. Paris: 1892 Heugel & Cie: Chants de la Vieille France. Julien Tiersot. Paris: 1904 Plon: Histoire de la Chanson Populaire en France. Paris: 1889 Wikipedia (Online): https://www.wikipedia.de

Kategorie	**√/X (vorhanden/ nicht vorhanden)**	**Ergebnisse**
Sprache		Englisch
Liedtitel		Banks Of Sweet Primroses
Metrum		3/2 (2/2)
Tempo		M.M. = 72
Takt-/Metrumwechsel	√	Metrum
Pausen	√	
Auftakt	√	
Erstes Intervall		↗ 5
Tonumfang, insgesamt		
Tonumfang, bezogen auf Tonika		
größtes Intervall und -bewegung		↘ 7
Richtung der Schlussphrase		↘
Schlussphrasenrichtung		↘ 2
Tonart		Dur
Stabilität der Tonart	√	
Schlusskadenz		V-I
Phrasenstruktur		A (2) B (2) A1 (2) C (2)
Individuelle Merkmale		vorwiegend 3/2, auch 2/2 in Teil C
Thema		Unglückliche Liebe
Bearbeitungsdatum		10.4.2020
bearbeitet von		IL
Quelle		Penguin Book of Folk Songs

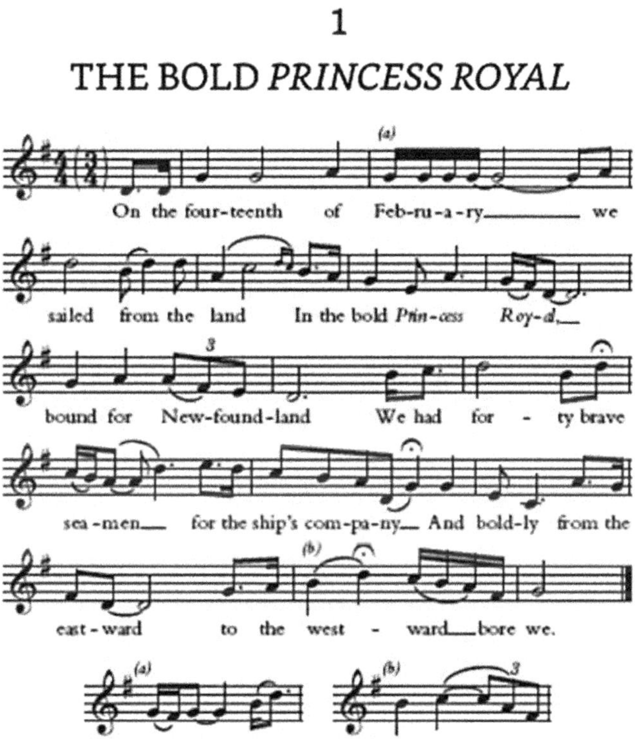
1
THE BOLD PRINCESS ROYAL
(a)
On the four-teenth of Feb-ru-a-ry we
sailed from the land In the bold Prin-cess Roy-al,
3
bound for New-found-land We had for - ty brave
sea-men for the ship's com-pa-ny And bold-ly from the
(b)
east-ward to the west - ward bore we.
(a)
(b)
3

Abbildung 1: Englisches Volkslied und Analysekategorien

Im nächsten Schritt wurden die tabellarischen Daten aller Volkslieder kodiert, um statistisch auswertbare Ergebnisse zu erzielen (s. Tabelle 2). In einer Excel-Tabelle wurde anschließend jedes Lied in einer Zeile und jedes musikalische Merkmal als kategoriale Variable (Spalte) aufgeführt. Den jeweiligen Ausprägungen eines Merkmals wurden Kodierungen mit den Werten 0, 1 oder 2 zugeordnet. Die Sprache des Liedes gilt dabei als abhängige Variable.

Tabelle 2: Gestaltungsmöglichkeiten der musikalischen Kategorien und quantifizierende Kodierung

Musikalische Kategorie	**Gestaltungsmittel**	**Kodierung**
Takt	2-er	0
	3-er	1
	abweichend oder beide	2
Takt/Metrumwechsel	nein	0
	ja	1
Pausen	nein	0
	ja	1
Auftakt	nein	0
	ja	1
Ambitus	9 Halbtonschritte (H.) oder	0
	weniger	1
	10 H. oder mehr	
Umfang des größten Tonsprungs	7 H. oder weniger	0
	8 H. oder mehr	1
Bewegungsrichtung des größten Tonsprungs	abwärts	0
	aufwärts	1
	beides	2
Bewegung des finalen Intervalls	abwärts	0
	aufwärts	1
	Tonrepetition	2
Tonart	modal	0
	diatonisch	1
Tonartstabilität	nein	0
	ja	1
Schlusskadenz	abweichend	0
	Dominante-Tonika (V-I)	1
Phrasenstruktur	asymmetrisch	0
	symmetrisch	1
Ungültige Daten (jede Kategorie)	ungültig	

Bei der folgenden statistischen Auswertung wurde ein induktives Verfahren gewählt. Für das induktive Verfahren wurde zunächst ein multinominales logistisches Regressionsmodell (vgl. Kersten 2016) angepasst und die relative Wahrscheinlichkeit (rW) für eine Zugehörigkeit zu den Sprachkategorien je nach Ausprägung der Variablen (musikalische Kategorien) errechnet. Für das induktive Verfahren wurde ein Modell mit allen vorhandenen Merkmalen aufgestellt. Anschließend wurde eine Rückwärtsselektion mithilfe des AIC (Informationskriterium nach Akaike) durchgeführt.[5] Das Modell wurde für kategoriale Variablen angepasst, die mehr als zwei Ausprägungen besitzen. Modelliert wurde die Wahrscheinlichkeit, dass eine Beobachtung aus der Kategorie j stammt, wenn die Prädiktoren X1, . . ., XK gegeben sind. In diesem Fall wird als abhängige Variable die Sprache und als Prädiktoren werden die zwölf musikalischen Kategorien betrachtet. Das AIC reduzierte sich nur ein wenig:

- AIC des vollen Modells: ## [1] 740.7433
- AIC des neuen Modells: ## [1] 736.494

Im multinominalen logistischen Modell wurde schließlich eine Referenzkategorie (Sprache) bestimmt, anhand welcher für die übrigen Kategorien ein eigener Satz an Parametern berechnet wird. In diesem Beispiel ergab sich die Sprache Tschechisch als passende Referenzkategorie. Die Teilmodelle hatten in groben Zügen diese Struktur:

$$ln\left(\frac{P(Sprache = Englisch)}{P(Sprache = Tschechisch)}\right) = \beta_{10}+\beta_{11}(Metre = 1)+\beta_{12}(Metre = 2)+\beta_{13}(Tempo = 1)+\beta_{14}(Tempo = 2)+\ldots$$

$$ln\left(\frac{P(Sprache = Französisch)}{P(Sprache = Tschechisch)}\right) = \beta_{20}+\beta_{21}(Metre = 1)+\beta_{22}(Metre = 2)+\beta_{23}(Tempo = 1)+\beta_{24}(Tempo = 2)+\ldots$$

$$ln\left(\frac{P(Sprache = Deutsch)}{P(Sprache = Tschechisch)}\right) = \beta_{30}+\beta_{31}(Metre = 1)+\beta_{32}(Metre = 2)+\beta_{33}(Tempo = 1)+\beta_{34}(Tempo = 2)+\ldots$$

Mit der Exponentialfunktion wurden die Teilmodelle dann zugunsten der besseren Interpretierbarkeit transformiert. Dadurch entstand beispielsweise die folgende Formel:

$$\frac{P(Sprache = Englisch)}{P(Sprache = Tschechisch)} = \exp(\beta_{10})\cdot\exp(\beta_{11})(Metre = 1)\cdot\exp(\beta_{12})(Metre = 2)\cdot\exp(\beta_{13})(Tempo = 1)\cdot\ldots$$

Auf der linken Seite der Formel befindet sich die relative Wahrscheinlichkeit. Die Wahrscheinlichkeit, dass ein Lied beispielsweise zur Sprachkategorie

5 In der Statistik ist ein Informationskriterium ein Kriterium zur Modellauswahl. Man folgt dabei der Idee, dass ein Modell nicht unnötig komplex sein soll und balanciert die Anpassungsgüte des geschätzten Modells an die vorliegenden empirischen Daten und dessen Komplexität, gemessen an der Anzahl der Parameter, aus. Dies erfolgt meist mit dem Informationskriterium nach Akaike (AIC). Das Kriterium ist negativ orientiert, d. h. bei einer Auswahl von möglichen Kandidaten für Modelle für die Daten ist das bevorzugte Modell dasjenige mit dem minimalen AIC-Wert.

‚Englisch' gehört, wird durch die Wahrscheinlichkeit, dass ein Lied zur Sprachkategorie ‚Tschechisch' gehört, dividiert. Es gilt: Ist der Quotient (die rW) kleiner als 1, ist die Wahrscheinlichkeit für die Sprache ‚Tschechisch' als abhängige Variable größer. Ist es größer als 1, ist die Wahrscheinlichkeit für ‚Englisch' größer. Daraus folgt: Je stärker die relative Wahrscheinlichkeit ansteigt, desto wahrscheinlicher wird eine Zuordnung des Liedes zur Kategorie ‚Englisch'. Dies ist auf alle anderen Teilmodelle und die Variablen (musikalische Kategorien) übertragbar. Zur Interpretation der Daten wurde die Erhöhung und Verringerung der relativen Wahrscheinlichkeit beobachtet, um damit Aussagen zu generieren. Schließlich wurde zusätzlich für die Einflussvariablen auch der p-Wert der erkannten Effekte bestimmt, um darzustellen, welche Effekte statistisch signifikant sind.

5.2 Ergebnisse: Multinominales logistisches Regressionsmodell

Im Folgenden werden die Ergebnisse der Studie unter Zuhilfenahme des multinominalen logistischen Regressionsmodells vorgestellt und diskutiert. Das Modell mit den zwölf Einflussvariablen (musikalische Kategorien) und den vier abhängigen Variablen (Sprachen) stellt sich als sehr komplex heraus. Bei der Auswertung führte dies dazu, dass für eine musikalische Kategorie ein signifikanter Effekt in einem Modell beobachtet wurde (d. h. in der Gegenüberstellung von zwei Sprachen, z. B. Deutsch-Tschechisch), jedoch für die anderen Sprachen nicht. Somit zeigt sich, dass sich zwei Sprachen in Bezug auf eine Variable voneinander abgrenzen lassen, bei den anderen Sprachen dies jedoch nicht der Fall ist. Signifikante Effekte der relativen Wahrscheinlichkeit lassen sich für die Parameter ‚Takt-/Metrumwechsel', ‚Auftakt', ‚Ambitus', ‚Umfang des größten Tonsprungs', ‚Tonartstabilität' und ‚Phrasenstruktur' feststellen.

Die Sprache Französisch kann in Bezug auf das Merkmal ‚Takt-/Metrumwechsel' von Tschechisch abgegrenzt werden. Die relative Wahrscheinlichkeit, dass ein französisches Lied vorliegt, steigt im Vergleich zu Tschechisch um den Faktor 64.8 ($p = .001$), sofern ein Takt- oder Metrumwechsel vorliegt. Es zeigt sich, dass französische Lieder, auch im Vergleich zu englischen und deutschen – jedoch ohne signifikanten Effekt – metrisch deutlich stärker variieren. Tschechische Lieder stechen als die metrisch am stärksten gebundenen heraus, französische Lieder als die metrisch instabilsten. Englisch und Deutsch liegen dazwischen (rW Englisch/Tschechisch = 10.5 bzw. Deutsch/Tschechisch = 3.8).

Die Effekte für den Parameter ‚Auftakt' sind in allen drei Teilmodellen signifikant ($p = < .001$) und stechen aus der gesamten Erhebung heraus. Hier lässt sich eine klare Rangfolge aufzeigen: Mit einer Erhöhung der relativen

Wahrscheinlichkeit um mehr als das 4254-fache entstammen Lieder mit einem Auftakt der Sprache Englisch. Danach folgen mit großem Abstand Deutsch und Französisch (rW Deutsch/Tschechisch = 100.8 bzw. Französisch/Tschechisch = 99.8). Tschechische Lieder haben somit mit der niedrigsten Wahrscheinlichkeit einen Auftakt.

Im Bereich des Merkmals ‚Ambitus' lässt sich ein signifikanter Effekt im Vergleich von Englisch und Tschechisch feststellen. Ein Tonumfang von zehn Halbtönen oder mehr liegt mit einer Erhöhung der relativen Wahrscheinlichkeit um das ca. sechsfache signifikant wahrscheinlicher bei englischen Liedern vor als bei tschechischen (p = .01). Auch wenn die folgenden Effekte nicht statistisch signifikant sind, haben französische Lieder mit großer Wahrscheinlichkeit einen niedrigeren Ambitus als alle anderen Sprachen, die relative Wahrscheinlichkeit ist negativ (rW Französisch/Tschechisch = -1). Deutsche Lieder ordnen sich hinsichtlich des Ambitus zwischen Tschechisch und Englisch ein (rW Deutsch/Tschechisch = 2).

Mit einer Signifikanz von p = .002 lässt sich für den Parameter ‚Umfang des größten Tonsprungs' ebenfalls Englisch von Tschechisch abgrenzen und mit p = < .001 Deutsch von Tschechisch. Hier zeigt sich der Effekt, dass die relative Wahrscheinlichkeit für die Sprachen Englisch und Deutsch um das ca. 5.5-fache steigt, wenn ein großer Sprung von einer kleinen Sexte (acht Halbtöne) oder mehr vorliegt. Für das Deutsche ist die Wahrscheinlichkeit mit dem Faktor 5.6 geringfügig größer als für Englisch mit dem Faktor 5.4. Damit grenzen sie sich deutlich von tschechischen Liedern ab, die zu kleineren Tonsprüngen neigen. Wenn auch ohne statistische Signifikanz, würde die Wahrscheinlichkeit für ein französisches Lied mit einem großen Tonsprung sogar noch weiter sinken (rW Französisch/Tschechisch = -0.6).

In Bezug auf die Tonart bzw. den Modus eines Liedes lassen sich signifikant Französisch und Deutsch von Tschechisch abgrenzen. Deutsche Lieder haben im Vergleich zu allen anderen Sprachen eine fünffach größere Wahrscheinlichkeit (p = .045) für eine diatonische Tonart (Moll oder Dur). Tschechisch liegt in der Rangfolge dahinter. Für ein französisches Lied hingegen sinkt die Wahrscheinlichkeit um den Faktor -1.3 (p = .001). Somit neigen französische Lieder eher zu modalen oder anderen Skalen. Auch wenn dies nicht statistisch signifikant ist, liegt ein ähnlicher Effekt für Englisch mit dem Faktor -0.7 vor.

Wenn ein Lied das Merkmal Tonartstabilität aufweist, was bedeutet, dass keine Modulationen in andere Tonarten auftreten oder beispielsweise Zwischendominanten und tonartfremde Töne verwendet werden, so ist es statistisch neunfach wahrscheinlicher (rW Englisch/Tschechisch = 9.2), dass es sich um ein englisches Lied handelt als um ein tschechisches Lied (p = .007).

Englische Lieder scheinen in Bezug auf ihre Tonart bzw. Skala außergewöhnlich beständig zu sein – gegensätzlich verhalten sich die tschechischen Lieder. Deutsche und französische Lieder gruppieren sich dazwischen ein, wenn auch statistisch nicht mit signifikantem Effekt (rW Deutsch/Tschechisch = 2.3), während es am unwahrscheinlichsten ist, dass ein französisches Lied in der Tonart bleibt (rW Französisch/Tschechisch = 0.8).

Auch für die Kategorie ‚Phrasenstruktur' lässt sich ein signifikanter Effekt feststellen. Sowohl im Vergleich Englisch/Tschechisch als auch im Vergleich Deutsch/Tschechisch neigen tschechische Lieder eher zu asymmetrischen Phrasen als deutsche und englische, die weitgehend symmetrisch aufgebaut sind. Hier sticht Englisch als die mehr als siebenfach stärker symmetrische Sprache heraus (rW Englisch/Tschechisch = 7.8; p = .002). Deutsche Lieder sind mit einer fünffach größeren Wahrscheinlichkeit im Vergleich zum Tschechischen symmetrisch gebaut (rW Deutsch/Tschechisch = 5.0; p = .001). Auch wenn der Effekt für französische Lieder sich nicht als signifikant herausstellte, so zeigen die Daten, dass die Wahrscheinlichkeit für ein französisches, symmetrisch geformtes Lied sogar um den Faktor -0.2 sinken würde. Somit erweisen sich Lieder dieser Sprache als die formal unregelmäßigsten.

Für die musikalischen Parameter ‚Metrum', ‚Schlussphrasen-Richtung' sowie ‚Schlusskadenz' konnten keine signifikanten Effekte im logistischen Modell aufgezeigt werden. Hierzu können jedoch durch die folgende deskriptive Auswertung Aussagen getroffen werden.

Im Weiteren folgt eine komprimierte Zusammenfassung der Auffälligkeiten im Sprachvergleich:

> Für die Merkmale der zeitlichen Gestaltung ‚Metrum', ‚Takt-/Metrumwechsel' und ‚Pausen' lassen sich Gruppierungen vornehmen. Auch wenn die Unterschiede gering sind, scheinen Tschechisch und Deutsch in Bezug auf Metrum und Pausen eine Gruppe (A) zu bilden und Englisch und Französisch eine zweite Gruppe (B). Gruppe A weist in der Gesamthäufigkeit weniger Lieder mit Auffälligkeiten wie zum Beispiel komplexe Metren (Mittelwert M = 5.5 Lieder) und Takt-/Metrumwechseln (M = 5) auf sowie weniger Pausen bzw. Unterbrechungen (M = 9.5). Die Lieder der Gruppe B dagegen variieren stärker in Bezug auf Takt und Metrum und enthalten mehr Pausen (komplexes Metrum: M = 19.5; Takt-/Metrumwechsel: M = 28; Pausen: M = 23).

Der Auftakt ist, wie auch schon oben beobachtet, die aussagekräftigste Kategorie der Erhebung. Hier ist ein markanter Unterschied zwischen Tschechisch und Englisch sichtbar. Tschechische Lieder beinhalten bis auf eine Ausnahme nie einen Auftakt auf einer unbetonten Zeit, englische Lieder dagegen fast immer. Das Französische zeigt eine 50:50-Verteilung, wohingegen das Deutsche, ähnlich wie Englisch, öfter zu Auftakten neigt.

Auf der melodischen Ebene lässt sich die Tendenz zu einem größeren Ambitus bei englischen und deutschen Liedern im Vergleich zu tschechischen und französischen Liedern beobachten. Der Mittelwert der Lieder mit einem großen Tonumfang (zehn Halbtöne oder mehr) beträgt für Englisch und Deutsch 92.5, für Tschechisch und Französisch liegt er bei 73.5.

Einen weiteren Anhaltspunkt für die melodische Gruppierung von Englisch/Deutsch und Französisch/Tschechisch liefern die ‚größten Intervallsprünge' in den Liedern. Mit einem Mittelwert von $M = 88.5$ Liedern haben französische und tschechische Lieder meist Intervallsprünge bis zu sieben Halbtönen und somit eine engere Spannweite. Deutsch und Englisch hingegen zeigen eine Verteilung von $M = 56$ Liedern mit bis zu sieben Halbtönen und $M = 44$ Liedern mit Sprüngen bis zu acht Halbtönen oder mehr. Somit erlauben sie ca. zur Hälfte eine größere melodische Weite.

Auf melodischer Ebene lässt sich ebenfalls ablesen, dass Englisch die einzige Sprache zu sein scheint, deren Lieder wiederholte Töne statt Auf- oder Abwärtsbewegung am Ende einer Phrase erlauben ($n = 13$ L.), was bei anderen Sprachen kaum der Fall ist ($M = 2$ L.). Es bestätigt sich jedoch die Regelmäßigkeit, dass Melodien unabhängig von der Sprache zu 70 – 80 % abwärtsgeführt werden ($n = 321$ L.).

Auf der melodisch-harmonischen Ebene zeigt sich, das französische Lieder zu 32 % mit dem unüblichen Fall von modalen Skalen auftreten und somit deutlich häufiger als Lieder anderer Sprachen. Deutsche Lieder verwenden diese fast nie (nur $n = 2$ L.). Bei englischen und tschechischen Liedern liegt der gemeinsame Mittelwert bei $M = 12.5$ Liedern mit modalen Skalen. Somit erweisen sich modale Skalen darin auch eher als eine Seltenheit.[6]

Die Daten zur Harmonik weisen im Vergleich mit den melodischen Aspekten auf einen Kontrast hin: Tschechisch und Französisch, die melodisch enger gefasst sind, scheinen auf der harmonischen Seite wieder eine Gruppe zugunsten der gegenläufigen Tendenz zu formen. Auch wenn es ein geringer Teil der Lieder ist (17 %), so weisen Lieder in den beiden Sprachen häufiger harmonische Freiheit in Form eines Ausbruchs aus der Ausgangstonart (Modulation, Ausweichung o.ä.) auf, während deutsche und englische Lieder mit einem gemeinsamen Mittelwert von $M = 7.5$ Liedern nur sehr vereinzelt solche Fälle besitzen.

6 Aufgrund der musikalischen Tradition sind Lieder ab ca. 1700 diatonisch geschrieben, weshalb die Mehrheit der Lieder insgesamt (85 %) diatonische Skalen (Dur- oder Molltonarten) aufweist. Im Detail beachtenswert sind im Französischen insbesondere die modalen Lieder, die nach 1700 entstanden sind.

Allgemein erscheint Deutsch als die harmonisch stabilste Sprache, da sie am häufigsten mit diatonischen Skalen versehen ist (98 L.), in der Ausgangstonart bleibt (91 L.) und zudem meist in der diatonischen V-I-Kadenz (Dominante-Tonika) endet (91 L.). Die anderen Sprachen erweisen sich mit einem Mittelwert von M = 23.3 Liedern mit anderen Schlusskadenzen als V-I als harmonisch flexibler.

Zuletzt offenbaren die Daten erneut eine Gruppierung von Deutsch und Englisch gegenüber Tschechisch und Französisch. Auch wenn der melodische Bereich und die Sprünge von französischen und tschechischen Liedern im Allgemeinen enger sind (s.o.), so enthalten sie spezifische Strukturen, die sie wiederum komplexer machen als deutsche und englische Lieder: mehr Pausen, häufigere harmonische Abweichungen und auf formaler Ebene auch deutlich mehr asymmetrische Phrasen (M = 35.5 L.). Deutsche und englische Lieder weisen hingegen durchschnittlich nur in 11.5 % der Fälle asymmetrische Phrasen auf. Eine grafische Gesamtübersicht der Ergebnisse liefern die Abbildungen 2 und 3.

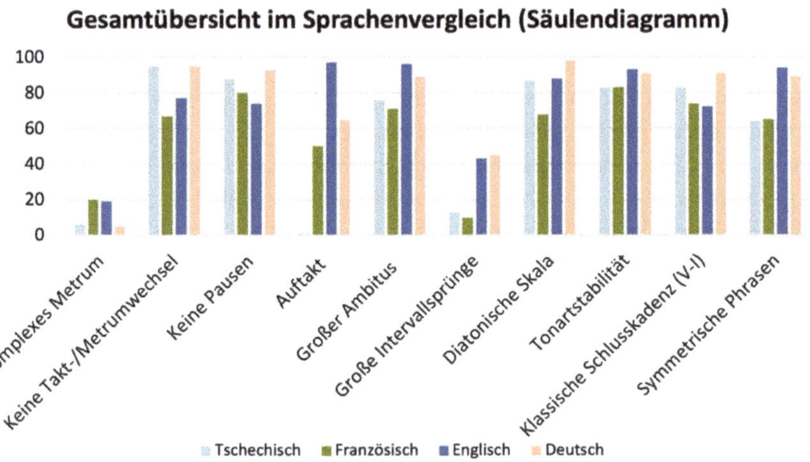

Abbildung 2: Gesamtübersicht der relevanten Ergebnisse im Sprachenvergleich (Säulendiagramm)

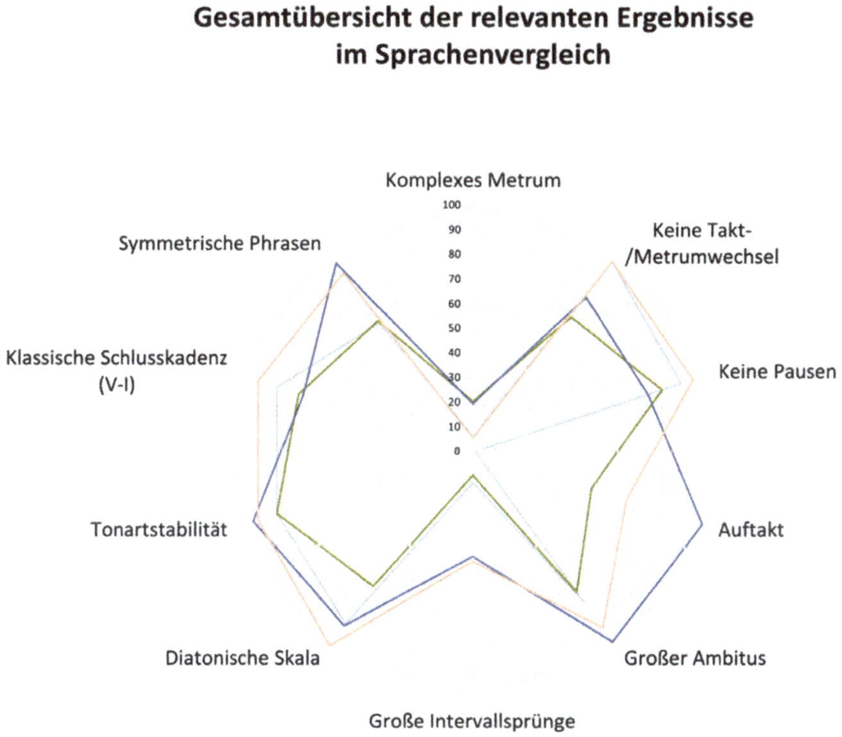

Abbildung 3: Gesamtübersicht der Ergebnisse im Sprachenvergleich (Netzdiagramm der Sprachenprofile)

6. Diskussion der Ergebnisse

Aus den oben dargestellten Ergebnissen kann gefolgert werden, dass sich sprachspezifische Unterschiede in den musikalischen Kategorien widerspiegeln. Somit ist anzunehmen, dass sprachliche Strukturen auch einen Einfluss auf die auditive Wahrnehmung und Verarbeitung sowie Rezeption von Musik ausüben könnten.

Am auffälligsten ist dieser Effekt für die musikalische Kategorie ‚Auftakt'. Die klare Abgrenzung des Tschechischen vom Englischen lässt sich vermutlich grammatikalisch begründen: Im poetischen und musikalischen Metrum erfüllt der Auftakt die Funktion einer kurzen Einleitung auf unbetonter Zeit und außerhalb der Phrase in Form weniger Noten bzw. Silben. Musikalische Auftakte werden daher in der Regel mit unbetonten Partikeln, Pronomina oder

Präpositionen, wie es im Englischen und Deutschen der Fall der ist, realisiert (z. B. in den Liedern „The sailor went to sea“; „One morning in the month of may“; „Ein Jäger aus Kurpfalz“ oder „Im Frühtau zu Berge“). Häufig treten Auftakte auch mit Adverbien auf wie bei dem Lied „Now the winter is gone“. Die semantische Funktion der Adverbien, die Umstände einer Handlung oder eines Geschehens näher zu beschreiben, geht mit der einleitenden Funktion eines Auftaktes einher. Dass tschechische Lieder in der vorliegenden Untersuchung keine Auftakte aufweisen, scheint damit zusammenzuhängen, dass die tschechische Sprache nicht über grammatikalisierte Kategorie des unbestimmten oder bestimmen Artikels verfügt. Die hochfrequente und obligatorische Verwendung von Artikeln im Deutschen und Englischen lässt folglich erklären, dass diese Lieder häufig Auftakte aufweisen. Das Französische bildet eine Zwischenform, was möglicherweise mit der phonologischen Verschmelzung von Artikeln und Nomen mit Anfangsvokal zusammenhängt, wie zum Beispiel bei „l'eau“. Im Französischen finden wir Auftakte häufig mit Adverbien, aber auch mit Substantiven und Personalpronomen wie bei den Liedern „Quand j'etois chez mon père“; „Là bas sur la montagne“ oder bei „Maman, j'ai-z'un amant“. Damit lässt sich das Französische in der Art der Verwendung des Auftaktes deutlich vom Englischen und Deutschen abgrenzen.

Für die Konzeptualisierungsstrategien von Auftakten kann angenommen werden, dass die tschechische Sprache dafür sorgt, dass ihre Sprecher*innen musikalisch weniger auditive Einbettung und Kontext benötigen, als dies bei englischen und deutschen Sprecher*innen mit einer deutlichen Präferenz für Auftakte und damit für Kontextualisierung zu verzeichnen ist. Da das Französische anderen Betonungsregeln folgt als die Vergleichssprachen, lässt dies vermuten, dass die auditiven Präferenzen sich in diesem Punkt für das Französische noch einmal unterscheiden. Ein eindeutiger Anhaltspunkt für Auftakte und ihre Konzeptualisierungsstrategien in den untersuchten Sprachen geht jedoch aus der Erhebung nicht hervor und muss weiter untersucht werden.

Mit der Synthese der deskriptiven und inferentiellen Daten lassen sich zudem erste Gruppierungen zugunsten der übrigen musikalischen Merkmale vornehmen: Durch statistische Unterschiede zeigt sich in metrisch--rhythmischer Hinsicht eine Gruppierung von je zwei Sprachen: So bilden Deutsch und Tschechisch eine Gruppe mit wenigen Abweichungen in den metrisch-rhythmischen Kategorien und weisen in den Liedern eine gewisse Geradlinigkeit auf. Da es sich bei Deutsch und Tschechisch um Sprachen zweier unterschiedlicher Familien handelt (slawische und germanische Sprachfamilie), lässt sich ein interessanter Querbezug dazu herstellen, dass sich allgemein typologische und konzeptuelle Veränderungen in der tschechischen Sprache durch den engen Sprachkontakt mit dem Deutschen seit dem 13. Jahrhundert nachweisen lassen.

In verschiedenen grammatikalischen und somit auch kognitiven Bereichen weisen die Sprachen kontaktlinguistische Ähnlichkeiten auf, insbesondere im Aspektsystem, was eng mit der Konzeptualisierung von Ereignissen zusammenhängt (vgl. Berger 2013, 2014; Mertins 2018). Um Schlussfolgerungen zur metrisch-rhythmischen Ebenheit in deutschen und tschechischen Liedern vorzunehmen, müssen weitere detaillierte vergleichende Studien zur Prosodie der Sprachen geleistet werden.[7] Die Bevorzugung einer holistischen Perspektive mit Fokus auf dem Endpunkt bei den beiden Sprachen könnte jedoch auch eine Erklärung für rhythmisch-metrische Zielorientiertheit und Beständigkeit in der Musik sein. Die Ähnlichkeit von Englisch und Französisch in rhythmisch-metrischer Hinsicht ist ebenfalls nicht einfach zu erläutern, da Englisch germanischen und Französisch romanischen Ursprungs ist. Patel et al. (2006) führten bereits eine umfangreiche Studie zum Vergleich von französischer und englischer Prosodie mit der Instrumentalmusik durch und fanden heraus, dass sich für die gesprochene Sprache beider Sprachen mithilfe der nPVI-Gleichung (normalized pairwise variability index‘[8]) ein eindeutiger Unterschied zwischen den Vokallängen feststellen lässt, wobei Englisch mehr Variabilität aufwies als Französisch. Dieser Unterschied konnte sich jedoch nicht in der Instrumentalmusik nachweisen lassen, wo die Sprachen eine ähnliche rhythmische Variabilität besaßen. Patel et al. folgerten, dass Musik zwar die Kontraste in der Tondauer von Sprachen wiedergeben kann, nicht aber die allgemeine zeitliche Variabilität (vgl. ebd.). Dieses Ergebnis lässt sich mit den vorliegenden Daten zur Vokalmusik unterstreichen, da sich hier ebenfalls Englisch und Französisch mit ihrer Tendenz zu mehr Flexibilität in Form von Taktwechseln, komplexen Metren etc. ähnlich variabel zeigen.

Gerade bei den Gruppierungen in metrisch-rhythmischer Hinsicht liegen bei Volksliedern historisch-kulturelle Einflussfaktoren nahe, die u.a. mit den

---

7 Bekannt ist lediglich, dass beide Sprachen die melodische und dynamische Wortakzentuierung kombinieren, dass aber im Deutschen die dynamische Betonung stärker ist als im Tschechischen (vgl. Skála 1981). Dieser Umstand trägt jedoch nicht zur Erklärung der o.g. Zusammenordnung bei.

8 Die nPVI-Gleichung (dt. „normalisierter paarweiser Variabilitätsindex“) wird zur Untersuchung und Quantifizierung der rhythmischen Variabilität von Musik und Sprache eingesetzt. Sie kann die durchschnittliche Differenz zwischen benachbarten Ereignissen in einer zeitlichen Sequenz (z.B. Noten in einer Melodie bzw. aufeinanderfolgende Vokale in einem gesprochenen Satz) quantifizieren (vgl. Daniele 2017).

regionalen Tänzen und deren (auch höfischen) Pflege einhergehen. Die Untersuchung dieser Einflüsse würde den Umfang dieses Beitrags übersteigen, ist jedoch in diesem Kontext von hoher Relevanz, da sie als möglicher Störfaktor der Daten miteinbezogen werden muss.

Auf der melodisch-harmonischen Seite erscheint ein anderes Gruppierungsbild als in rhythmischer Hinsicht: Deutsche und englische Lieder weisen insgesamt häufiger große Intervallsprünge auf, haben oft einen großen Ambitus und fallen daher durch ihre melodische Weite auf, gleichzeitig aber auch durch harmonische Stringenz (wenig Modulationen und Abweichungen, häufig diatonische Skalen). Tschechische und französische Lieder hingegen sind in ihrem Tonumfang mehrfach begrenzt und neigen ebenso wenig zu großen Tonsprüngen, was von melodischer Begrenzung zeugt. Auf der harmonischen Ebene jedoch eröffnen diese Lieder mehr Räume durch Modulationen, Tonartwechsel und modale Skalen.

Übertragen auf die Sprachintonation wurde bereits belegt, dass die französische Sprache im Gegensatz zur englischen nachweislich eine geringere Tonhöhenvariabilität aufweist und dass sich dies ebenso in deren Instrumentalmusik niederschlägt (vgl. Patel et al. 2006). Das heißt, wenn die Stimme bei gesprochener Sprache von einem Vokal zum nächsten wechselt, ist die Größe der Tonhöhenänderung im Französischen kleiner als im Englischen. Die ermittelte Variabilität der Intervalle, gemessen an der akustisch beobachtbaren Grundfrequenz (F0), ist bei französischer Musik signifikant geringer als bei englischer Musik. Dieses Ergebnis konnten die Daten der vorliegenden Studie für die Vokalmusik bestätigen und liefern die Erkenntnis, dass die tschechische Sprache sich in diesem Merkmal dem Französischen annähert, so wie die deutsche Sprache dem Englischen.

Insgesamt legen neuere theoretische und empirische Arbeiten zur Intonationsphonologie nahe, dass gesprochene Tonintervalle tatsächlich wichtig für die mentale Repräsentation der Intonation sein können, auch wenn gesprochene Sprache sich nicht an feste Frequenzverhältnisse hält (vgl. Dilley 2004). Wenn dies der Fall ist, dann ist in Kombination mit den Ergebnissen von einer linguistischen Relativität für die auditive Wahrnehmung von musikalischen Intervallmustern auszugehen und kann für den Bereich der Intonation bzw. Tonhöhe bestätigt werden. Interessant erscheint der Umstand, dass sich Tschechisch und Französisch hier ähneln, obwohl für die tschechische gesprochene Sprache noch keine solch geringe Intervallvariabilität nachgewiesen wurde. Es erscheint auf Grundlage der Daten evident, dass tschechische und französische Lieder eher harmonische als melodische Variabilität aufweisen. Für deutsche und englische Lieder gilt das Gegenteil.

Sollen die vielfältigen obigen Interpretationsversuche nun auf konzeptuelle Präferenzen übertragen werden, so erscheint das Prinzip ‚harmonische statt melodischer Weite' (im tschechischen und französischen) als eine Tendenz zu mehr Prozesshaftigkeit, die der Verlaufsperspektive in der Raumkognition ähnelt. Diese könnte sich auch mit den asymmetrischen Phrasen in den o.g. zwei Sprachen belegen lassen. Deutsche Lieder, ähnlich wie englische, erscheinen demgegenüber sowohl harmonisch als auch im Phrasenbau als sehr zielorientiert und wenig flexibel, spiegeln jedoch mit größeren Intervallkontrasten auch reichlich sprachliche Intonationsunterschiede und somit melodische Weite wider.

Die rhythmische Gruppierung von Deutsch und Tschechisch versus Englisch und Französisch weicht jedoch von diesen Schlussfolgerungen ab. Hier offenbart sich bereits, dass rhythmisch-metrische Aspekte von Sprache und Musik zwar eng mit der melodisch-harmonischen Ebene verflochten sind, jedoch stets eine differenzierte Betrachtung erfordern. Generalisierende Aussagen bewegen sich also an dieser Schnittstelle immer auf einem schmalen Grat. Da französische Lieder neben mehr harmonischer Vielfalt ebenso auch in die Gruppe der Lieder mit mehr rhythmischer Variabilität fallen, erscheint Französisch in der vorliegenden Studie die Sprache mit den ungewöhnlichsten bzw. flexibelsten Strukturen zu sein. Allein am Klangbild der gesprochenen französischen Sprache, mit ihrem melodischen Fluss durch den fehlenden bzw. sehr unregelmäßigen Wortakzent, lässt sich diese Auffälligkeit nachvollziehen. Hiermit unterscheidet sich die Sprache deutlich von sehr metrischen Sprachen wie Deutsch und Englisch, aber auch von Sprachen mit vielen Konsonanten wie dem Tschechischen. Es erscheint plausibel, dass für das Französische auch musikalisch abweichende Regeln und Strukturen gelten, die weiter zu erörtern sind. Die musikalischen und sprachlichen Ähnlichkeiten von Französisch und Tschechisch stellen sich als eine unerwartete Entdeckung der Untersuchung heraus, die spannende Forschungsperspektiven aufwirft. Die Ähnlichkeiten von deutschen und englischen Liedern sind im Vergleich dazu einfacher und augenscheinlicher zu begründen, nämlich mit dem gemeinsamen Ursprung in der germanischen Sprachfamilie.

7. Zusammenfassung und Forschungsausblick

Die vorliegende Erhebung bestätigt in weiten Teilen die Annahme, dass Sprachen einen Einfluss auf die Komposition und Gestaltung von Musik haben können.

Im Fokus dieses Beitrags steht die kognitive Schnittstelle von Sprache und Musik. Die Zielsetzung lautete, die Schnittstelle in Bezug auf die Relevanz der ‚Thinking for Speaking'-Hypothese und damit in Bezug auf die linguistische Relativität für die auditive Wahrnehmung von Musik ins Auge zu fassen und in einer explorativen Studie eine erste Datengrundlage für Hypothesen zu einer möglichen ‚Listening for Speaking'-Theorie zu schaffen. Eine zentrale Frage war dabei, ob musikalische Werke mit ihren Gestaltungsmerkmalen quasi auch „sprachspezifisch" angelegt sind und ob dies von den muttersprachlichen Einflüssen der Musikschaffenden herrührt. Eine einschlägige Beantwortung dieser Frage ist hier (noch) nicht möglich. Vielmehr lassen sich die Ergebnisse als eine erste empirische Grundlage für weitere darauf aufbauende Forschungsarbeiten betrachten.

Da es bislang keine Studien gibt, die einen konkreten Anhaltspunkt für empirische Erhebungen des sprachspezifischen Musikhörens bereitgestellt haben, haben wir uns hier einfachen, vergleichbaren musikalischen Werken in verschiedenen Sprachen gewidmet, um mögliche Unterscheidungsmerkmale herauszuarbeiten, die erste Anhaltspunkte liefern. Innerhalb der Stichprobe von 400 Volksliedern der tschechischen, englischen, französischen und deutschen Sprache konnten jeweils zwölf musikalische Merkmale analysiert, quantifiziert und statistisch verglichen werden. Es stellt sich heraus, dass sich allein durch den vorhandenen bzw. nicht vorhandenen Auftakt signifikante Abgrenzungen zwischen den Sprachen vornehmen ließen, jedoch fehlt die empirische Grundlage für die Interpretation dieser Unterschiede zugunsten der konzeptuellen Strukturen. Hier konnten deshalb nur erste Vermutungen über den Zusammenhang des Auftaktes mit der Verwendung von Wortarten wie Artikeln in den jeweiligen Sprachen angestellt werden. Für die weiteren Merkmale konnten im Vergleich der Sprachen ebenfalls signifikante Unterschiede festgestellt werden und es ließen sich interessante Gruppierungen von jeweils zwei Sprachen zugunsten einiger musikalischer Tendenzen vornehmen. Jedoch sind diese nicht statistisch haltbar und die Interpretation dieser Unterschiede bleibt noch spekulativ. Der Vergleich der Sprachprofile in den untersuchten Volksliedern zeigt, dass sich die Sprachen durchaus musikalisch unterscheiden, dass ihre Profile sich jedoch im Gros weiterhin ähneln.

Insgesamt erscheint die metrisch-rhythmische Ebene von Sprache und Musik wissenschaftlich erkenntnisreich zu sein. Es erscheint uns ein aufschlussreicher Weg zu sein, Ansätze wie die von Patel et al. weiterzuverfolgen und beispielsweise die nPVI-Gleichung deutlich umfassender auf Lieder und ihre Ursprungssprachen anzuwenden sowie auf andere Merkmale auszuweiten. Ergänzend dazu sollten phonotaktische Überlegungen in der strukturellen

Formung der betreffenden Sprachen deutlich ausgeweitet werden, da sie sich eben häufig aufgrund der prosodischen Struktur mit musikalischen Aspekten in Verbindung bringen lassen.

Um einen weiteren Schritt in Richtung der Betonungsstrukturen in Liedern zu unternehmen, ist die quantitative Erschließung der Verteilungen der Wortarten auf musikalische Strukturen in der Vokalmusik im Vergleich zu Äußerungen gesprochener Sprache vorzunehmen, um dort etwaige Muster festzustellen. Zudem ist es erstrebenswert, Methoden zu finden, die tiefer in die melodisch-harmonische Ebene und ihre Bedeutung bzw. Analogien in Sprachen eintauchen.

Die zukünftige Forschung hat somit die Aufgabe, musikalische Merkmale zu isolieren und diese im Sprachvergleich mit einer großen Datenfülle im Detail zu untersuchen, um statistisch signifikante Evidenz für oder gegen die skizzierten Tendenzen zu erhalten. Dieser Beitrag liefert dazu Anstöße: Es bietet sich an, mit Merkmalen der niedrigsten kognitiven Ebene, also prosodischen Strukturen wie Rhythmus und Tonhöhe zu beginnen. Es erscheint uns als ein gewinnbringender Weg, beispielsweise die nPVI-Gleichung deutlich umfassender anzuwenden. Wünschenswert ist es, solche Quantifizierungen beispielsweise für Tonhöhenintervalle oder rhythmische Werte mit deutlich mehr Liedern, auch anderer musikalische Gerne z. B. Werke klassischer Musik, mit den jeweiligen Vergleichssprachen vorzunehmen. Anschließend ließe sich die Anwendung der Gleichung auch auf Merkmale höherer kognitiver Ebenen ausweiten, zum Beispiel auf Wortarten und musikalische Motive. Wie bereits dargestellt, sind allgemein deutlich mehr phonotaktische Überlegungen auf der linguistischen Seite der betreffenden Sprachen nötig, um Aussagen zu prosodischen Strukturen in Verbindung mit musikalischen Aspekten bringen zu können. Wenn signifikante Daten mit diesen kleinteiligen Erhebungen zusammengestellt werden, können Hypothesen in Bezug auf konzeptuelle Präferenzen verschiedener Muttersprachler*innen aufgestellt und diese in experimentellen Settings mit großen Stichproben getestet werden.

Zudem sind mehr Studien zur rhythmischen Differenzierung von Sprache und Musik durchzuführen, da der Sprachrhythmus eher als Begleiterscheinung von Betonung und phonotaktischen Strukturen auftritt, während er in der Musik ein maßgeblich ordnendes und konstituierendes Prinzip ist. Auch hierbei können Präferenzen einzelner Sprachen in Erscheinung treten, die dann auf das Musikhören anwendbar sind.

Zuletzt sei noch eine Anmerkung zur Relevanz dieser Forschungsrichtung angeschlossen: In einer Zeit, in der sich anhand der Mehrsprachigkeitsdebatte zeigt, dass Sprachen zu kognitiven Ressourcen werden können (vgl. Bialystok

1999), während sich Armut und Bildungsferne sogar neuronal niederschlagen und damit kognitive Barrieren hervorbringen können (vgl. Hanson et al. 2013), ist dafür zu sorgen, dass gerade in der Frühförderung das Augenmerk auf die größtmögliche Stärkung der Ressourcen gelegt wird. Bilingualität kann den möglichen Nachteil von Kindern aus armen Familien ggf. ausgleichen (vgl. Engel de Abreu et al. 2012). Musik ähnelt der Verwendung von mehreren Sprachen, da ihre Verarbeitung und Produktion ebenso Paradebeispiele für komplexe mentale Prozesse sind, die kognitive Flexibilität schlichtweg erfordern, um sie überhaupt durchführen zu können. Der auditive Kanal scheint also für solche wichtigen Prozesse eine ansehnliche Rolle zu spielen. Gerade wenn zu einigen nachteiligen Faktoren noch die gegenwärtige exzessive Nutzung von Bildschirmen hinzukommt und dadurch die reale soziale Interaktion mit ihrem auditiven Input sinkt (Riedel & Büsching 2017; Anitha et al. 2021), wird das Hören umso mehr vernachlässigt. Man kann hier von einer „auditiven Armut" sprechen. Die stärkere Förderung und Forderung des auditiven Kanals bedürfen auch Daten, die ihre Wichtigkeit, gerade für das Lernen, stützen. Solche Daten kann die Forschung in diesem Bereich liefern, nicht nur weil sie allgemein Aufschluss über die Bedeutung von Sprachen und Musik in der menschlichen Kognition gibt. Denn sofern bekannt ist, welchen Einfluss Sprachen auf die auditive Wahrnehmung haben, so ist auch mehr darüber bekannt, wie wichtig die beidseitige Beziehung von Sprache und Musik für die auditive Entwicklung – gerade von Kindern – ist, und inwiefern das Musikhören, genauso wie das Denken, ohne Sprache(n) kaum vorstellbar ist.

8. English summary: Connections between language, music and cognition

Connections between language, music and cognition: an exploratory study of language-specific features in German, French and English folk songs
In linguistic and musicological research, music and language are regarded as universal human forms of expression and means of communication that are temporally-organized and culturally-specific acoustic events. Both are independently existing syntactic systems that use complex, hierarchically structured sequences. In the case of music, the emphasis lies on the acoustic-emotional level of phonetic expression (sounds). Through the close relationship between musical elements and emotions, feelings such as tension, relaxation, sadness and joy can be expressed. In language, on the other hand, the meaning-bearing side of phonetic expression (lexical words) is central. Phonological units are arbitrarily interpreted as lexical words and subordinated to a

propositional world-structuring syntactic system. The connections between language, music, and cognition represent a broad interdisciplinary field of research. So far, only very few studies have dealt with linguistic relativity in relation to the composition and especially the reception of music. Psycholinguistic research shows that linguistic structures shape individual thinking, resulting in language- and culture-specific conceptualizations, and thus also sociocultural diversity. However, it has not yet been sufficiently researched whether language-specific conceptualization schemes underlie auditory processes. To date, there are no studies that investigate the question of whether melodic-rhythmic structures of different first languages have an influence on the structures of perception of musical stimuli. Also, very few studies exist that address the way in which linguistic relativity might relate to listening to music. In the present study we assume that musical achievements, such as folk songs, from different cultural and epochs show not only individual features of composers but also specific linguistic structural features in the form of different rhythmic-melodic structures, which can be distinguished from each other like linguistic structural features of different languages. The authors present a study on language-specific features in German, Czech, French, and English folk songs. In a sample of 400 folk songs, musical features such as pitch and pitch intervals, rhythm and meter, were analyzed. The sample includes 100 songs in each language from different historical periods from the 13th to the 20th century and from different geographical regions. The sample includes different musical forms, such as dance and hunting songs as well as children's songs and lullabies, in which themes common to all cultures and close to life are taken up. The language of the song was considered the dependent variable. A multinominal logistic regression model was applied in the analysis and the relative probability (rW) for belonging to the language categories was calculated depending on the characteristics of the selected musical categories. It could be shown that in some musical areas – such as the use of an upbeat – language-specific differences are reflected in the musical categories. For example, Czech and English differ significantly: All Czech songs but one do not contain an upbeat on an unaccented beat, whereas English songs almost always do. French songs show a 50:50 distribution, whereas German, like English, tends to have upbeats more frequently. In addition, a significant effect was found for the category 'phrase structure': Czech songs tend more towards asymmetrical phrases than German and English, which are largely symmetrical in structure. English stands out here as the more symmetrical language. German songs are also more likely to be built symmetrically compared to Czech.

For some musical variables, such as the presence of an upbeat, the preference for one meter over another, and the overall pitch range the study provide evidence for language-specific effects on music. Given these findings, we can stipulate that linguistic structures intrinsically exert an influence on the auditory perception and processing as well as reception of music. With the synthesis of the descriptive and inferential data, initial groupings can then be made in favor of the other musical features: Statistical differences reveal a grouping of two languages each in metric-rhythmic terms: Thus, German and Czech form a group with few deviations in the metric-rhythmic categories and show a certain regularity in the songs. Since German and Czech are languages of two different families, an interesting cross-reference can be made to the fact that typological and conceptual changes in the Czech language in general can be traced through close language contact with German since the 13th century.

A central question of the present paper was whether the creative features of musical works are also language-specific and whether this stems from the native-language influences of the musicians. A definite answer to this question is not (yet) possible at this point. However, our findings allow a preliminary conclusion that language-specific differences are reflected in the musical categories.

Literaturverzeichnis

Altenmüller, E. (2018). *Vom Neanderthal in die Philharmonie. Warum der Mensch ohne Musik nicht leben kann*. Berlin: Springer Verlag.

Anitha, F. S., Narasimhan, U., Janakiraman, A., Janakarajan, N., & Tamilselvan, P. (2021). Association of digital media exposure and addiction with child development and behavior: A cross-sectional study. *Ind Psychiatry J, 30,* 265–71.

Beauchemin, M., Gonzalez-Frankenberger, B., Tremblay, J., Vannasing, P., Martínez-Montes, E., Belin, P., & Lassonde, M. (2011). Mother and stranger: An electrophysiological study of voice processing in newborns. *Cerebral cortex, 21*(8), 1705–1711.

Berger, T. (2013). Eine Ungewöhnliche Verwendung Des Aspekts Im Tschechischen – Der Imperfektive Aspekt in Handlungssequenzen. *Zeitschrift Fur Slawistik*. doi: 10.1524/slaw.2013.0002.

Berger, T. (2014). The convergence of Czech and German between the years 900 and 1500. In *Congruence in contact-induced language change: Language families, typological resemblance, and perceived similarity,* 184–198.

Besson, M., Barbaroux, M., & Dittinger, E. (2017). Music in the brain. In R. Ashley & R. Timmers (Eds.), *The Routledge companion to music cognition* (pp. 37–48). New York, London: Routledge.

Bialystok, E. (1999). Cognitive complexity and attentional control in the bilingual mind. *Child Development, 70*(3), 636–44. doi: 10.1111/1467-8624.00046.

Brown, S. (2001). The "Musilanguage" model of music evolution. In N. Wallin, B. Merker, & S. Brown (Eds.), *The origins of music* (pp. 271–300). Cambridge, MA: MIT Press.

Brown, S. (2017). A joint prosodic origin of language and music. *Frontiers in Psychology, 8*. doi: 10.3389/fpsyg.2017.01894.

Carus-Verlag: Liederprojekt, abgerufen am 23.11.2022, unter: https://www.liederprojekt.org

Clouzot. (1895). *Chansons Populaires des Provinces de l'Ouest*. Jérome Bujeaud.

Cross, I. (2001). Music, cognition, culture, and evolution. *Annals of the New York Academy of Sciences, 930*(1), 28–42.

Dahlem, M. (2008). *Untersuchung akustischer Eigenschaften spontaner Lautäußerungen japanischer Neugeborener: ein Beitrag zur Erarbeitung sprachuniverseller Frühindikatoren für Sprachentwicklungsstörungen bei Säuglingen mit orofazialen Spalten*. Würzburg. Deutsche digitale Bibliothek, abgerufen am 04.05.2022, unter: https://www.deutsche-digitale-bibliothek.de/item/DGRY75OZWBLXAENLUVOXDXTMIR2DOGRB

Daniele, J. R. (2017). A tool for the quantitative anthropology of music: Use of the NPVI equation to analyze rhythmic variability within long-term historical patterns in music. *Empirical Musicology Review*. doi: 10.18061/emr.v11i2.4893.

DeCasper, A. J. & Spence, M. J. (1986). Prenatal maternal speech influences newborns' perception of speech sounds. *Infant behavior and Development, 9*(2), 133–150.

Die Liederkiste, abgerufen am 23.11.2022, unter: https://www.liederkiste.com

Dilley, L. C. (2004). The phonetics and phonology of tonal systems. *Electrical Engineering, Doktorarbeit*. Massachusetts Institute of Technology.

Dolscheid, S., Shayan, S., Majid, A., & Casasanto, D. (2013). The thickness of musical pitch: Psychophysical evidence for linguistic relativity. *Psychological Science, 24*(5), 613–21. doi: 10.1177/0956797612457374.

Dolscheid, S., Çelik, S., Erkan, H., Küntay, A., & Majid, A. (2020). Space-Pitch Associations differ in their susceptibility to language. *Cognition*. doi: 10.1016/j.cognition.2019.104073.

Engel de Abreu, P. M. J., Cruz-Santos, A., Tourinho, C. J., Martin, R., & Bialystok, E. (2012). Bilingualism enriches the poor: Enhanced cognitive control in low-income minority children. *Psychological Science*. doi: 10.1177/0956797612443836.

Fikkert, P. (1994). *On the acquisition of prosodic structure*. Dordrecht: Holland Institute of Generative Linguistics.

Fletcher, P. & Garman, M. (Eds.). (1986). *Language acquisition: Studies in first language development*. Cambridge: Cambridge University Press.

Griffiths, T. D. (2003). The neural processing of complex sounds. In *The cognitive neuroscience of music* (pp. 168–202). Oxford: Oxford University Press.

Hanson, J. L., Hair, N., Dinggang, G., Shen, F., Gilmore, J. H., Wolfe, B. L., & Pollak, S. D. (2013). Family poverty affects the rate of human infant brain growth. *PLoS ONE*. doi: 10.1371/journal.pone.0080954.

Heugel & Cie. (1892). *Chansons populaires* [Vincent d'Indy collection]. Paris: Julien Tiersot.

Heugel & Cie. (1904). *Chants de la Vieille France*. Paris: Julien Tiersot.

Historisch-kritisches Liederlexikon der Albert-Ludwigs-Universität Freiburg, abgerufen am 23.11.2022, unter: https://www.liederlexikon.de

Honing, H., ten Cate, C., Peretz, I., & Trehub, S. E. (2015). Without it no music: Cognition, biology and evolution of musicality. *Philosophical Transactions of the Royal Society B: Biological Sciences*, *370*(1664), 20140088.

Horák, J. & Hutter, J. (1940). *Naše Písně*. Školní nakladatelství pro Čechy a Moravu.

Jespersen, O. (1922). *The woman. Language: Its nature, development and origin* (pp. 237–254). London: Allen and Unwin.

Jusczyk, P. W. (1997). *The discovery of spoken language*. Cambridge MA: MIT Press.

Kisilevsky, B. S./ Hains, S. M. J./ Jacquet, A. Y./ Granier-Deferre, C./ Lecanuet, J. P. (2004). Maturation of fetal responses to music. *Developmental science 7*(5), 550–559.

Kersten, N. (2016). Multinominale, Ordinale Und Stereotype Logistische Regression – Eine Einführung In Die Regressionsanalyse Kategorialer Zielvariablen. *GMS Medizinische Informatik, Biometrie Und Epidemiologie, 12*(1), 1–14. doi: 10.3205/mibe000163.

Kölsch, S. (2013). *Brain and music*. Hoboken, NJ: Wiley-Blackwell.

Leimbrink, K. (2016). *Kommunikation von Anfang an. Die Entwicklung von Sprache in den ersten Lebensmonaten*. Tübingen: Stauffenburg.

Mampe, B., Friderici, A., Christophe, A., & Wermke, K. (2009). Newborns' cry melody is shaped by their native language. *Current Biology, 19*(23), 1994–1997.

Mannion, C./ Sanatullova-Allison, E./ Sanatullov, M. (2012). Applying the Theory of Linguistic Relativity to Music: An Initial Exploration'. Hellenic Journal of Music, Education and Culture Vol. 3. Article 4, 53–70.

Mertins, B. (2018). *Sprache und Kognition: Ereigniskonzeptualisierung im Deutschen und Tschechischen*. Berlin, Boston: De Gruyter. https://doi.org/10.1515/9783110615746

Mithen, S. (2005). *The singing Neanderthals: The origins of music, language, mind and body*. London: Weidenfeld & Nicholson.

Oller, D. K. (2000). *The emergence of the speech capacity*. New York, Psychology Press. https://doi.org/10.4324/9781410602565.

Papoušek, M. & Papoušek, H. (1981). Musical elements in the infant's vocalization: Their significance for communication, cognition, and creativity. *Advances in Infancy Research, 1*, 163–224.

Parncutt, R. (2009). Prenatal development and the phylogeny and ontogeny of music. *The Oxford handbook of music psychology*, 219–228.

Partanen, E., Kujala, T., Tervaniemi, M., & Huotilainen, M. (2013). Prenatal music exposure induces long-term neural effects. *PLoS ONE, 8*(10), e78946. doi: 10.1371/journal.pone.0078946.

Patel, A. D. (2008). *Music, language, and the brain*. Oxford: Oxford University Press.

Patel, A. D., Iversen, J. R., & Rosenberg, J. C. (2006). Comparing the rhythm and melody of speech and music: The case of British English and French. *The Journal of the Acoustical Society of America*. doi: 10.1121/1.2179657.

Reclam Verlag. (Ed.) (2006). *Deutsche Volkslieder. Texte und Melodien*. Stuttgart Reclam.

Riedel, R. & Büsching, U. (2017). *BLIKK-Medienstudie 2017*. Berlin: Bundesministerium für Gesundheit.

Rölleke, H. (1993). *Das Volksliederbuch*. Köln: Kiepenheuer & Witsch.

Saffran, J. R. (2003). Statistical language learning: Mechanisms and constraints. *Current Directions in Psychological Science, 12*, 110–114.

Sallat, S./ Jentschke, S. (2015). Music perception influences language acquisition: melodic and rhythmic-melodic perception in children with specific language impairment. *Behavioural Neurology*, 2015. 1–10. http://dx.doi.org/10.1155/2015/606470

Skála, E. (1981). Diachronische Und Synchronische Aspekte Der Deutsch-Tschechischen Interferenz. *Zeitschrift Für Germanistik, 2*(4), 389–403.

Slobin, D. (1996). From "Thought and Language" to "Thinking for Speaking". In J. J. Gumperz & S. C. Levinson (Eds.), *Rethinking linguistic relativity* (pp. 70–96). Cambridge, MA: Cambridge University Press.

Tiersot, J. (1889.). *Histoire de la chanson populaire*. Paris: E. Plon, Nourrit, et Cie.

Trehub, S. E. (2000). Human processing predispositions and musical universals. In N. Wallin, B. Merker & S. Brown (Hg.). *The Origins of Music*, 427–448.

Vihman, M. M. (1985). Language differentiation by the bilingual infant. *Journal of Child Language, 12*(2), 297–324.

v. Humboldt, W. (2015). Über Das Vergleichende Sprachstudium In Beziehung Auf Die Verschiedenen Epochen Der Sprachentwicklung (1820). In A. Leitzmann (Ed.), *Gesammelte Schriften (1820–1822)* (pp. 1–34). Berlin: De Gruyter.

Webb, A. R., Heller, H. T., Benson, C. B., & Lahav, A. (2015). Mother's voice and heartbeat sounds elicit auditory plasticity in the human brain before full gestation. *Proceedings of the National Academy of Sciences, 112*(10), 3152–3157.

Wermke, K. & Mende, W. (2009). Musical elements in human infants' cries: In the beginning is the melody. *Musicae Scientiae, 13*(2_suppl), 151–175.

Wermke, K. & Mende, W. (2011). From emotion to notion: The importance of melody. In J. Decety & J. T. Cacioppo (Eds.), *The Oxford handbook of social neuroscience* (pp. 624–648). Oxford: Oxford University Press.

Wermke, K. & Mende, W. (2013). Am Anfang war die Melodie – Wie Babys ihre Muttersprache erlernen. *Kreativität, Struktur und Emotion*. Würzburg, Königshausen & Neumann, 41–49.

Wermke, K., Teiser, J., Yovsi, E., Kohlenberg, P. J., Wermke, P., Robb, M., & Lamm, B. (2016). Fundamental frequency variation within neonatal crying: Does ambient language matter? *Speech, Language and Hearing, 19*(4), 211–217.

Whalen, D. H., Levitt, A. G., & Wang, Q. (1991). Intonational differences between the reduplicative babbling of French-and English-learning infants. *Journal of Child Language, 18*(3), 501–516.

Williams, R. V. & Lloyd, A. L. (1959). *The Penguin book of English folk songs*. London: Penguin Books.

Wray, A. (1998). Protolanguage as a holistic system for social interaction. *Language and Communication, 18*(1), 47–67.

Anna Marklová and Barbara Mertins

Perception of goal-oriented locomotion events in monolingual and bilingual adults – a free-viewing eye-tracking study

Abstract: The current study explores the influence of language-specific conceptual perspectives on the visual perception of goal-oriented motion events. Three groups of participants (n = 112) participated in an eye-tracking study: German monolinguals, whose language showed a preference for emphasizing an endpoint (holistic perspective), a mixed-monolingual group of speakers of languages which conceptualize motion events as a process, without emphasis on an endpoint (phasal perspective), and bilingual speakers of German and a "phasal" language (Russian, Turkish, English). Eye-movements were recorded for six seconds during the presentation of pictures depicting goal-oriented motion events. No memory or verbalization task followed the presentation of stimuli. The results indicate that in a situation where neither language nor memory is prompted, the underlying conceptual perspective is not activated. This study is one of few studies aiming to investigate the effects of conceptual perspectives on visual perception without prompting language use or its unnatural suppression.

Keywords: linguistic relativity, eye-tracking, goal-oriented motion events, seeing for speaking, bilingualism

1. Introduction

In his famous article "From 'Thought and Language' to 'Thinking for Speaking'" (1996), Slobin formulated the idea that during preparation for speaking, speakers are selecting different aspects of an event they want to describe, according to structural properties of their mother tongue or, if they are multilingual, of their mother tongues. Verbalization of events thus differs across languages, since there are different obligatory categories in each of them. Slobin describes language as a highly selective and conventionally schematic map, which leads speakers to focus on particular details of the real-world experience and leave others out. The same situation is described differently with respect to options of the grammatical encoding of a particular language. "Utterances are not verbal film clips of events. An event cannot be fully represented in language: linguistic expression requires schematization of some sort" (Slobin 2003, p. 159). The so-called "thinking for speaking" process "involves picking those characteristics that a) fit some conceptualization of the event, and b) are readily encodable in the language"

(Slobin 1987, p. 435). Similarly, Levelt in his production/comprehension model assumes that preparation of a (pre)verbal message is "tuned" according to a target language because speakers are required to use language-specific conceptual features (1989).

Slobin stated in one of his early studies that "we will probably never succeed in demonstrating the effects of grammar on world view or nonlinguistic behavior" (Slobin 1987, pp. 435–436). However, in the past two decades attempts have been made to explore the extent of language influence on non-linguistic behavior. Cognitive processes such as categorizing and memorizing have been examined, and comparative studies suggest that in some situations, these processes are influenced by language (Choi et al. 1999; Choi & Bowerman 1991; Filipović & Jaszczolt 2012; Levinson et al. 2002; Majid et al. 2004; Papafragou et al. 2008; Schmiedtová 2001; Stutterheim et al. 2012; Trueswell & Papafragou 2010). The question of the extent of language influence has still not been fully answered (Goldin-Meadow & Gentner 2003; J. A. Lucy 2016; Malt & Wolff 2010).

The "seeing for speaking" hypothesis (Carroll et al. 2004) proposes that linguistic categories shape our thoughts not just in the process of preparing content for verbalization, but also during the observation of a scene we are going to describe or memorize. The process of memorization is not non-linguistic per-se, since tacit use of language is still possible. For this reason, we cannot classify language differences found in memory tasks as a proof of language influence on purely non-linguistic cognition. In Stutterheim et al. (2012), eye-movements were recorded and a memory task was employed in an experiment examining the encoding of goal-oriented motion events. In the description of such events, two main preferences have been observed: the phasal perspective encoding the process of an event, and the holistic perspective focusing on an endpoint/outcome. The preferences were led by grammatical features of the participant's mother tongue. In Stutterheim et al. (2012), the differences which were found in a verbalization task were also identified in the visual perception of native speakers of different languages (Arabic, Czech, English, Russian, Spanish, Dutch, and German). As hypothesized, these perceptual differences reflected the holistic perspective of Czech, German, and Dutch, and phasal perspective of Arabic, Russian, English, and Spanish. Athanasopoulos et al. (2005) found a similar pattern in German and English speakers when examining similarity judgment tasks.

In our current research, we are further exploring the effects of grammatical categories on conceptual perspectives and investigating the scope of such effects. In the previous research on this topic, a verbalization or memory task always followed a stimuli presentation. We are now investigating whether the conceptual perspective (phasal or holistic) influences the eye-gaze behavior when watching pictures representing goal-oriented motion events while the participants are not being prompted to verbalize or memorize. This idea arose from the principle that categories which are deeply anchored in the grammar of our language cause an automatization in thinking (conceptualization) about particular situations. Since speakers must use obligatory grammatical categories in verbalization, they are unconsciously trained to focus on them, which may lead to a greater sensitivity to these particular features even in a not explicitly linguistic context. To explore this idea, we created a new experiment which included neither verbalization nor memory tasks to examine the extent of the effect language has on cognition.

Lucy (1996) proposed a set of requirements for studies examining linguistic relativity. He argues that such research "should assess the cognitive performance of individual speakers aside from explicitly verbal contexts and try to establish that any cognitive patterns that are detected also characterize everyday behavior outside of the assessment situation" (Lucy 1996, p. 48). In our present research, the experiments have been designed in line with these requirements. That is, we did not prompt the use of language and at the same time we assured the participants that neither language nor memory tasks would follow the stimuli presentation, but in turn every step of the experiment would be presented in complete silence. This assurance was part of the instruction. In line with the second requirement formulated by Lucy, we made the effort to simulate everyday life situations and avoid an over-artificiality of the task and thus we did not include any distractive task during the stimuli presentation to impede the use of tacit language.

To sum up, the findings of research into conceptual perspectives in goal-oriented motion events show: (1) different linguistic experience causes differences in linguistic behavior; (2) different linguistic experience causes differences in preverbal conceptualization ("thinking for speaking"); (3) different linguistic experience causes differences in cognitive processes such as memorizing and perception before verbalization ("seeing for speaking"). We want to take a further step in this line of research and test whether (4) different linguistic experience causes differences in perception, without verbalization being activated.

2. Previous studies

Motion events have been in the focus of linguistic relativity research for a long time. They are an important semantic domain across languages which exhibits different lexicalization patterns (Slobin 2003). Talmy (1985) offered a basic characteristic of motion events: A "basic motion event consists of one object (the

„Figure") moving or located with respect to another object (the referent-object or „Ground")" (Talmy 1985, 61). This characteristic described both static (location) and dynamic events (motion). In the following section, we only consider representation of the dynamic event and therefore the terminology in this paper is based on that used in studies on dynamic motion events (Schmiedtová 2011; Schmiedtová et al. 2011; Stutterheim et al. 2012). Moreover, we examine a specific type of these events, so-called goal-oriented motion events. A goal-oriented, or, telic, motion event is "the continuing motion of entities (animate or inanimate objects) towards an endpoint. In a situation of this type, speakers may refer to the motion event in holistic terms, i.e., including motion + goal, or they may select a beginning, intermediate or final phase of the motion event" (Schmiedtová, Stutterheim & Carroll 2011, p. 69).

Linguistic research has been exploring motion events and their representation in language and cognition (for an overview see Filipović & Ibarretxe-Antuñano Iraide 2015). A lot of studies have been based on the theory of lexicalization patterns (Talmy 1985) and the distinction between satellite-framed and verb-framed languages. These languages differ in how they encode the manner of motion and the path of motion in the sentence structure. While satellite-framed languages encode the manner of motion in the main verb and the path of motion in other arguments, verb-framed languages encode this information the other way around (Slobin 1991, 1996, 2004, 2006). These patterns have been systematically examined (e.g. Kita & Özyürek 2003; McNeill 2001; Özyürek et al. 2005; Ozcaliskan 2005; Caballero 2017; Ellis & Cadierno 2009; Han & Cadierno 2010). The application of the thinking for speaking hypothesis on motion events has been further explored in psycholinguistic research (e.g. Filipović 2011; Filipović & Geva 2012; Finkbeiner et al. 2002; Gennari et al. 2002; Papafragou et al. 2002).

In the area of goal-oriented motion events, the phenomenon of goal-over-source asymmetry has been observed in many languages and it was assessed as universal by some researchers (e.g. Dirven & Verspoor 2004). It is described as a tendency to pay more attention to the goal of an action rather than to its source. Empirical studies (e.g. Landau & Zukowski 2003; Lakusta & Landau 2005; Johanson et al. 2009; Papafragou 2010) found evidence of this asymmetry in different languages and in different age groups. However, even considering this asymmetry, the preference for endpoints (or "goals") does not have the same strength across languages, as has been shown in the studies below.

In von Stutterheim and Nüse (2003), German and English native speakers (17 per group) were presented a short film ("Quest") and were asked to retell the content while watching. The results showed that English speakers often used bare verb phrases (e.g. "He runs", "He jumps") without additional information about the endpoint or the direction. On the other hand, German native speakers preferred mentioning the endpoint and rarely used bare verb phrases. Note that in this task, present tense was predominantly used in descriptions (Stutterheim & Nüse 2003). After performing further experiments with typologically different languages, the authors hypothesized about the influence of the category of aspect on event conceptualization. The grammaticalized category of aspect was connected to the tendency to parse event sequences into small units (Stutterheim & Nüse 2003). That is, as aspect is marked in the predicate, speakers prefer the phasal perspective under which events "are hooked up to a deictic center" (Stutterheim & Nüse 2003, p. 873). These findings were corroborated by Carroll et al. (2004), who argued that the particular principles of encoding events were developed during first language acquisition.

Schmiedtová et al. (2011) further explored the topic of grammaticalized aspect as a main cause of the difference between the holistic and the phasal perspective. They carried out a series of studies which focused on the process of conceptualization of goal-oriented motion events. Languages with grammaticalized aspect – MS (Modern Standard) Arabic, Czech, Russian, English, and Spanish -, as well as non-aspectual languages – German, Norwegian – were represented.

Grammaticalized aspects signify if the event is either ongoing (imperfective, progressive) or completed (perfective). As an example, take the Russian and Czech languages, which both have grammaticalized perfective and imperfective. The use of perfective in a goal-oriented motion event itself can have the feature of a holistic perspective, because it often requires the addition of an endpoint (Schmiedtová et al. 2011). Another option both Russian and Czech speakers have is to use the so-called simplex imperfective form of a verb during the description of goal-oriented motion events. Such a form can (but does not necessarily have to) be complemented with another argument, and if an argument is added, it does not have to be an endpoint.

Both Czech and Russian thus have a grammaticalized form to mark completion (perfective aspect), or ongoingness (imperfective aspect). These are used to express either a holistic or phasal perspective. Simplex imperfect is used differently in descriptions of video clips depicting unfinished goal-oriented motion events by Russian and Czech speakers. While Russian speakers very often use a bare phrase with an imperfective verb form, Czech speakers express a possible endpoint in describing such situations, often by using the perfective form of a verb. Moreover, Czech allows the use of perfective for expression of present tense ("here-and-now-reading"), which is not possible in Russian. These findings show that even typologically related languages can display different preferential patterns for event construal.

In Schmiedtová (2011), the influence of the conceptual perspective of the native language was observed in language production data and in memory tasks, and moreover, also in allocation of attention during observing the scenes. Czech and Russian native speakers with high proficiency in German as well as German native speakers were tested. The eye-tracking data showed the difference in focusing on an endpoint in three measurements – fixation counts, the overall probability of speakers looking at least once in the area of endpoint (or area of interest = AoI), and the probability of speakers looking in the AoI during the first two seconds. The Russian learners of German focused on an endpoint systematically less than the Czech speakers of German and German native speakers. In conclusion, these findings have shown that differences in the linguistically-mediated conceptualization of motion events lead to differences in the amount of attention which is paid to different parts of such events. A goal-oriented motion event can be conceptualized from a holistic perspective, emphasizing an endpoint, or from a phasal perspective, focusing on the process (Schmiedtová 2011).

A further cross-linguistic study was carried out by Stutterheim et al. (2012), who investigated the influence of conceptual perspectives in seven groups – native speakers of German, Dutch, Czech, MS Arabic, Russian, English, and Spanish (n = 20 per group). Eye-tracking, a memory task and a language production task were employed. The results showed a clear preference in German, Dutch and Czech to focus on an endpoint (a holistic perspective), in contrast to MS Arabic, Russian, English, and Spanish.

In a study by Schmiedtová (2013), the influence of the holistic perspective was also found in Czech native speakers with a high level of English proficiency. In language production tasks carried out in English, they produced a significantly higher number of endpoints than English native speakers. It was concluded that even highly proficient L2 speakers followed the perspective of their native language while speaking in L2 (Schmiedtová 2013).

Flecken et al. (2014) explored the perception of motion events by German and MS Arabic. Data from 20 German and 20 MS Arabic speakers were collected. The participants were shown six sets of seven video clips and while the sound of ocean waves was simultaneously played in the background. In some of the scenes the participants heard a specific additional sound. After the set of seven video clips ended, seven screen shots of the clips appeared on the screen and participants were asked to select the screen shots of the clips in which they had heard the additional sound. The authors claimed that the distractor task was strong enough to allow observation of non-verbal event-processing. However, we cannot be sure that in such a situation, the language is not still used tacitly as a strategy for the forthcoming task. The participants' eye-movements were recorded during the whole experiment and the eye-tracking data did not display any significant effect of language on the cumulative fixation duration on the endpoints. (Flecken et al. 2014, p. 60).

The study by Athanasopoulos et al. (2015) examined conceptual perspectives in a non-linguistic context. It studied the role of language context during a similarity judgment task. They worked with groups (n = 15 per group) of English monolinguals, German monolinguals, English-German bilinguals in an English context, and English-German bilinguals in a German context. All the bilinguals were native speakers of German with English as their L2. Nineteen triads of video clips were used as stimuli. Participants were instructed to tell the experimenter whether they thought Clip X, which appeared last, was more similar to Clip A or to Clip B. All the target stimuli (Clip X) included an endpoint. The two alternative clips offered a version with and without an endpoint. The analysis showed that German monolinguals and German-English bilinguals in a German context chose motion-completion alternates significantly more often than English monolinguals and German-English bilinguals in an English context. In the second experiment, a verbal interference task was added (repeating a string of three two-digit numbers). While there were no significant differences between the groups when the numbers were repeated in English, the preference for motion-completion alternates was higher compared to the situation in which they were repeated in German. It was concluded that the verbal interference task blocked the effect of that language on the similarity judgment task. Thus, in the case of monolingual speakers, no language influence took place. In the case of bilingual speakers, their second language which was not a language of the verbal interference task, was still accessible and influenced the similarity judgments task.

A study by Papafragou et al. (2008) was based on cross-linguistic differences in lexicalization patterns. Greek speakers and English speakers were presented with videoclips with motion events either depicting an endpoint or without an endpoint in two different conditions: linguistic in which speakers were instructed to describe the clips afterwards, and non-linguistic in which the participants were told that after they watch all the clips, a memory task would follow. Eye-tracking data was recorded and each separated second of presentation was analyzed. The results from the analysis were mixed: Greek speakers focused on the endpoint more than English speakers in linguistic conditions in the first second of presentation, but the opposite was found in the third second of presentation: English speakers focused on an endpoint more than Greek speakers. In the non-linguistic condition, English speakers fixated an endpoint more than Greek speakers. Overall, Greek speakers were more likely than English speakers to arrive first at an endpoint area in a linguistic condition, but this pattern was not found in the non-linguistic condition. Total fixation time did not show any differences between speakers in linguistic or in non-linguistic conditions. The question arises of how reliable the differences found in the separated seconds are. Meaning, if the interpretation of the results is reliable. Since there were no previous hypotheses about the behavior in each separate second, the interpretation and theories were made post-hoc, working with the existing results. We should be careful with over-interpreting such mixed patterns, especially when they seem to contradict each other. In our study, we relied on only two main measurements (total cumulative fixation time and entry time) for the whole six seconds of viewing, and then did an additional analysis of the first three seconds of viewing. We did not want to conduct a statistical analysis for each second separately, since the chance that we would find a random, unpredicted pattern would be high.

Papafragou continued with exploring the patterns found in Papafragou et al. (2008) in a study by Trueswell and Papafragou (2010) where they reported the effect of language on the visual fixations which they called "reverse-Whorfian effect". This effect directs the attention of the viewer to aspects of a scene which are encoded in the language as "details" and not as a "core", thus speakers need to focus on them more to remember them.

The results of the studies (Athanasopoulos et al. 2015; Papafragou et al. 2008; Trueswell & Papafragou 2010) indicate the complexity of the potential language effect on cognitive processes. Different conditions of the same task (as co-occurrence of a distractive task of linguistic or non-linguistic kind) have an influence on the results. However, we see a problem with making strong claims based on relatively small samples and inconsistent analyzes. We would like to address a feature of all three studies which we see as problematic, namely the small number of participants per group. In both studies by Papafragou's group (Papafragou et al. 2008; Trueswell & Papafragou 2010), there were a maximum of 10 participants per group. The effects found in their experiments were mixed (reverse-Whorfian effect, different patterns of eye-movements for each separate second) and they need to be proven by repeating the study with more participants.

As discussed above, there is convincing evidence that the effect of conceptual perspectives is connected to the grammatical category of aspect and that speakers of languages with different aspectual systems differ in their attention towards the endpoint of a motion event in verbalization, memory tasks and seeing for speaking (i.e. in visual attention towards the endpoint while preparing for a memory task). In our current study, our research team has focused on other questions which have emerged, namely on the role of bilingualism and the extent of language effects on visual perception. New groups of participants have been recruited and new experiments have been designed.

Moreover, in our current experiment, we have pushed the "seeing for speaking" hypothesis even further. We are interested in examining whether the differences in emphasis on the endpoint appear even when there is no verbalization or memory task following the stimuli presentation. Our goal was to set up a task which simulates how events and scenes are naturally perceived in real-world situations. Thus, we did not want to artificially oppress tacit language (neither did we encourage it). This makes our research unique and the first of its kind. In the following section, we are presenting the first insight into our analysis of the new data.

3. Research questions

In the current experiment, we created three groups of participants, according to conceptual perspectives of their language(s): a group of speakers of a phasal language, a group of speakers of a holistic language, and a group of bilingual speakers of a phasal and a holistic language (detailed description in the Methodology section). In our sample of participants, the holistic language in all cases was German, but we collected speakers of different phasal languages. We considered languages without grammaticalized aspectual categories (perfective and imperfective) to belong to the "phasal" group. We formulated the following research questions:

1. Does the visual perception task trigger an influence of the phasal or holistic perspective on attention towards an endpoint in motion events?
2. What language-specific preferences are manifested in bilingual speakers while they free-view motion event drawings?

In line with the previous studies (Schmiedtová 2011, 2013; Stutterheim et al. 2012), we expected speakers of the holistic language to have an earlier entry time into AoI (endpoint) and longer fixation time in that area than phasal-language speakers. Additionally, we expected the bilingual speakers to behave differently in comparison to the other two groups. However, there was a reason to expect that, since German is the dominant language for them all, their behavior might be close to the behavior of German monolingual speakers, similar to other analyzes of bilingual speakers (Filipović 2019; Filipović & Hawkins 2019).

We wanted to find out if conceptual perspectives manifest themselves in a simple free-watching non-verbal task. This kind of task has not been proved yet to reveal language preferences. Because of that, we collected data from monolingual speakers of languages with different perspectives. We wanted to find out if the phasal and holistic perspectives would be reflected on eye-movements under the conditions of such a task. Moreover, we wanted to incorporate a group of bilingual speakers to establish a better image of how the perspectives work in their complexity, instead of adding the variable of bilingualism later in the research.

4. Methodology

4.1. Data coding and analysis

One area of interest (AoI) was pre-defined for each critical stimulus. It contained the endpoint for each kind of stimulus. The spatial dimensions of the areas differed, since the naturality of the scenes was emphasized. Two main measurements were analyzed: entry time into the AoI, and total cumulative fixation duration time in the AoI. We considered these measurements as the most suitable indicators of the conceptualization of the motion event because the speed with which the participants look at the AoI for the first time can indicate the automatic processes behind the eye-movement, and the total fixation duration time can indicate how important the AoI is for the viewer. We did an analysis for the whole six seconds of viewing, and then we additionally analyzed the first three seconds of viewing. We wanted to control whether the eye-gaze behavior changes with time of viewing of the stimulus progressing. We cannot expect that eye-movements reflect the same kind of cognitive behavior during all six seconds of stimulus presentation. It has already been shown that the first phase of observation after the stimulus onset is dedicated to fast-mapping of the scene (so-called ambient mode) while the concentration on details takes place later (so-called focal mode) (Helo et al. 2014; Pannasch & Velichkovsky 2009; Unema et al. 2005; Vincent et al. 2008). There was a possibility that with the increasing time of the presentation, the automatization of the eye-movement processes would decrease (Castelhano et al. 2009; Castelhano & Henderson 2005; Henderson & Hollingworth 1998; Vincent & Tatler 2008). Thus, the eye movements during the sixth second of the presentation could be more voluntarily driven than the ones in the first second. Therefore, we wanted to verify if the first half of the presentation time has the same or different patterns than the whole six seconds of the presentation.

In eye-tracking research, several conventional measurements are used very frequently, namely fixation duration time or dwell time, and fixation count.

We did not analyze the fixation count since we did not consider it as a suitable measurement for revealing the influence of conceptual perspectives. The study by Flecken et al. (2014) analyzed the number of fixations on endpoints in the verbal and non-verbal tasks. It is hard to interpret what exactly this piece of information tells us. We cannot easily formulate a plausible hypothesis about language influence on the number of fixations on endpoints because fixating an area of interest does not provide sufficient amount of information to expect, for example, that German speakers should have a higher number of fixations on endpoints. To formulate such an expectation, additional information such as fixation length or the number of revisits made to the relevant area of interested would be required. In other words, the number of fixations itself does not reflect how much attention was paid to a particular critical area.

Additionally, we made a qualitative analysis of saccadic behavior. Saccades are rapid eye movements from one fixation to another (Holmqvist 2011, p. 560) and we expected that they could be a suitable indicator of the attention shift from one part of the scene to another.

4.2. Participants

In the present study, three groups of participants were examined. The total number of participants was 112.

The German group consisted of 55 German adults (47 females, 8 males; age range from 18 to 29, M=24,24, SD=2,36) who were raised in a monolingual German environment and who use German on a daily basis. All of them were undergraduate students of the TU Dortmund.

The mixed monolingual (phasal language) group consisted of 23 adult speakers (11 females, 12 males; age range from 16 to 30, M=23,78, SD=3,88) of a phasal language who were raised in the environment of the phasal language(s) (12 English, 7 Arabic, 1 Albanian, 1 Urdu, 1 Ukrainian, 1 Italian). They were recruited in courses and events organized by the TU Dortmund (A1 German language courses, English speakers recorded in York during a cooperation with the University of York).

The bilingual group consisted of 34 adult bilinguals (28 females, 6 males; age range from 17 to 29, M=22,53, SD=2,96) who were raised either in a bilingual setting with German and a phasal language (16 Turkish, 5 Polish, 5 Russian, 3 English, 1 Chinese, 1 Bulgarian, 2 Spanish, 1 Arabic) or acquired the second language later in their life and have used both languages on a daily basis for longer than 6 years. All of them were undergraduate students at TU Dortmund.

All participants had B1-proficiency in English but they did not speak English on a daily basis (except the English monolingual group). For all bilingual participants, German was their dominant language at the time of the data recording and although they had different language backgrounds, they constituted a fairly homogenous group. For the Turkish-German speakers, German was acquired in early childhood and Turkish was a heritage language they spoke at home. For the rest, German was acquired later in life and became their main language of communication. On the basis of the linguistic system of Albanian, Bulgarian and Urdu in which grammatical aspect is expressed, we assume that these languages use the phasal perspective when encoding goal-oriented motion events.

4.3. Material

Eighteen different images were used as stimuli. 6 of these were critical items, the other 12 served as fillers. The critical stimuli depicted an animal performing a motion event. There were three kinds of critical stimuli, as shown in Figure 1. Each kind of stimuli was used two times. The critical stimuli were used in an experiment employing a verbalization task and it was observed that all were steadily interpreted as motion events. This time we were not interested in the differences between the types of stimuli according to salience of the endpoint in particular, instead, we were interested in the area of an endpoint and the cross-linguistic differences in attention paid to it among the speakers. Thus, we treated the stimuli as one group. The fillers depicted one or more animals which were not performing any motion event. The stimuli were presented for six seconds. The fixation cross appeared between each two stimuli and it was activated by 250 ms of uninterrupted eye-gaze. The stimuli were presented in semi-randomized order (with a critical stimulus preceded by two fillers as a control).

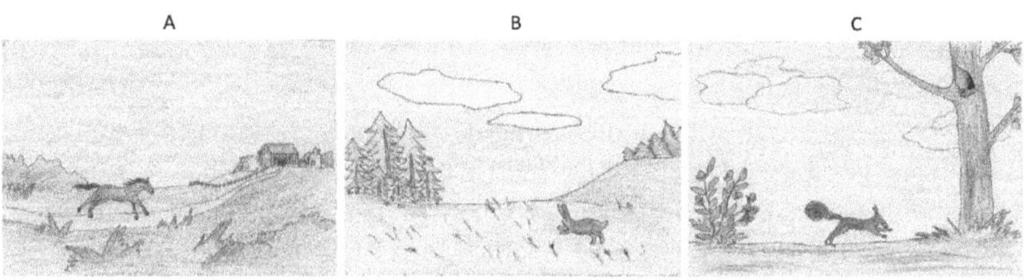

Figure 1: Example of stimuli. (A) an animal heading towards an obvious endpoint; (B) an animal heading towards a not very obvious endpoint; (C) an animal heading from a starting point (source) towards an endpoint

A remote eye tracking device with SMI Technology was used for recording the eye gaze. The sampling rate was 250 Hz. The monitor was 40″ with 16:10 ratio. Calibration was carried out for each participant before the experiment. BeGaze software was used for an analysis of eye-gaze. The SMI Experiment Center recorded eye movement time-locked.

The participants were given oral instructions in German (for German monolinguals) or in English (for bilinguals and phasal language monolinguals). The reason for English instruction was that we did not want to activate either of the two languages the bilinguals spoke, but there was also a pragmatic reason for choosing English in interaction with the phasal-language speakers – the experimenters did not speak all the languages which were spoken by the participants fluently. For this reason, English was picked since all the participants were proficient in this language and so were the experimenters. We expected their native language(s) to be accessible and we chose a language in which all of them had a school level (B1) proficiency, but which they did not list as a language of daily use. We were interested if the influence of the native language(s) would be observable in such situation. We are aware that the local language environment could skew the influence of the native language(s) perspectives.

The participants were instructed to watch a series of pictures on a computer screen. They were told to observe the pictures silently and pick their favorite one in the end. They were explicitly told that no other task will follow and that they will see all the pictures again in one screen in the end, so there was no need for participants to memorize them. We were not interested in the results of this question, since it served only experimental purposes, namely keeping attention of the participants and reassurance about unnecessity to memorize the pictures. The instruction was designed to suppress a possible preparation for verbalization or memorizing of the content of the pictures.

The participants were seated in front of the monitor at a distance of approximately 60–65 cm. After the instructions were given, participants were given the chance to ask for clarification if needed. Then the calibration phase started. Immediately afterwards, the presentation of the stimuli began. After the experiment, the participants filled in a questionnaire asking about their language(s), education and family situation. For most participants, the participation in the experiment was part of their requirements for a university course.

5. Results

We applied two statistical methods for our dataset, which will be explained below. The statistics are calculated in the software R (R Core Team 2018).

5.1. Linear mixed effects model

In order to quantify patterns of eye-movement, we analyzed the fixation duration and the entry time to the AoI (endpoint). For all measurements, data were analyzed using linear mixed effect models. For fitting the models, the package lme4 (Bates, Mächler, Bolker & Walker 2015) was used. For each measurement, the language was used as a fixed effect, and the stimulus and the participant were included as random effects. For both models (fixation duration time and entry time), the phasal-language group was set as a reference group.[1] The significance level of 5 % was used for the calculation of entry time, and the significance level of 2,5 % was used for the calculation of fixation time, since two tests were conducted – one for six seconds of viewing and one for three seconds of viewing.

Table 1 depicts the results of the linear mixed model of the entry time into the endpoint area (AoI). In this model, we did not find a significant effect of language on the entry time. That means that there was no effect of language on the speed in which participants entered the endpoint area.

Table 1: Fixed effect of the linear mixed model of the entry time into the endpoint area for six seconds

	Estimate	Std. Error	t value	p-value
(Intercept)	1930.6	265.5	7.271	<0.05
German	34.2	146.4	0.234	0.81
Bilingual	-178.4	159.8	-1.116	0.26

Table 2 depicts the results of the linear mixed model of the fixation time on the endpoint area over six seconds. We did not find a significant effect of language on the fixation duration in this model. That means that there was no significant difference between speakers' groups in the total time of looking at the area of the endpoint.

1 This decision has been made at random and it does not have an influence on the results of the analysis.

Table 2: Fixed effect of the linear mixed model of the fixation time on the endpoint area in six seconds

	Estimate	Std. Error	t value	p-value
(Intercept)	781.799	161.290	4.847	<0.05
German	30.403	76.571	0.397	0.69
Bilingual	4.508	83.516	0.054	0.95

We did the same test for the fixation time on the endpoint area over the first three seconds of viewing. The results are depicted in the Table 3. In this model, the significant effect of language was not found.

Table 3: Fixed effect of the linear mixed model of the fixation time on the endpoint area in three seconds

	Estimate	Std. Error	t value	p-value
(Intercept)	580.75	73.33	7.920	<0.05
German	78.23	47.00	-1.664	0.09
Bilingual	-35.30	50.52	0.699	0.48

5.2. Chi-square test

In addition to the linear mixed effects model, the chi-square test was applied to explore if there was a difference in noticing the area of the endpoint – in other words, if there is a dependency between performing a fixation in the area of endpoint and the language group. We were working with binary parameters: there is a fixation on the AoI versus there is no fixation on the AoI. The significance level of 2.5 % was used, since two tests were conducted – one for six seconds of viewing and one for three seconds of viewing.

For the measurement of the presence of fixation in the AoI in six seconds of viewing, the p-value of the Chi-square test is 0.06 (>0.025) and not significant. We did not find any difference of fixation appearance between the language groups.

The same test was done for the first three seconds of viewing. The p-value of the Chi-square test is 0.26 (>0.025) and thus not significant. Thus, as well as in the measurement after six seconds of viewing, we did not find any difference of fixation appearance between the language groups for three seconds of viewing.

5.3. Analysis of saccadic behavior

In a qualitative analysis of saccadic behavior, different patterns were found among German speakers and the mixed-monolingual group of phasal-language speakers. Direct saccades between a figure and an endpoint were analyzed. We expected that this measurement could indicate that the participant makes a conceptual connection between the two fixation areas, since the semantic connection between a moving figure and an endpoint already exists. Thus, this measurement has a potential to carry an additional piece of information which fixation duration time itself cannot provide. There were a number of direct saccades observed between a figure and an endpoint in three seconds of viewing and then in six seconds of viewing. The saccades were considered to be direct if there was no fixation between the fixation on the figure and the fixation on the endpoint. We manually counted the number of direct saccades for each trial. We analyzed how the number increased in time in each participant group and for each stimulus. We analyzed each item separately. The results are presented in Table 4. The table presents a percentage of speakers whose numbers of direct saccades increased after an additional three seconds of viewing. The percentage of German speakers was constistently higher than phasal-language speakers in all six stimuli and thus the comparison of these two groups showed a solid pattern. This tendency is supported by the results from the linear mixed effect model. As shown in the Tables 2 and 3, the German speakers had the lowest fixation duration time on the area of an endpoint in comparison to the other two groups after three seconds of viewing. After six seconds of viewing, this group had the highest fixation duration time. This information alone is not very remarkable, since there were no significant effects in the test. However, this tendency could reflect the saccadic behavior explained above. Bilingual speakers, on the other hand, manifested mixed behavioral patterns. It is worth noting that they showed the same pattern in the same kind of stimuli: among the three groups, in unambiguous endpoint stimuli they had the lowest percentage performing additional direct saccades; in source-endpoint stimuli their direct saccades increase was between the German speaker group and the phasal language group, and in unclear endpoint stimuli, they had very similar saccadic patterns to the German speaker group.

Table 4: Percentage of speakers whose numbers of direct saccades increased after additional three seconds of viewing

	Unambiguous endpoint stimuli		**Source-endpoint stimuli**		**Unclear endpoint stimuli**	
	Dog	**Horse**	**Mouse**	**Squirrel**	**Stork**	**Rabbit**
German	40 %	52,73 %	49,09 %	25,45 %	21,82 %	41,82 %
Phasal	34,78 %	43,48 %	34,78 %	17,39 %	13,04 %	26,09 %
Bilinguals	26,47 %	41,18 %	47,06 %	32,35 %	20,59 %	41,18 %

5.4. Control analysis of the participants' groups

We were aware of the fact that the lower homogeneity of the groups of participants could bring noise into the data and thus into the analysis. We explored this possibility by an additional descriptive analysis. Sixteen participants from the bilingual group were Turkish-German bilinguals, growing up in a Turkish-speaking household. We compared the overall entry time and fixation duration time measurements of this sub-group with the rest of the group with descriptive methods. We looked at the box plots (see Figures 2 and 3) and there is no visible difference between the two subgroups for entry time and the fixation duration time. Thus, we can assume that the heterogeneity of the group did not cause a distortion of the results.

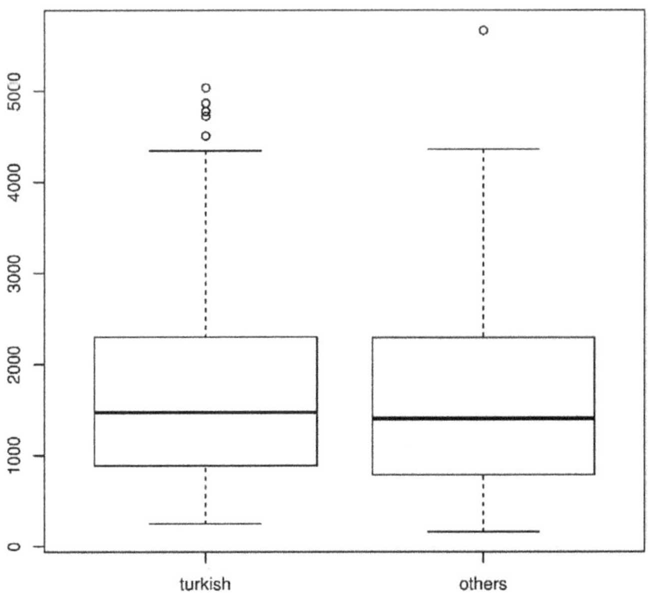

Figure 2: Box plots comparing the entry time of the Turkish-German Bilingual Group to all other bilingual speakers

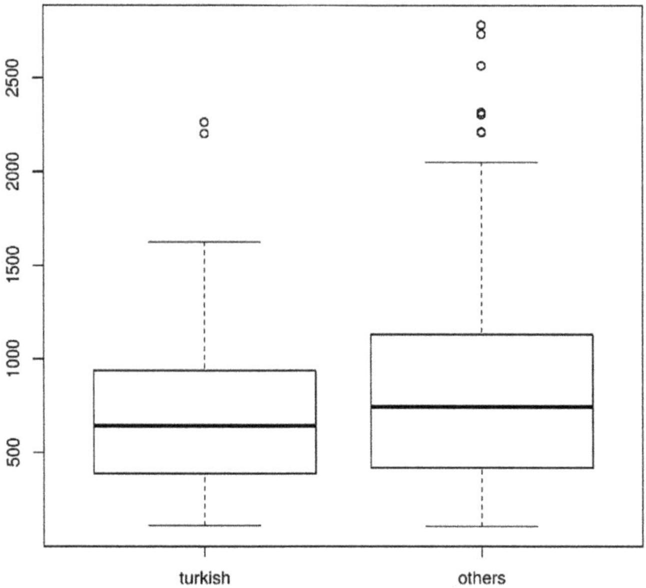

Figure 3: Box plots comparing the fixation time of the Turkish-German Bilingual Group to all other bilingual speakers

We followed the same procedure with the data from the phasal-language group. Twelve participants from this group were English monolinguals. Box plots in Figures 4 and 5 display the comparison of overall entry time and fixation duration time in this sub-group with the rest of the group. The descriptive analysis again did not show any significant differences.

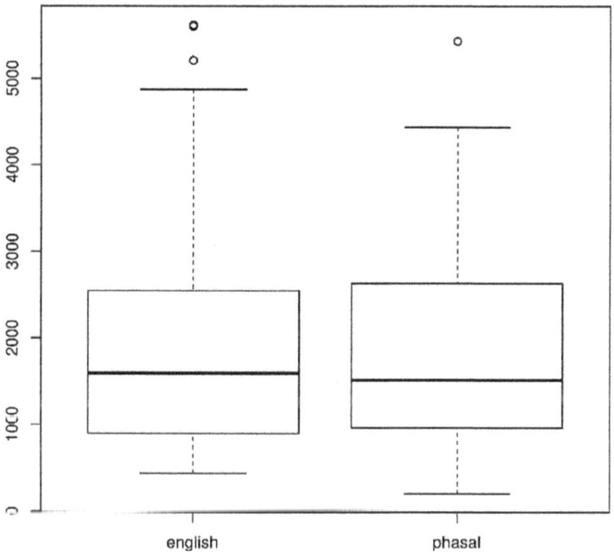

Figure 4: Box plots comparing the entry time of English speakers to all other Phasal language speakers

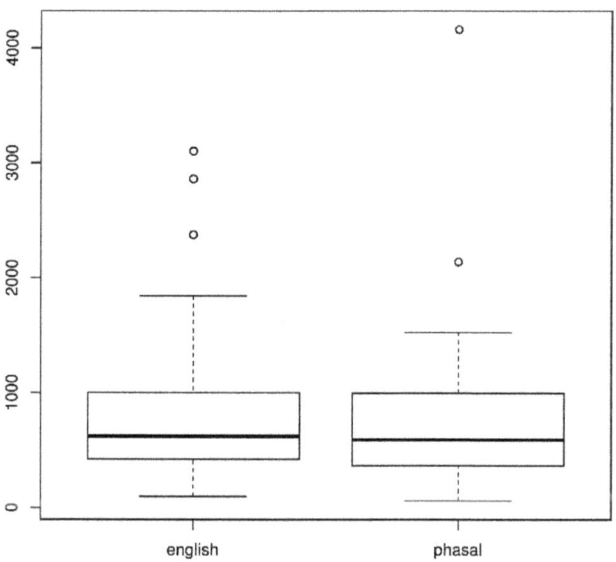

Figure 5: Box plots comparing the fixation time of English speakers to all other Phasal language speakers

6. General Discussion

In the current experiment, we investigated the scope of linguistic relativity, testing it in an experiment with a non-linguistic task. We presented a picture stimulus depicting a motion event to speakers of languages with different conceptual perspectives and analyzed the entry time into the area of the endpoint and the fixation duration time in this area. In previous experiments with stimuli of a similar kind (goal-oriented motion events), the differences between monolingual speakers were observed in eye-movements. However, the majority of the previous experiments included either a verbalization task after picture presentation, or a memory task. Some previous research also conducted experiments without explicit language or memory use, but incorporated rather unnatural tasks (as in Athanasopoulos et al. 2015).

In previous studies broaching the same subject, i.e., the influence of language-specific categories on non-verbal cognition, different patterns were found. After the analysis of data from a small number of participants, Trueswell and Papafragou (2010) concluded that a reverse-Whorfian phenomenon can be observed in eye-movements, but just in a particular phase of stimuli observation. Athanasopoulos et al. (2015) concluded that while a language-interference task is taking place during stimuli presentation, one of the languages bilingual speakers are speaking is blocked and thus only the second language has an influence on the similarity judgment task. We argue that these results could be a product of over-usage of statistical analysis on the same dataset, and the effect of a small number of participants per group.

In our study, we favor a higher number of participants per group over their homogeneity, since a low number of participants has been a constant feature of previous studies (Athanasopoulos et al. 2015; Papafragou et al. 2008; Trueswell & Papafragou 2010). The heterogeneity of the groups is the limitation of this study. We willingly took the risk of studying less represented languages in order to explore their behavioral traits. We employed additional statistical tests to reassure that the heterogeneity of our groups does not have an effect, but replicating the study on more homogeneous groups is an important task for the future.

In the current experiment, we also limited an immediate influence of language by way of a carefully designed experiment, which was focused exclusively on looking at pictures. In this specific setting, the influence of conceptual perspectives on perception without speaking was not observed. There was no significant difference between the three groups of participants.

In our design, we used still pictures which were previously tested in a verbalization task and which were consistently described as motion events.

There is an undeniable difference between presenting still pictures and videoclips, which were used in the previous research. We cannot exclude that the effect might appear while observing videos presenting motion events in more dynamic manner. However, visual inspection of the saccadic behavior in the critical stimuli showed us that the eye gaze of the participants "followed" the suggested movement of the figure in the picture and participants presumably did connections between the figure, the direction of its movement, and potentially the endpoint. Our assessment is supported by comparison of the eye movements on the critical stimuli with the eye movements on fillers, where the main focus of the eye gaze stayed on the figure and then continued with scanning of the scene as a whole, instead of continuing in one preferred direction of the eye gaze from the figure.

We came to the conclusion that in a situation where participants free-watch pictures representing motion events without additional prompts to describe the events, the influence of language is either not present, or too small to manifest itself in the given number of trials and participants. So far, the effect of holistic and phasal perspective has not been shown in a free-watching task. The effects reported in verbalization or memory tasks were observable, but not overwhelmingly robust. It is possible that this effect disappears when a scene is simply observed and no other task prompting the use of language follows. In our task, we did not distract participants in any way to suppress the possibility of tacit language, so the task was as close to an every-day natural situation as possible. Still, we could not find any effect of language.

Nevertheless, some interesting patterns were identified in a qualitative analysis of saccadic behavior of our data. These patterns lead us to the conclusion that we should question if the measurements frequently used in eye-tracking research (such as fixation count, or fixation duration) are suitable for analysis of the complexity of cognitive processes behind eye-movements. For future research, we should question the sufficiency of these measurements for the investigation of such processes. These processes are very dynamic and we cannot expect that eye-movements reflect the same kind of cognitive behavior during all six seconds of stimulus presentation. We cannot expect that the already mentioned difference between ambient and focal mode is the only differentiation of cognitive behavior during free-viewing. Our qualitative analysis of saccadic behavior indicates that patterns can in part stay hidden due to the insistence on conventional measurements.

A more systematic research on bilingual speakers is also needed. While our study did not find significant differences between the three groups, the patterns in eye-movements of bilingual speakers showed mixed behavior in the qualitative analyzes according to a particular stimulus. Further research is needed for a better understanding of the interaction between language and cognition in bilingual speakers. More experiments simulating real world situations are necessary to explore the influence a language can have in real world situations, not just in specific experimental settings.

References

Athanasopoulos, P./Bylund, E./Montero-Melis, G./Damjanovic, L./Schartner, A./Kibbe, A./Riches, N./Thierry, G. (2015). Two languages, two minds: Flexible cognitive processing driven by language of operation. *Psychological Science,* 26, 518–526.

Bates, D./Mächler, M./Bolker, B./Walker, S. (2015). Fitting linear mixed-effects models using lme4. *Journal of Statistical Software,* 67, 1–48.

Caballero, R. (2017). Metaphorical motion constructions across specialized genres. In I. Ibarretxe-Antuñano (ed.), *Human cognitive processing* (vol. 59): *Motion and space across languages*, pp. 229–254. Amsterdam: John Benjamins.

Carroll, M./Stutterheim, C. von/Nüse, R. (2004). The language and thought debate: A psycholinguistic approach. In T. Pechmann/C. Habel (eds.), *Multidisciplinary approaches to language production* (vol. 13), pp. 183–219. Berlin: Mouton de Gruyter.

Castelhano, M./Henderson, J. (2005). Incidental visual memory for objects in scenes. *Visual Cognition,* 12, 1017–1040.

Castelhano, M. S./Mack, M. L./Henderson, J. M. (2009). Viewing task influences eye movement control during active scene perception. *Journal of Vision,* 9, 1–15.

Choi, S./Bowerman, M. (1991). Learning to express motion events in English and Korean: The influence of language-specific lexicalization patterns. *Cognition: International Journal of Cognitive Science,* 41, 83–121.

Choi, S./McDonough, L./Bowerman, M./Mandler, J. M. (1999). Early sensitivity to language-specific spatial categories in English and Korean. *Cognitive Development,* 14, 241–268.

Dirven, R./Verspoor, M. (2004). *Cognitive linguistics in practice (vol 1): Cognitive exploration of language and linguistics.* Amsterdam: John Benjamins.

Ellis, N. C./Cadierno, T. (2009). Constructing a second language: Introduction to the special section. *Annual Review of Cognitive Linguistics,* 7, 111–139.

Filipović, L. (2011). Speaking and remembering in one or two languages: Bilingual vs. monolingual lexicalization and memory for motion events. *International Journal of Bilingualism,* 15, 466–485.

Filipović, L. (2019). *Bilingualism in action: Theory and practice.* Cambridge: Cambridge University Press.

Filipović, L./Geva, S. (2012). Language-specific effects on lexicalization and memory of motion events. In L. Filipović/K. Jaszczolt (eds.), *Human cognitive processing (vol. 36): Space and time in languages and cultures: Language, culture, and cognition*, pp. 269–282. Amsterdam: John Benjamins.

Filipović, L./Hawkins, J. A. (2019). The complex adaptive system principles model for bilingualism: Language interactions within and across bilingual minds. *International Journal of Bilingualism,* 23, 1223–1248.

Filipović, L./Ibarretxe-Antuñano, I. (2015). Motion. In E. Dabrowska/D. Divjak (eds.), *Handbook of cognitive linguistics*, pp. 527–546. Berlin: Mouton De Gruyter.

Filipović, L./Jaszczolt, K. (eds.). (2012). *Human cognitive processing (vol 36): Space and time in languages and cultures: Linguistic diversity.* Amsterdam: John Benjamins.

Finkbeiner, M./Nicol, J./Greth, D./Nakamura, K. (2002). The role of language in memory for actions. *Journal of Psycholinguistic Research,* 31, 447–457.

Flecken, M./Stutterheim, C. von/ Carroll, M. (2014). Grammatical aspect influences motion event perception: Findings from a cross-linguistic non-verbal recognition task. In *Language and Cognition: An Interdisciplinary Journal of Language and Cognitive Science.* Advance online publication.

Gennari, S./Sloman, S. A./Malt, B. (2002). Motion events in language and cognition. *Cognition,* 83, 49–79.

Goldin-Meadow, S./Gentner, D. (eds.). (2003). *Language in mind: Advances in the study of language and thought.* Cambridge, MA: MIT Press.

Han, Z./Cadierno, T. (2010). *Second language acquisition (vol. 50): Linguistic relativity in SLA: Thinking for speaking.* Bristol, UK: Multilingual Matters.

Henderson, J. M./Hollingworth, A. (1998). Eye movements during scene viewing. In G. Underwood (ed.), *Eye guidance in reading and scene perception*, pp. 269–293. Amsterdam: Elsevier.

Hickmann, M./Hendriks, H. (2010). Typological constraints on the acquisition of spatial language in French and English. *Cognitive Linguistics,* 21, 189–215.

Hickmann, M./Hendriks, H./Harr, A.-K./Bonnet, P. (2018). Caused motion across child languages: A comparison of English, German, and French. *Journal of Child Language,* 45, 1247–1274.

Holmqvist, K./Nyström, M./Andersson, R./Dewhurst, R./Jarodzka, H./Van de Weijer, J. (2011). *Eye tracking: A comprehensive guide to methods and measures*. Oxford: Oxford University Press.

Ji, Y./Hendriks, H./Hickmann, M. (2011). How children express caused motion events in Chinese and English: Universal and language-specific influences. *Lingua*, 121, 1796–1819.

Johanson, M./Selimis, S./Papafragou, A. (2009). Cross-linguistic biases in the semantics and acquisition of spatial language. In J. Chandlee (ed.), *Proceedings of the 33rd annual Boston University conference on language development*, pp. 256–265. Somerville, MA: Cascadilla Press.

Kita, S./Özyürek, A. (2003). What does cross-linguistic variation in semantic coordination of speech and gesture reveal? Evidence for an interface representation of spatial thinking and speaking. *Journal of Memory and Language*, 48, 16–32.

Lakusta, L./Landau, B. (2005). Starting at the end: The importance of goals in spatial language. *Cognition*, 96, 1–33.

Landau, B./Zukowski, A. (2003). Objects, motions, and paths: Spatial language in children with Williams syndrome. *Developmental Neuropsychology*, 23, 105–137.

Levelt, W. J. M. (1989). *Speaking: From intention to articulation. ACL-MIT Press series in natural-language processing*. Cambridge, MA: MIT Press.

Levinson, S. C./Kita, S./Haun, D. B. M./Rasch, B. H. (2002). Returning the tables: Language affects spatial reasoning. *Cognition*, 84, 155–188.

Lucy, J. (1996). The scope of linguistic relativity: An analysis and review of empirical research. In J. J. Gumperz/S. C. Levinson (eds.), *Studies in the social and cultural foundations of language: Rethinking linguistic relativity*, pp. 37–69. Cambridge: Cambridge University Press.

Lucy, J. A. (2016). Recent advances in the study of linguistic relativity in historical context: A critical assessment. *Language Learning*, 66, 487–515.

Majid, A./Bowerman, M./Kita, S./Haun, D. B. M./Levinson, S. C. (2004). Can language restructure cognition? The case for space. *Trends in Cognitive Sciences*, 8, 108–114.

Malt, B. C./Wolff, P. M. (eds.) (2010). *Words and the mind: How words capture human experience*. Oxford: Oxford University Press.

McNeill, D. (2001). Analogic/Analytic representations and cross-linguistic differences in thinking for speaking. *Cognitive Linguistics*, 11, 43–60.

Ozcaliskan, S. (2005). Metaphor meets typology: Ways of moving metaphorically in English and Turkish. *Cognitive Linguistics*, 16, 207–246.

Ozyurek, A./Kita, S./Allen, S./Furman, R./Brown, A. (2005). How does linguistic framing of events influence co-speech gestures? Insights from crosslinguistic variations and similarities. *Gesture*, 5, 219–240.

Papafragou, A. (2010). Source-goal asymmetries in motion representation: Implications for language production and comprehension. *Cognitive Science*, 34, 1064–1092.

Papafragou, A./Hulbert, J./Trueswell, J. (2008). Does language guide event perception? Evidence from eye movements. *Cognition*, 108, 155–184.

Papafragou, A./Massey, C./Gleitman, L. (2002). Shake, rattle, 'n' roll: The representation of motion in language and cognition. *Cognition*, 84, 189–219.

Pulverman, R./Golinkoff, R. M./Hirsh-Pasek, K./Buresh, J. S. (2008). Infants discriminate manners and paths in non-linguistic dynamic events. *Cognition*, 108, 825–830.

R: A language and environment for statistical computing [Computer software]. (2018). R Foundation for Statistical Computing. Vienna, Austria.

Schmiedtová, B. (2011). Do L2 speakers think in the L1 when speaking in the L2? *Vigo International Journal of Applied Linguistics*, 8, 139–179.

Schmiedtová, B. (2013). Traces of L1 patterns in the event construal of Czech advanced speakers of L2 English and L2 German. *International Review of Applied Linguistics in Language Teaching*, 51, 87–116.

Schmiedtová, B./Stutterheim, C. von/Carroll, M. (2011). Language-specific patterns in event construal of advanced second language speakers. In A. Pavlenko (ed.), *Thinking and speaking in two languages*, pp. 66–107. Bristol: Multilingual Matters.

Slobin, D. I. (1987). Thinking for speaking. *Annual Meeting of the Berkeley Linguistics Society*, 13, 435–445.

Slobin, D. I. (1991). Learning to think for speaking. *Pragmatics*, 1, 7–25.

Slobin, D. I. (1996). From 'Thought and Language' to 'Thinking for Speaking'. In J. J. Gumperz/S. C. Levinson (eds.), *Studies in the social and cultural foundations of language (vol. 17): Rethinking linguistic relativity*, pp. 70–96. Cambridge: Cambridge University Press.

Slobin, D. I. (2003). Language and thought online: Cognitive consequences of linguistic relativity. In S. Goldin Meadow/D. Gentner (eds.), *Language in mind: Advances in the study of language and thought*, pp. 157–191. Cambridge, MA: MIT Press.

Slobin, D. I. (2004). The many ways to search for a frog: Linguistic typology and the expression of motion events. In S. Stromqvist/L. Verhoven/R. Berman/D. Slobin (eds.), *Relating events in narrative (vol. 2): Typological and contextual perspectives*, pp. 219–257. Hillsdale, NJ: Lawrence Erlbaum Associates.

Slobin, D. I. (2006). What makes manner of motion salient? Explorations in linguistic typology, discourse, and cognition. In M. Hickmann/S. Robert (eds.), *Typological studies in language (vol. 66): Space in languages: Linguistic systems and cognitive categories*, pp. 59–81. Amsterdam: John Benjamins.

Stutterheim, C. von/Andermann, M./Carroll, M./Flecken, M./Schmiedtová, B. (2012). How grammaticized concepts shape event conceptualization in language production: Insights from linguistic analysis, eye tracking data, and memory performance. *Linguistics,* 50, 833–867.

Stutterheim, C. von/Nüse, R. (2003). Processes of conceptualization in language production: language-specific perspectives and event construal. *Linguistics,* 41, 851–881.

Talmy, L. (1985). Lexicalization patterns: Semantic structure in lexical forms. In T. Shopen (ed.), *Language typology and syntactic description (vol. 3): Grammatical categories and the lexicon*, pp. 57–149. Cambridge: Cambridge University Press.

Trueswell, J. C./Papafragou, A. (2010). Perceiving and remembering events cross-linguistically: Evidence from dual-task paradigms. *Journal of Memory and Language,* 63, 64–82.

Vincent, B. T./Tatler, B. W. (2008). Systematic tendencies in scene viewing. *Journal of Eye Movement Research,* 2, 1–18.

Christopher J. Hall

English as a Lingua Franca as an expression of linguistic diversity: A cognitive perspective

Abstract: My focus here is English as a Lingua Franca (ELF), as a global manifestation of diverse Englishes and as an outcome of SLA. I first discuss defining features of ELF from a cognitive perspective, concluding that ELF mode is characterized by (a) heterolingual participants, (b) using English alongside other linguistic resources, (c) in the absence of (expectations of) shared norms. I call attention to the inherent diversity in ELF and propose a number of key dimensions along which the resources, processes, and outcomes of ELF usage can vary. This raises the issue of what, if anything, is *distinctively diverse* about ELF, compared with other domains of L2 English usage. I explore this question through the lens of the second language assessment framework of "CAF" (complexity, accuracy, and fluency). I argue that accuracy is neither a coherent nor a relevant dimension of ELF performance, and that it is here that the distinctive diversity of ELF resides. I move on to consider the potential contribution of psycholinguistics to a theoretical account of ELF diversity, concluding that although studies of structural priming are relevant, the prospects for a psycholinguistic account of ELF are limited. I argue that the theoretical framework of Usage-based Linguistics offers a better cognitive fit with ELF. Within this approach, I show how the phenomenon of ELF obliges us to reconfigure traditional ontologies of English in terms of the individual resources that diverse language users deploy in usage events. I conclude by highlighting implications for social justice and pedagogy.

Keywords: ELF (English as a Lingua Franca), CAF (complexity, accuracy, fluency), idiolect, Usage-based Linguistics, language ontology

1. Introduction

Linguistic diversity is the principal focus of sociolinguistics (*within* languages) and typological linguistics (*between* languages), but it has largely been glossed over or "abstracted out" in psycholinguistics and other cognitive approaches to language (cf. Hall 2018b). A major exception to this is developmental psycholinguistics, and particularly Second Language Acquisition (SLA). Several subfields of SLA are concerned centrally with diversity as a core feature of the developmental processes and outcomes involved (e.g. cross-linguistic influence, interlanguage, and individual learner differences). In line with this volume's aim to explore diversity and cognition through the lens of language, my focus here is English as a Lingua Franca, as a global manifestation of diverse Englishes and as an outcome of SLA. My rationale is based on the following key observations. First, that internal linguistic diversity can shed as much light on human cognition as cross-linguistic comparison can. Second, that all languages exhibit great internal diversity. Third, that some languages are more internally diverse than others, with English more so than most. And fourth, that language contact, and therefore L2 learning and use, can be a major determinant of this diversity.

One measure of the inherent internal diversity of a language is the number of people who have acquired it in infancy. English, like Mandarin, Spanish, Bengali, and Hindi, has over 300 million native speakers. But perhaps more important than sheer size of the speech community is its geographical distribution. Unlike the other big languages, English is the native tongue of several large and many small national populations across the five major continents. Within and across these L1 groups, English varies according to the community using it, the context it is used in, and the purpose of its use. Moreover, its diversity inevitably increases through extended contact with speakers of other languages. The global distribution of L1 English through conquest and trade beginning in the early modern period resulted in language contact on an unprecedented scale, leading to even greater numbers of multilingual learners and users. Interaction between L1 and L2 users has reshaped the language many times over around the globe, to the extent that treating English as a single monolithic entity is no longer tenable for most academic and practical purposes.

The field of World Englishes (cf. Saraceni 2021) has explored the diversity of the language as a global phenomenon, especially in the many postcolonial settings in which, aside from the interpersonal, it also plays a significant role in political, economic, educational, and cultural affairs. Users in Kachru's postcolonial "Outer Circle" (Kachru 1985) have generally developed their knowledge of the language in what is called an "English as a Second Language" (ESL) context, where formal learning is accompanied and followed by regular experiences with the language outside the classroom. In some respects the ESL route to English resembles that taken by L2 learners situated within Kachru's "Inner Circle" of native anglophone contexts, although here they are less likely to have a common L1. A numerically much larger group develop the language in the "English as a Foreign Language" (EFL) contexts of Kachru's "Expanding Circle", where English does not figure so prominently in public life and learners tend to share the same L1. But however the language is learned, it is *used* globally, and one of the widest uses is in lingua franca communication, where L1 users are absent or in a minority (cf. Jenkins et al. 2018). Language knowledge and use in its multifarious manifestations is a prime example of unity and diversity in human cognition, involving the development, deployment, and dynamic restructuring of millions of sets of complex mental resources. What does interaction in L2 Englishes tell us about these resources? Why does this matter? Yet mainstream understandings of language, both lay and professional, tend to deny or downplay linguistic diversity. English is viewed as a fixed, monolithic system, existing as an ideal abstraction, which can be taught and tested like other school subjects, and which L1 and L2 users alike generally fail to acquire correctly (Hall 2020). In this chapter, I explore the linguistic diversity of English as a Lingua Franca (ELF) from a cognitive perspective, with a view to ultimately challenging harmful monolithic beliefs about the language and its heterogeneous users.

The chapter is organized as follows. In Section 2, I discuss defining features of ELF from a cognitive perspective and conclude that ELF mode is characterized by (a) heterolingual participants, (b) using English alongside other linguistic resources, (c) in the absence of (expectations of) shared norms. In Section 3, I call attention to the inherent diversity in ELF and propose a number of key dimensions along which the resources, processes, and outcomes of ELF usage can vary. I conclude this section by raising the issue of what, if anything, is *distinctively diverse* about ELF, compared with other domains of L2 English usage. Section 4 explores this question through the lens of the second language assessment framework of "CAF" (complexity, accuracy, and fluency). I argue that accuracy is neither a coherent nor a relevant dimension of ELF performance, and that it is here that the distinctive diversity of ELF resides. Section 5 considers the potential contribution of psycholinguistics to a theoretical account of ELF diversity. I conclude that although studies of structural priming are relevant, the prospects for a psycholinguistic account of ELF are limited. In Section 6, I argue that the theoretical framework of Usage-Based Linguistics offers a better cognitive fit with ELF. Within this approach, I show in Section 7 how the phenomenon of ELF obliges us to reconfigure traditional ontologies of English in terms of the individual resources that diverse language users deploy in usage events. Section 8 concludes by highlighting implications for social justice and pedagogy.

2. Defining English as a Lingua Franca

Although a distinct scholarly field and paradigm named ELF has emerged this century, disseminating research in annual conferences, a journal, a handbook, several monographs and many edited volumes, the ontological status of the phenomenon has remained somewhat ambiguous (cf. Hall 2020). Most ELF researchers are (applied) sociolinguists, and in line with their principal disciplinary identity and epistemological commitments, they have adopted the position that ELF is a communicative mode or setting, or a social practice, in which different L2 Englishes figure. For others, in contrast, ELF refers to the *form(s)* of English used by non-native speakers and writers when they interact with users who have a different L1. Whether more emphasis is placed on social practices or linguistic forms, however, it is use rather than user group which is the more central feature of ELF: although the linguistic identity of users is a fundamental element, they are only "ELF users" or "ELF speakers" in certain interactional contexts. This is not to say that some L2 users of English do not themselves identify as (predominantly) ELF users. As Ehrenreich (2018, p. 47) points out, "[f]or many speakers [ELF] clearly [...] serves a range of identificatory purposes in their global interactional spaces". But it is the interplay between interlocutors with different L1s in English-medium encounters which defines ELF as a communicative mode rather than a shared system or code. Accordingly, Seidlhofer (2011, p. 7) defines ELF as "any use of English among speakers of different first languages for whom English is the communicative medium of choice, and often the only option". The same speakers interacting in English with co-linguals or L1 users would not usually be taken to be engaging in ELF mode. Although it is not explicit in Seidlhofer's definition, it is assumed that L1 users of English, if involved at all, are not viewed as providing or modeling the linguistic norms for the interaction – hence the often reported sense of common identity between non-native speakers (NNSs) with different L1s in ELF encounters (cf. Baker 2015). But the commonality does not extend to the *forms* they use in these encounters – i.e. it is not seen as a uniform "international variety" of English. Even for scholars who implicitly present ELF as a resource rather than a mode of use, its formal diversity is a fundamental feature: for Cogo and House (2018, p. 210), for example, "ELF is an "open-source phenomenon", which is constantly adapted by its users and varies according to the context where it is used".

There has been little work on ELF which adopts or refers explicitly to cognitive models of language. Studies that do so have tended to concentrate on what are understood to be qualitative differences between L1 and L2 users. This has had the unfortunate consequence of perpetuating a view of "ELF users" as inherently less competent than L1 users, because of the distinct cognitive challenges they are assumed to have faced in the SLA process. For instance, Alptekin (2011, p. 159) argues that ELF performance is different from L1 English performance because it "stem[s] from different cognitive resources and [is] the outcome of different cognitive processes". And Mauranen contends that "[f]rom a cognitive point of view, we would expect ELF speakers to *approximate* English forms because this would allow them to attain reasonable economy in processing while securing a good chance of achieving comprehension" (2012, p. 57, my emphasis).

For Mauranen, approximations are forms which differ from Standard English, such as *categoration*, *discuss on*, *from other point of view*. They generally do not cause any communication breakdown, but are viewed as defective: expressions which "ELF speakers tend to get [...] slightly wrong" (p. 144). Yet a definition of ELF as a cognitive phenomenon does not require reference to, or comparison with, L1 users. I have described ELF as "an exercise in joint cognition to which individual heterolingual participants bring repertoires of mentally-represented [English] linguistic resources which they have constructed on the basis of prior experience (including L1 influence)" (Hall 2018a, p. 76). This definition, to be elaborated further in what follows, recognizes that ELF is first and foremost a function of particular usage events, in which diverse L2 English resources are deployed and reshaped.

From a cognitive perspective, then, ELF involves the comprehension and production of utterances constructed from L2 English resources in heterolingual contexts. Based on this, the argument I wish to pursue here is that, crucially, the absence or decentring of L1 English users and usage in these contexts has the effect of compromising one of the central (psycho)linguistic principles of language knowledge and use: namely, the conventionality of the code (e.g. Clark 1996). According to Lewis (1969), conventions are coordination devices which emerge in a particular community to determine preferred outcomes in joint activities between members of the community. Clark (1996) applies this understanding of convention to language, defining separate languages as "signalling systems" of mappings between linguistic forms and meanings which constitute part of a community's "common ground" (Clark 1996, pp. 70–77). Knowledge and understanding of social conventions, including their applicability to all members of a community, emerge early. Rakoczy and Tomasello (2009), for example, demonstrate that children of around three years old not only follow linguistic conventions, but also adopt normative behaviors towards others who violate those conventions. Ambridge et al. (2012) review studies on how children "retreat from overgeneralization", i.e. start to conform to the often idiosyncratic conventions of the adult community system. Children acquiring English, for example, come to understand that even though the word *cooker* should mean "one who cooks" on the basis of the regular addition of the agentive suffix *-er* to verbs, for adult members of the community they grow up in it happens to refer to the appliance used for cooking. The authors conclude that underpinning the mechanisms which cause the retreat is a "necessary pre-condition that motivates children to respect adult conventions in the first place" (2012, p. 11). That precondition is attenuated in the use and ongoing development of English by participants in ELF interactions.

So, ELF contexts differ from native speaker (NS) ones because in the former the interactants do not belong to a single community and there is therefore no "assumption of predetermined community conventions" (Hall 2018a, p. 80). Yet like L1 users, L2 users in non-ELF contexts take for granted that communication will be governed by conventional forms, or *norms* to use the sociolinguistic term. In EFL and many ESL contexts, the norms are those of L1 users of standard varieties from the Inner Circle, but they equally might have arisen as "indiginized varieties" in the Outer Circle. Shared forms do not necessarily reflect conventional norms, however: interaction between L2 users from the same or similar L1 background may also conform to the non-conventional but shared regularities which arise from parallel learning trajectories modulated by common processes of cross-linguistic influence. Spanish L1 users of English, for example, will typically pronounce words like *stop* and *sleep* with an epenthetic initial [e], and omit pronominal subjects (e.g. "Is easy"), due to L1 influence. Mauranen has referred to such shared sets of L2 features as "similects" and has helpfully defined ELF as "second-order language contact" in which users of *different* English similects interact (2012, p. 29). The blurring of language boundaries within a single individual reflected in similects is a fundamental feature of bilingualism, of course. We know from studies of bilingual processing and mental representation that during monolingual performance in one language, be it L1 or L2, a speaker's other language is not completely supressed (Kroll et al. 2012). It is increasingly being recognized that typical language use by bi- and multilinguals taps into all a speaker's linguistic resources, regardless of socially constructed "named language" boundaries – in other words, the phenomenon of *translanguaging* (García & Li Wei 2014). Indeed, there is much discussion in the ELF literature about the inherently bilingual nature of the phenomenon (Jenkins 2015). We return to this issue in Section 7.

Figure 1 summarizes the typical characteristics of ELF which emerge from this initial discussion. The three characteristics each highlight an aspect of diversity: (a) ELF interactions feature participants who do not share a common L1; (b) ELF interactions feature the deployment of resources from multilingual repertoires; (c) ELF interactions unfold in the absence of an expectation of shared norms.

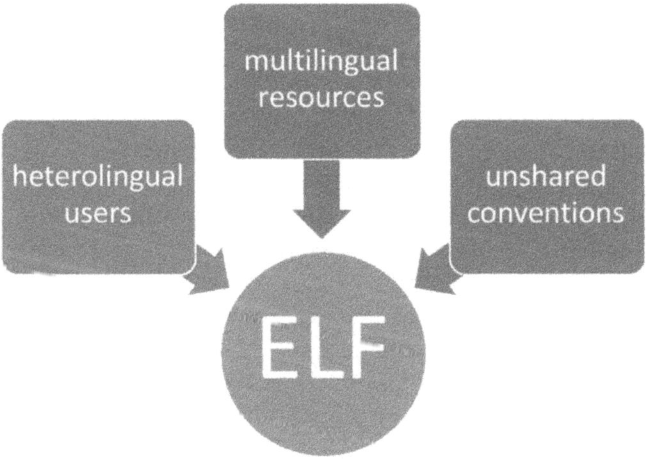

Figure 1: Typical characteristics of ELF from a cognitive perspective

These three characteristics do not exhaust the diversity found in ELF, however. The scope and extent of this diversity is the topic of the following section.

3. Dimensions of ELF diversity

ELF usage as defined in the foregoing admits huge intra- and inter-personal variation, which we can map along several continua, including the dimensions of diversity (henceforth "DD"s) listed in Table 1.

Table 1: Some dimensions of ELF diversity (DDs)

Dimension	From		To
(a) Lexico-grammatical complexity	Elaborate	↔	Simple
(b) Norm dependence	Localized, unstandardized, innovative, or idiosyncratic usage	↔	Inner Circle standard variety usage
(c) Translanguaging	Lots	↔	None at all
(d) Automaticity	Unconscious, rapid access	↔	Deliberate, labored search; or careful crafting
(e) Effective meaning-making/sharing	Full alignment	↔	Misalignment or breakdown

Consider, for example, the following scenarios (fictitious, but inspired by actual encounters that I have observed or that have been reported to me). In one, a L1 Kannada-speaking woman from Bangalore in India has traveled the 200 miles to Chennai to consult with L1 Tamil-speaking doctors in one of the specialist hospitals there. In another, a group of postgraduate students from several different countries are attending a research seminar in Luxembourg. In a third, elderly Japanese tourists ask a couple of kids selling beer on a Mexican beach about where they can try the best local fish. The Indian healthcare scenario is characterized by the use of highly localized Indian English accents (DD-b), with the doctor using quite elaborate vocabulary in complex sentences to which the patient responds with much simpler forms (DD-a). This contrast in English proficiency initially leads to mutual misunderstanding (DD-e). They proceed to draw on their shared knowledge of Hindi (DD-c), code-switching to compensate for the patient's effortful English (DD-d) and to facilitate mutual comprehension (DD-e again). At the Luxembourg seminar, the lecturer initially uses complex, carefully crafted English (DD-a and DD-d) following Inner Circle norms (DD-b), with no other languages involved (DD-c). The students engage their own Englishes to understand the talk with considerable ease (DD-e). Afterwards, lecturer and students shift to casual, unplanned, relatively simple English as they chat with each other on their way to get coffee (DD-a and DD-d). On the Mexican beach, the Japanese tourists use a limited English vocabulary with prominent Japanese phonetic features and little grammatical structure (DD-a and DD-b). They also switch frequently to Japanese and use gesture liberally (DD-c). Their search for English words is laborious, but the kids respond with effortless, quick-fire English (DD-d), most of it simple, pre-fabricated phrases and schemas (DD-a again), delivered in highly colloquial American English acquired from US visitors and popular culture (DD-b). The exchange is enjoyed by both parties, but ends with the tourists none the wiser about the local fish (DD-e). Note that these dimensions cover the resources (Englishes and others) that users bring to the usage event (DD-a, DD-b, DD-c), as well as the processes (DD-c, DD-d), and outcomes (DD-e) associated with it. Note too that often the same users can vary on different dimensions, depending on circumstances: the doctor can operate in monolingual or multilingual mode, for example, and the lecturer can carefully self-monitor or engage in spontaneous talk.

The diversity is immense, but all of this usage counts as ELF. This raises the question of what is *distinctively* diverse about ELF. All the dimensions of diversity we have considered so far are, for example, witnessed equally in EFL and ESL usage, where the typical characteristics of ELF are absent or infrequent. Consider, for example: a Kannada-L1 patient interacting in English with monolingual

English-L1 health workers in a UK hospital (a case of ESL); Spanish-L1 students at a postgraduate seminar in Spain where English is the medium of instruction (EFL); or young learners of English doing a tourist role-play activity at a high school in Japan (again, EFL). One can imagine such interactions being plotted anywhere along the five DDs listed in Table 1. Although much of the situation- and participant- dependent variation in our imagined ELF, EFL, and ESL scenarios is shared and can be accounted for from a sociolinguistic perspective, the distinctive interplay between the different DDs in ELF can only be isolated by adopting a cognitive vantage point. In the next section I demonstrate this by considering the distinction made in SLA between complexity, accuracy and fluency (CAF), and showing that "accuracy" is not a meaningful dimension for ELF.

4. ELF and CAF dimensions of L2 performance

Michel (2017, p. 50) provides a standard definition of CAF as dimensions of L2 performance:

> "Complexity refers to the size, elaborateness, richness, and diversity of the L2 performance. Accuracy is a measure for the target-like and error-free use of language. Fluency refers to the smooth, easy, and eloquent production of speech with limited numbers of pauses, hesitations, or reformulations". Following Housen and Kuiken (2009, p. 462), I take CAF as "principal epiphenomena of the psycholinguistic mechanisms and processes underlying the acquisition, representation and processing of L2 knowledge". Conceptualized thus, the "C" and "A" of CAF relate to the cognitive *resources* of English (mentally represented knowledge) and "F" to the *use* of those resources in interaction (processing).

What is perhaps most notable about the global population of L2 users of English is the diversity in breadth and depth of the *resources* they bring to usage events. Those with richer (more extensive and entrenched) resources will naturally be capable of greater complexity. As an epiphenomenon of acquisition and processing mechanisms as well as mentally represented knowledge, increased complexity will often be accompanied by increased fluency, as more constructions become entrenched and therefore proceduralized. From a usage-based perspective, both dimensions are associated with developing procedural knowledge (Ullman 2015) in a way that attention to accuracy is not. This is because, in parallel to and beyond the instructional and assessment contexts in which accuracy is a key goal, learning happens implicitly in usage events (Ellis 2005, 2017; Ellis & Wulff 2015). Learners are always also users, inevitably exposed to input from a diverse set of other users including co-lingual and heterolingual peers, NNS and NS teachers, and people with unstandardized accents and dialects. The input can be experienced in a range of usage event genres, including transactional and interactional, formal and casual, written and spoken, online and face-to-face (cf. Thorne & Reinhardt 2008; Hellermann et al. 2019). A considerable amount of the input will contain NNS and unstandardized NS features (i.e. "errors"), and a subset of this will serve as intake, contributing to the learner's developing repertoire. These features will be reinforced through recycling in output and often also by the existing, highly entrenched, L1 system. In other words, some of the resources entrenched in procedural memory through frequent encounters in usage events will diverge from the norms of "accuracy" developed in declarative memory through instruction and deliberate learning. A key cognitive mechanism through which such repeated exposure and use can result in learning is long-term structural priming (cf. Jackson 2017), which we take up in section 5.

Although some in SLA argue that the "A" in CAF should be taken to include appropriateness and acceptability as well as accuracy (Housen et al. 2012, p. 4), success in learning English is still generally understood in terms of the extent to which NS grammatical norms are accurately reproduced (cf. "target-like" and "error-free" in Michel's [2017] definition). For example, in their influential review of studies on the effectiveness of L2 instruction, Norris and Ortega (2000) uncontroversially assume "target-like levels of ultimate attainment" (p. 419) as the instructional goal; there is no question that the learning target is defined by anything other than NS standardized norms. This is despite the very well-attested (and uncontested) fact that "accurate" use of many grammatical constructions is unnecessary for meaningful interaction, serving more as a NS social identity marker (Widdowson 1994). Take, for example, "incorrect" countable use of nouns like *advice* and *furniture* in EFL or ESL, a notable and widespread feature of NNS (including ELF) usage (Hall et al. 2013). Despite the prominent attention paid to "correct" application of countability in teaching materials, NNS pluralization of such nouns poses no obstacle to comprehension (Björkman 2008). Of course, some NNS usage can cause or contribute to communication breakdown; crucially, though, it is not its divergence from NS norms (i.e. accuracy) *per se* which causes the problems. Indeed, similar issues arise also within NS-NS interaction. I think we can conclude, therefore, that given that accuracy is a coherent and relevant dimension only in contexts where NS conventions are taken to be the yardstick, it is not relevant for ELF.

Let us now return to the role of fluency and complexity in ELF. Understood as ease of processing, fluency has not figured at all in the definition of ELF we have been contemplating thus far. SLA research (Skehan 1998) has demonstrated how fluency and accuracy can be inversely correlated, such that an emphasis on accuracy in performance will often result in impaired fluency, and increased fluency will often incur a "cost" to accuracy (the so-called "trade-off hypothesis"). But when accuracy is understood as adherence to norms, and ELF is characterized by the unsettling of those norms, then the threat to fluency is diminished. This is because in ELF, meaningful interaction, not "correctness", is the goal. ELF scholars have tended to concentrate on participants in ELF interactions whose English resources are sufficiently entrenched to be accessible and usable fluently for effective/successful communication, e.g. in business (Nickerson 2005) and higher education (Jenkins 2014). They have observed how the prioritization of fluency over accuracy results in NNS forms, which can be viewed as innovations, i.e. expressions of creativity (Cogo & Dewey 2012). In ELF, complexity can thus involve diversity and richness of form and function which goes beyond the monolithic model taught and tested in the L2 classroom. If accuracy is removed from the equation, complexity can be developed and deployed with less attention to output (i.e. self-monitoring and self correction). When ELF becomes the default mode of usage, as it is for increasing numbers of L2 users, this can result in the unfettered entrenchment, and fluent deployment, of NNS forms, because in such scenarios, NNS repertoires develop independently of NS norms.

The vantage point afforded by CAF thus helps us isolate the *distinctive diversity* of ELF: by exposing the inapplicability of "accuracy" as a relevant factor in typical ELF usage events, we can begin to see how the phenomenon is one which has become unmoored from the traditionally assumed tenets of linguistic communication, in which success is governed by an expectation of shared norms (Langacker 1987; Clark 1996; Croft 2000; Verhagen 2015). Once native speakers are decentred, and no other single community of users steps in to replace them as norm providers, then common ground regarding form-meaning mappings is reduced and diversity escalates. This loosening of the constraints of conventionality can result in increased linguistic creativity, but it also induces a need for heightened attention to pragmatic strategies and negotiation of meaning (Pitzl 2012; Cogo & House 2018). In sum, at the heart of the ELF phenomenon from the cognitive perspective is the interplay between distinct heterolingual individual language resources. These can reach high levels of complexity, may be fluently accessed and deployed, but are not necessarily shared. How to approach this distinctive ELF diversity from a theoretical perspective is the subject of the next section.

5. Theorizing distinctive ELF diversity

Accuracy as a construct relies on the idealization that languages are fixed codes shared by all (legitimate) members of a speech community, such that usage which diverges from the code is inaccurate (or "incorrect": Milroy & Milroy 2012, p. 30). Harris (1981, p. 10) has argued that mainstream linguistics distorts the reality of language use as a result of implicit subscription to a "fixed code fallacy", which he describes in the following terms:

> Individuals are able to exchange their thoughts by means of words because [...] they have come to understand and to adhere to a fixed public plan for doing so. The plan is based on recurrent instantiation of invariant items [...]. Being invariant, sentences are context-free, and so proof against the vagaries of changing speakers, hearers and circumstances, rather as coin of the realm is valid irrespective of the honesty or dishonesty of individual transactions.

It is certainly the case that mainstream, cognitively-oriented linguistic theory assumes invariance, abstracting away from diversity. Jackendoff (2011, p. 587), in discussing speaker knowledge of the conventional form-meaning mappings of a language, asserts that "[t]wo speakers are mutually intelligible if their own personal mappings are close enough to enable them to achieve mutual understanding on the basis of exchanged signals". He goes on to observe that "[w]e typically idealize this situation by assuming that the mental systems in the members of a speech community are uniform and thereby can be regarded as a single language". He does acknowledge that the abstraction is not appropriate for all circumstances, however, pointing out that "we readily drop the idealization when dealing with differences of vocabulary, dialect, and register. We also drop the idealization, almost without noticing, when dealing with young children's speech, which only approximates adult language." In other words, the idealization is not tenable in sociolinguistics and developmental psycholinguistics. But if we wish to examine ELF as an expression of internal linguistic diversity from a cognitive rather than a sociolinguistic perspective, and in *usage* rather than *learning*, then we need to look beyond mainstream linguistic and psycholinguistic theory.

Notoriously, 20th-century psycholinguistic theory was concerned almost exclusively with mental representation and processing in monolinguals, mostly English speakers, and speakers of Standard English at that. The past couple of decades have, gratifyingly, seen an increasing amount of neuropsychological research with bi- and multilingual people (e.g. Nicol 2001; Grosjean & Li 2013; Schwieter 2019). Yet this multilingual turn in psycholinguistics has not been applied to ELF. Given its dimensions of diversity and status as a mode of use rather than an international variety, it is hard to imagine how language processing in ELF could be studied in the controlled, replicable conditions required for experimentation. Having said that, one psycholinguistic phenomenon relevant to the diversity of ELF usage which has been subjected to significant empirical scrutiny over the past decade or so is structural priming (Jackson 2018). Structural priming refers to the effect whereby exposure to a linguistic construction in input enhances the likelihood of its use in output. So, for example, having just heard or read a passive construction will make it more probable that you will use one yourself. This occurs because the mental representation of the construction in memory receives activation during receptive processing and so is more available in ensuing productive processing. In a review of the phenomenon, Pickering and Ferriera (2008) suggest that structural priming serves two important functions: (a) to promote alignment between interlocutors in dialogue; and (b) as an implicit learning mechanism. The former recognizes the shared natural environment in which structural priming occurs, as conversational participants tune their communicative behavior – both linguistic and non-linguistic – to enhance cooperation and understanding. The latter explains longer-lasting restructuring of mental representations, which happens automatically and unconsciously, on the basis of persistent repetition of constructions in usage.

Both of these functions of structural priming have heightened significance for ELF. With lowered expectations of shared linguistic norms, participants in ELF interactions need to be as resourceful as possible, exploiting opportunities to signal their cooperation and facilitate mutual understanding. Tacitly establishing what we might call "micro-conventions" on the fly by accommodating to one's interlocutors' distinctive linguistic forms is one way of doing this (cf. Hynninen 2016). The cognitive mechanism involved in achieving this formal alignment is structural priming. If ELF induces micro-conventions which override the mainstream conventions taught and tested in EFL and ESL, they may also become entrenched through repetition at the individual level, and this "alternative learning" can help explain the diversity of linguistic forms with which ELF is associated. There is even some experimental evidence from structural priming for the possibility that usage can lead to the entrenchment of micro-conventions which contravene wider community norms, although it is limited and not from ELF contexts. Luka and colleagues (Luka & Barsalou 2005; Luka & Choi 2012) demonstrate how reading aloud repeated instances of sentences in English by NSs can lead subsequently to higher judgments of grammaticality on structurally identical sentences compared with controls. This "structural preference effect" was found after a delay of seven days by Luka and Choi (2012). Increases in judgments of grammaticality were particularly strong for sentences which had been rated as only "moderately grammatical" by naive native speakers. Luka and Choi (2012) conclude that this is evidence that "incremental adjustments to the language processing system occur on a continuous basis and may extend to acquisition of novel syntactic structures" (p. 355). This may be what is happening with the entrenchment of originally transient micro-conventions, including "inaccurate" NNS forms, when experienced in ELF interactions and repeated across ELF usage events. But it is unclear how this could be modeled in an experimental context.

These observations suggest that psycholinguistic models based on behavioral and neuropsychological data will not, at least in any direct way, be sufficient for theorizing the linguistic/cognitive diversity of ELF. This is because psycholinguistic theory assumes that what is being processed, and what is mentally represented, is conventional (shared) linguistic code. Despite some precedents in the literature on processing in the context of L1 dialect variation (Loudermilk 2013), psycholinguistic theory is not set up to handle the distinctive diversity involved. But the conclusions drawn about implicit learning from the work on structural priming do point to a cognitively-oriented theoretical framework that can better accommodate ELF: the family of approaches known as Usage-Based Linguistics (UBL), to which we now turn.

6. Usage-based linguistics and individual linguistic resources

Usage-Based Linguistics addresses two main issues: development and systematicity. In other words: (a) how language develops in infants, in adults, and across the lifespan (i.e. processes of *usage* and *entrenchment*); and (b) how it is socially structured in shared systems for meaningful communication, and how those systems change over time (i.e. processes of *conventionalization*). In UBL, language is conceptualized as a cognitive resource constructed and continuously developing in individual minds on the basis of implicit analyzes of the frequency and distribution of form-meaning pairings in the input experienced during usage events (Langacker 2000; Tomasello 2003; Goldberg 1995; Ellis & Wulff 2015). Systematic patterns of language are not determined "top-down," as rules conforming to hard-wired universal principles. Neither are they monolithic sets of fixed social conventions to which individual speakers have (greater or lesser) access. Rather, they emerge "bottom-up" in individual minds on the basis of variable, socially-contextualized, experience. Essentially, the message of UBL is that people construct and entrench form-meaning regularities on the basis of what they are frequently exposed to (and go on to deploy) in meaningful usage.

For adult language learners in educational contexts, this means that implicit learning occurs independently of what they are instructed in, and are expected to learn, in classrooms. Moreover, in ELF, as we have seen, people are exposed to diverse manifestations of English in conditions in which shared norms cannot be assumed, and where the focus is on effective sharing of meaning rather than adherence to a monolithic set of formal conventions. In UBL, constructional accounts are increasingly being applied to SLA (Ellis & Wulff 2015), although the emphasis is implicitly on "target (NS) constructions", i.e. the pursuit of accuracy. But such approaches can equally explain how NNS forms may become entrenched as constructions across learning and usage. One way is through the constructional notion of abstract schemas (Tomasello 2003). These are mental representations which include slots that can be filled with specific items, e.g. the phrasal type *let's [V]* and the morphological type *[ADJ]-ness*. For NNSs, open slots in schemas they have constructed may be filled by items which NS norms disallow. For example, although all children acquiring L1 Inner Circle English end up adhering to the adult norm which prevents non-count nouns like *advice* and *furniture* plural from appearing in the schema *[N]-s*), some NNSs do not acquire the filter and, for them, constructions like *advices* and *furnitures* become entrenched. In other words, L2 learning and usage conditions may foreclose any "retreat from overgeneralization" as discussed by Ambridge et al. (2012). As we have seen, ELF favors such conditions, given the compromised principle of conventionality it involves. Furthermore, constructional schemas strongly entrenched in the NNS's L1 may also attract English L2 lexical material, leading to NNS forms traditionally accounted for in SLA by models of cross-linguistic influence.

UBL therefore provides an appropriate theoretical framework for understanding and explaining the distinctive diversity involved in ELF. Although the phenomenon has not been discussed in the mainstream UBL literature, ELF scholars have addressed its cognitive dimensions almost uniquely from a UBL perspective (e.g. Alptekin 2013; Hall et al. 2017; Hall 2018a; Mackenzie 2014; Mauranen 2012; Vetchinnikova 2015, 2019; Vetchinnikova & Hiltunen 2020). Of greatest relevance to the issue of ELF and diversity is the centrality in UBL of entrenchment in individuals as a result of their participation in usage events. Entrenchment has mostly been studied on the basis of cross-sectional corpus data (Stefanowitsch & Flach 2017). Yet given the emphasis placed on entrenchment as a result of subjective experience in unique usage events, it is perhaps surprising that the individual level has not been focused on more. Dąbrowska (2016), for example, points out that Cognitive Linguistics (a usage-based framework) has ignored the individual level, particularly as pertains to individual differences, which she has documented in several publications (e.g. Dąbrowska 2012). And Blumenthal-Dramé (2012) criticizes UBL for its "assumption that the gap between the individual-mental and the collective-behavioural levels can be bridged via statistical generalizations over [cross-sectional] corpus data" (p. 31).

Focusing on individual language users and their idiolectal resources is not very common in any brand of linguistics, although the individual mind is the locus of language for most of them. For Chomsky (1986), the proper object of analysis in linguistics is the construct he termed "I-language", an individual's internalized knowledge of their language. And the assumption is not restricted to generativism: Hall Jr (1985, p. 353), a critic of Chomskyan linguistics, asserts that "all phenomena of language exist only in the 'know-how'... of individual speakers, i.e., in their idiolects . . . Each idiolect exists only in the brain of the speaker who uses it". UBL too holds that language knowledge, both form and meaning, resides in individual minds. Croft (2000) states unambiguously that grammar is "a real, individual, psychological entity, not an abstraction that does not have a psychological (or physical) existence" (p. 27). Langacker (2008, pp. 30) asserts that "[f]or purposes of studying language as part of cognition, an expression's meaning is first and foremost its meaning for a single (representative) speaker". And Östman and Trousdale (2013) entertain the possibility of "shift[ing] the focus away from social and cultural categories like 'language' and 'dialect' in order to foreground the individual speaker, his or her internal linguistic network, and the social and cultural knowledge s/he associates with particular forms" (p. 482). Yet, beyond authorship identification studies in literary criticism (e.g. Love 2002) and forensic linguistics (e.g. Coulthard 2004), there are very few studies of individual L1 idiolectal usage. All that I know of use corpus data. One is Mollin's (2009) investigation of the collocational preferences of Tony Blair on the basis of a corpus of transcripts of his public speaking. Another is Barlow's (2013) UBL-framed study of the idiolectal features of several White House press secretaries. There is also Schmid and Mantlik's (2015) examination of a single construction across historical literary corpus data, including that of individual authors, which shows the interplay between idiolectal patterns of entrenchment and communal patterns of conventionalization.

There have been several studies of individual L2 learning trajectories in classroom contexts, some within UBL. Notably, Eskildsen (2009, 2012, 2015) has charted the development of a variety of English constructions by two learners who have L1 Spanish, using longitudinal classroom corpus data. In one study, Eskildsen (2009) shows how a learner, Carlos, developed knowledge of modal *can* in an incremental fashion, through experience and then productive use of the form with a succession of main verb exemplars. Tammelin-Laine and Martin (2016) chronicle the development of the Finnish negative construction by four adult nonliterate L2 learners. Like Eskildsen, and as predicted by UBL accounts, they observe exemplar-driven development of the construction, with gradual accretion of complexity, and the learning trajectories and outcomes they tracked were marked by significant individual differences. These studies of idiolectal SLA demonstrate how learning can happen piecemeal through participation in unique usage events, rather than the application across the board of learned rules.

But there has been only very limited work on the individual resources brought to, deployed in, and shaped by, ELF usage (i.e. independently of learning). Vetchinnikova (2015) is, I believe, the first study by an ELF scholar to use the UBL framework to analyze individual usage data. In this study, Vetchinnikova examines multi-word units in thesis drafts from different disciplines written in English by five NNS Master's students at a Finnish university. She compares these "production samples" with multi-word units used in: (a) an "exposure sample" of the publications each student had referred to, and (b) a reference sample of the publications referred to by one of the other students from a different discipline. She found that the multi-word units used by each individual coincided to a much greater degree with those used in the publications they cited (average 64 %), compared with those cited by other students (26 %). She interprets this as evidence for idiolectal profiles shaped by prior experience with linguistic input, just as predicted by UBL. But the ELF status of the data is debatable. Vetchinnikova (2019) describes the thesis drafts as belonging to "a typical academic English as a lingua franca (ELF) environment", citing one of the students who told her that they were writing their thesis for Swedish as well as Finnish colleagues. Yet academic writing is formal and highly normative. The samples of English they have been exposed to in this genre are from published sources which are likely to have been written according to NS Standard English norms, and furthermore, to have been copy-edited and style-corrected to ensure greater conformity to these norms (Jenkins 2014). Nevertheless, Vetchinnikova's careful analysis demonstrates how idiolectal L2 patterns tend to emerge from the language that users are exposed to.

In a similar study which more closely resembles typical ELF interaction, Vetchinnikova (2017) examines samples of individual commenters on blog postings from a NNS blogger. The corpus covers interactions on the blog over the course of seven years, involving over 4,000 commenters in addition to the blog author. Analysis of lexical preferences associated with the *it is [ADJ] that* construction for the author and five prolific commenters shows significant individual differences in comparison to a reference corpus constituted by a sample of text from less frequent commenters. Vetchinnikova uses the individual and cross-sectional corpora to represent language on the "cognitive plane" and the "communal plane" respectively, concluding that in the former case entrenched lexical preferences result in significantly different idiolectal profiles. The claim is reinforced by a type/token analysis of four-word lexical bundles across the two types of corpora, which shows that individuals have a greater variety and larger number of lexical bundles, reflecting individual preferences.

Finally, colleagues and I (Hall et al. 2017) conducted a corpus study of a single NNS user of English who uses the language in an ELF context. We examined a collection of emails sent by Antonio, a multilingual (Italian-L1) manager in a South African company, over an 18-month period. In Vetchinnikova's terms, this was the production corpus, reflecting the cognitive plane. Focusing on the *Can you/Could you [V]?* construction alternation used in requests, we compared Antonio's usage of the alternation with that in: (a) emails he had received over the period and 18 months prior to it (the "exposure corpus"); and (b) the massive EnronSent mail corpus of emails from a multinational corporation (Styler 2011), as a general reference corpus for the genre. Both of these latter corpora represent usage of the alternation on the "communal plane". The first reflects the usage Antonio experienced in the multilingual context of his online daily business interactions, where around 60 % of his 292 individual correspondents were L2 English users. Given its size and scale, the EnronSent corpus was taken to reflect global usage norms for the genre as a whole. We found that Antonio has an overwhelming preference for *can* over *could* in this construction (84 % vs 16 %), differing significantly from the usage in the reference corpora, where *could* is used in over 40 % of requests he experienced in emails directed to him and in 35 % of requests in the genre as a whole. We explored the possibility that the preference was due to Antonio's initial learning experience and/or differences in his construal of the constructions' pragmatics, but concluded that neither alone was able to account for the high numbers of *can*. Detailed examination of the distribution of token frequencies of verb types occurring in the constructions' frames reveal that a single verb, *assist*, although relatively uncommon in the overall genre, is particularly common in the input Antonio received. This seems to be the source of Antonio's structural preference, attracting to the schema slot a broad range of other main verbs. This exemplar-driven entrenchment of patterns is precisely what UBL proposes as the motor of development and usage (cf. Griess 2005, on the special role of verbs in this process).

7. An ontological perspective

What emerges from these studies is a view of language as overlapping but non-identical sets of individual resources which users deploy and develop in usage events. In the ontological framework I have been developing over the past few years (Hall 2013, 2020), English construed in this way may be defined as a set of resources "represented in the minds of individuals, in different quantities and degrees of entrenchment, which allows them to use certain linguistic features and constructions meaningfully with individuals who have sufficiently similar sets of resources" (Hall 2020, p. 23). The framework theorizes other ways in which English can be understood to exist as an ontological category, with a fundamental distinction drawn between conceptualizations of English as sociopolitical construction on the one hand and as sociocognitive phenomenon on the other. The former is a monolithic conceptualization, identified with "Standard English" as a component of (originally English) national identity. Like a monolith, English in this view is a single object, with a fixed form and shape, distinct from others. It is essentially this view that Harris (1981) asserts has led to the "fixed code fallacy" in linguistics. The latter view is a "plurilithic" one (Pennycook 2007), in which English is composed of multiple resources, processes, and products, is uncontained by defined borders, is formally and functionally diverse, and undergoes constant dynamic restructuring. It is this view that I have been pursuing here.

Adapting Chomsky's (1986) term "I-language" (where the "I" indicates individual, internal, intensional), I call the cognitive resources involved "I-Englishes" (Hall 2020). Furthermore, to acknowledge the situational contingency of their formal and functional diversity, I posit that I-Englishes are indexed in language users' minds to "I-registers" (Hall 2013), i.e. subsets of lexico-grammatical resources which become associated with certain external contextual conditions. In bi- and multilinguals, some I-registers will draw on resources associated with a particular named language. So, for example, Antonio's I-registers will include: resources of Italian activated in phone calls to family and friends in Italy; resources of English activated with family and friends in South Africa; limited Afrikaans co-activated with English in interaction with other friends there; and a set of rather formal English resources, including the *Can you [V]* construction, in business emails. A similar approach to this diversity of linguistic resources has been recognized also by scholars of translanguaging. Otheguy et al. (2015), for example, adopt an idiolectal approach in which separate named languages are social constructions, ontologically distinct from language understood as a cognitive phenomenon. This renders cognitively untenable the view of bilingualism as "dual competence" in two separate language systems. They distinguish the ontological categories and associated naming practices thus:

> [I]n accepting terms like 'language', 'a language,' 'monolingual', and 'bilingual', we are using categories that have nothing to do with individuals when seen from their own

> internal linguistic perspective, categories that have nothing to do, that is, with the billions of the world's idiolects, which exist in a separate, linguistically unnamed and socially undifferentiated mental realm. (p. 293)

In erasing the borders between named languages in the mental realm, their idiolectal view of translanguaging is consistent with the perspective on ELF developed here. The disregard for monolithic "named language" boundaries typifies both phenomena. Neither translanguaging nor ELF are consistent with the mainstream ontology of English as a single, fixed system. The argument I have pursued here suggests that such a conceptualization is an ideologically imbued social construct, and that what we call English is better understood as a set of plurilithic resources, processes, and products. But unlike scholars who have reached a similar conclusion from a critical, non-cognitivist perspective (e.g. Canagarajah 2020; Pennycook 2020), the idiolectal view locates the diversity of resources involved at the level of cognition, in individual language users' minds.

8. Implications and conclusions

In this chapter I have explored linguistic diversity through a cognitive lens, focusing on English and its use as a lingua franca in global contexts. This focus allowed me to critically examine the status of community norms in mainstream assumptions about what constitutes a (named) language, and to problematize the associated construct of "accuracy" in SLA. I concluded that the distinctive diversity of ELF resides in the absence of an expectation of shared norms in the habitual interactions between heterolingual L2 users which characterize the lingua franca mode. According to this view, the diversity is best explained in terms of patterns of usage and entrenchment at the cognitive, idiolectal level, as theorized in UBL. Understood thus, English is conceptualized not in terms of a single ontological category, as a monolithic abstract system, but rather as distributed across millions of sets of plurilithically-constituted mental resources which are deployed in, and modified through, usage events. Adopting this radical ontological commitment presents both opportunities and challenges for applied linguists and others who seek to expose and resist the social injustices which arise from language ideologies based on monolithic thinking.

Ideologies of monolithic English (and other named languages) dominate public discourse and are perpetuated by educational processes (Lippi-Green 2012). In denying the diversity of English resources and practices that exist on the cognitive and communal planes, such ideologies result in social injustices for both native and non-native speakers (Piller 2016). As I have argued elsewhere (e.g. Hall & Cunningham 2020; Hall 2021), ontological clarity is a vital component of efforts to contest harmful language ideologies. It is widely acknowledged that sociolinguists have contributed to this clarity and have challenged the pernicious effects of monolithic thinking about named languages by demonstrating the systematicity and the legitimacy of unstandardized NS varieties (cf. Labov 1982) and indigenized NNS varieties (cf. Kachru 1985). But on their own, such efforts are insufficient. Applied and critical sociolinguists have pointed out that they need to be complemented by greater understanding of the power of language ideologies. As Snell (2018, p. 370) observes with regard to NS dialectal prejudice: "[b]efore we can counter dangerous beliefs about language we first have to understand how they are socially produced and accepted as convincing and effective […]." This stance is equally true of NNS contexts and associated injustices, yet the way forward is less clear. In NS contexts, the discriminatory beliefs and practices involved can be transparently linked to the extralinguistic prejudices of racism (Flores & Rosa 2015) and class positioning (Snell 2013), and this should make them somewhat easier to expose and challenge. NNSs in L2 classrooms or in interaction with NSs, however, may be stigmatized solely by virtue of being users of NNS linguistic forms, independently of intersectional factors. This is due in part to the ingrained assumption that the principle of conventionality should necessarily apply in NNS contexts. The assumption manifests in TESOL and SLA as the powerful, prevailing belief that there must be a single learning model and target and that only so-called "standard" English forms can fulfill that role.

The dominant response to this in recent applied linguistics has been to shift the focus away from linguistic forms, associated as they are with accuracy, and instead to recast English as a social (local or translingual) practice (Pennycook 2010; Canagarajah 2013). This ontological shift, although welcome, has unfortunately been accompanied by the downplaying of English as cognitive resource (Canagarajah 2020; Pennycook 2020). Given what UBL is revealing about the ineluctably diverse and dynamic nature of L2 resources, and given how the approach complements rather than conflicts with sociolinguistic perspectives (Ortega 2018; Eskildsen 2020), this marginalization of the cognitive seems unwarranted. A recognition of the cognitive instantiation of language actually enriches the strategies that can be developed to promote ontological clarity about English, and therefore to contest monolithic ideologies (Hall 2021). Wicaksono and Hall (2020) argue that an ontology of English should be *useful* for teachers, learners, and users. As I have argued in this chapter from the perspective of ELF, an ontology which balances the cognitive with the social is useful because it explains how linguistic diversity, instead of leading to Babel, is a normal and inevitable input to, and outcome of, usage-based learning.

Teachers of English tend not to be easily convinced by arguments which might undermine their own investment in mastering the NS standard variety, and many have strong beliefs about grammatical accuracy which will not be overturned by appeals to English as a social practice alone (Hall 2021). It is here that a plurilithic conceptualization of English, emerging from a cognitive understanding of ELF, can play an important role in challenging monolithic thinking. The distinctive linguistic diversity found in ELF usage emerges naturally from the way the human mind constructs I-language resources from usage events. An understanding of this might go some way towards loosening the attachment of educators to unjust and unattainable learning targets. To help global learners participate felicitously in the diverse ELF scenarios they will find themselves in after they have left the classroom, educators will ultimately need to adapt their pedagogical practices towards the development of appropriate I-language resources, rather than knowledge of "accurate" forms.

References

Ambridge, Ben/Pine, Julian M./Rowland, Caroline F./Chang, Franklin/Bidgood, Amy: "The retreat from overgeneralization in child language acquisition: Word learning, morphology, and verb argument structure". *Wiley Interdisciplinary Reviews: Cognitive Science*, 4(1), 2012, 47–62.

Barlow, Michael: "Individual differences and usage-based grammar". *International Journal of Corpus Linguistics*, 18(4), 2013, pp. 443–78.

Björkman, Beyza: "English as the lingua franca of engineering: The morphosyntax of academic speech events". *Nordic Journal of English Studies*, 7, 2008, pp. 103–22.

Blumenthal-Dramé, Alice: *Entrenchment in usage-based theories. What corpus data do and do not reveal about the mind.* De Gruyter Mouton: Berlin, 2012.

Canagarajah, Suresh: *Translingual practice: Global Englishes and cosmopolitan relations.*Routledge: London, 2013.

Canagarajah, Suresh: "English as a resource in a communicative assemblage: A perspective from Flat Ontology". In Hall, Christopher/Wicaksono, Rachel (eds.), *Ontologies of English. Conceptualising the language for learning, teaching, and assessment.* Cambridge University Press: Cambridge, 2020, pp. 295–314.

Chomsky, Noam: *Knowledge of language.* Praeger: New York, NY, 1986.

Clark, Herbert H.: *Using language.* Cambridge University Press: Cambridge, 1996.

Cogo, Alessia/House, Juliane: "The pragmatics of ELF". In Jenkins, Jennifer/Baker, Will/Dewey, Martin (eds.), *Routledge handbook of English as a Lingua Franca.* Routledge: London, 2018, pp. 210–223.

Coulthard, Malcolm: "Author identification, idiolect, and linguistic uniqueness". *Applied Linguistics*, 45(4), 2004, pp. 431–447.

Croft, William: *Explaining language. An evolutionary approach.* Longman: London, 2000.

Dąbrowska, Ewa: "Different speakers, different grammars. Individual differences in native language attainment". *Linguistic Approaches to Bilingualism* 2(3), 2012, pp. 219–253.

Dąbrowska, Ewa: "Cognitive linguistics' seven deadly sins". *Cognitive linguistics*, *27*(4), 2016, pp. 479–491.

Ehrenreich, Susanne: "Communities of practice and English as a lingua franca". In In Jenkins, Jennifer/Baker, Will/Dewey, Martin (eds.), *Routledge handbook of English as a Lingua Franca*. Routledge: London, 2018, pp. 37–50.

Ellis, Nicholas C.: "Construction grammar and second language acquisition". In Hoffmann, Thomas/Trousdale, Graeme (eds.), *The Oxford handbook of construction grammar*. Oxford University Press: Oxford, 2013.

Ellis, Nicholas C.: "Cognition, corpora, and computing: Triangulating research in usage-based language learning". *Language Learning*, 67(1), 2017, pp. 40–65.

Ellis, Nicholas/Wulff, Stefanie: "Usage-based approaches to SLA". In VanPatten, Bill/Williams, Jessica (eds.), *Theories of second language acquisition: An introduction* (2nd edn). Routledge: London, 2015, pp. 75–93.

Ellis, Rod: "Measuring implicit and explicit knowledge of a second language: A psychometric study". *Studies in Second Language Acquisition*, 27, 2005, pp. 141–172.

Eskildsen, Søren, W.: "Constructing another language – Usage based linguistics in second language acquisition". *Applied Linguistics*, 30(3), 2009, pp. 335–357.

Eskildsen, Søren, W.: "Negation constructions at work". *Language Learning*, 62, 2012, pp. 335–372.

Eskildsen, Søren, W.: "What counts as a developmental sequence? Exemplar-based L2 learning of English questions". *Language Learning*, 65(1), 2015, pp. 33–62.

Eskildsen, Søren, W.: "From constructions to social action: The substance of English and its learning from an interactional usage-based perspective". In Hall, Christopher/Wicaksono, Rachel (eds.), *Ontologies of English. Conceptualising the language for learning, teaching, and assessment*. Cambridge University Press: Cambridge, 2020, pp. 59–79.

Flores, Nelson/Rosa, Jonathan. "Undoing appropriateness: Raciolinguistic ideologies and language and education". *Harvard Educational Review*, 27(2), 2015, pp. 110–128.

García, Ofelia/Li Wei: "Translanguaging: Language, bilingualism and education". Palgrave Macmillan: London, 2014.

Goldberg, Adele: *Constructions. A construction grammar approach to argument structure*. Chicago University Press: Chicago, 1995.

Grosjean, François/Li, Ping: *The psycholinguistics of bilingualism*. Wiley: Chichester, 2013.

Hall, Christopher J.: "Cognitive contributions to plurilithic views of English and other languages". *Applied Linguistics*, 34, 2013, pp. 211–231.

Hall, Christopher J.: "Cognitive perspectives on English as a Lingua Franca". In Jenkins, Jennifer/Baker, Will/Dewey, Martin (eds.), *Routledge handbook of English as a Lingua Franca*. Routledge: London, 2018a, pp. 74–84.

Hall, Christopher J.: "The psycholinguistics of English". In Seargeant, Philip/Hewings, Ann/Pihlaja, Stephen (eds.), *Routledge handbook of English language studies*. Routledge: London, 2018b, pp. 406–419.

Hall, Christopher J.: "An ontological framework for English." In Hall, Christopher/Wicaksono, Rachel (eds.), *Ontologies of English. Conceptualising the language for learning, teaching, and assessment*. Cambridge University Press: Cambridge, 2020, pp. 13–36.

Hall, Christopher J.: "Incorporating ontological reflection into teacher education about English for global learners: A rationale and some guiding principles." In Bayyurt, Yasemin (ed.), *Bloomsbury world Englishes*, Volume 3: *Pedagogy*. Bloomsbury: London, 2021, pp. 11–26.

Hall, Christopher J./Cunningham, Clare: "Educators' beliefs about English and languages beyond English: From ideology to ontology and back again." *Linguistics and Education*, 57, 2020, pp. 1–14.

Hall, Christopher J./Schmidtke, Daniel/Vickers, Jamie: "Countability in world Englishes". *World Englishes*, 32(1), 2013, pp. 1–22.

Hall, Christopher J./Joyce, Jack/Robson, Christopher: "Investigating the lexico-grammatical resources of a non-native user of English: the case of *can* and *could* in email requests". *Applied Linguistics Review*, 8(1), 2017, pp. 35–59.

Harris, Roy: *The language myth*. Duckworth: London, 1981.

Hellermann, John/Eskildsen, Søren W./Doehler, Simona P./Piirainen-Marsh, Arja (eds.): *Conversation analytic research on learning-in-action: The complex ecology of second language interaction 'in the wild'*. Springer: Dordrecht, 2019.

Housen, Alex/Kuiken, Folkert: "Complexity, accuracy, and fluency in second language acquisition". *Applied Linguistics*, 30(4), 2009, pp. 461–473.

Housen, Alex/Kuiken, Folkert/Vedder, Ineke: "Complexity, accuracy and fluency. Definitions, measurement and research". In Housen, Alex/Kuiken, Folkert/

Vedder, Ineke (eds.), *Dimensions of L2 performance and proficiency: Complexity, accuracy and fluency in SLA*. John Benjamins: Amsterdam, 2012, pp. 1–20.

Hynninen, Niina: *Language regulation in English as a lingua franca*. De Gruyter: Berlin, 2016.

Jackendoff, Ray: "What is the human language faculty? Two views." *Language*, 87(3), 2011, pp. 586–624.

Jackson, Carrie N.: "Second language structural priming: A critical review and directions for future research". *Second Language Research*, 34(4), 2018, pp. 539–552.

Jenkins, Jennifer: *English as a lingua franca in the international university: The politics of academic English language policy*. Routledge: London, 2014.

Jenkins, Jennifer: "Repositioning English and multilingualism in English as a Lingua Franca". *Englishes in Practice,* 2(3), 2015, pp. 49–85.

Jenkins, Jennifer/Baker, Will/Dewey, Martin (eds.): *Routledge handbook of English as a Lingua Franca*. Routledge: London, 2018.

Kachru, Braj: "Standards, codification and sociolinguistic realism: The English language in the outer circle". In Quirk, Randolph/Widdowson, Henry G. (eds.), *English in the world. Teaching and learning the language and literatures*. Cambridge University Press: Cambridge, 1985, pp. 11–30.

Kroll, Judith F./Dussias, Paola E./Bogulski, Carrie A./Valdes Kroff, Jorge R.: "Juggling two languages in one mind: What bilinguals tell us about language processing and its consequences for cognition". *Psychology of Learning and Motivation*, 56, 2012, pp. 229–262.

Labov, William: "Objectivity and commitment in linguistic science: The case of the Black English trial in Ann Arbor". *Language in Society*, 11(2), 1982, pp. 165–201.

Langacker, Ronald W.: *Foundations of cognitive grammar: Theoretical prerequisites. Volume I*. Stanford University Press: Stanford, CA, 1987.

Langacker, Ronald W.: "A dynamic usage-based model". In Barlow, Michael/Kemmer, Suzanne (eds.), *Usage-based models of language*. CSLI Publications: Stanford, CA, 2000, pp. 1–63.

Langacker, Ronald W.: *Cognitive grammar: A basic introduction*. Oxford University Press: Oxford, 2008.

Larsen-Freeman, Diane: "Second language acquisition, WE, and language as a complex adaptive system (CAS)". *World Englishes*, 37, 2018, pp. 80–92.

Lippi-Green, Rosina: *English with an accent: Language, ideology and discrimination in the United States* (2nd edn). Routledge: London, 2012.

Loudermilk, Brandon C.: "Psycholinguistic approaches". In Bayley, Robert/Cameron, Richard/Lucas, Ceil (eds.), *The Oxford handbook of sociolinguistics*. Oxford University Press: Oxford, 2013.

Luka, Barbara J./Barsalou, Lawrence W.: "Structural facilitation: Mere exposure effects for grammatical acceptability as evidence for syntactic priming in comprehension". *Journal of Memory and Language*, 52(3), 2005, pp. 436–459.

Luka, Barbara J./Choi, Heidi: "Dynamic grammar in adults: Incidental learning of natural syntactic structures extends over 48 h.". *Journal of Memory and Language*, 66(2), 2012, pp. 345–360.

Mackenzie, Ian: *English as a Lingua Franca. Theorizing and teaching English*. Routledge: London, 2014.

Mauranen, Anna: *Exploring ELF. Academic English shaped by non-native speakers*. Cambridge University Press: Cambridge, 2012.

Mollin, Sandra: ""I entirely understand" is a Blairism. The methodology of identifying idiolectal collocations". *International Journal of Corpus Linguistics*, 14(3), 2009, pp. 367–392.

Motha, Suhanthie: *Race, empire, and English language teaching: Creating responsible and ethical anti-racist practice*. Teachers College Press: New York, NY, 2014.

Nickerson, Catherine: "English as a lingua franca in international business contexts". *English for specific purposes*, 24(4), 2005, pp. 367–380.

Nicol, Janet L.: *One mind, two languages: Bilingual language processing*. Blackwell: Oxford, 2001.

Ortega, Lourdes: "Ontologies of language, second language acquisition and world Englishes". *World Englishes*, 37(1), 2018, pp. 64–79.

Östman, Jan-ola/Trousdale, Graeme: "Dialects, discourse, and construction grammar". In Hoffmann, Thomas/Trousdale, Graeme (eds.), *The Oxford handbook of construction grammar*. Oxford University Press: Oxford, 2013.

Otheguy, Richard/García, Ofelia/Reid, Wallis: "Clarifying translanguaging and deconstructing named languages: A perspective from Linguistics". *Applied Linguistics Review*, 6 (3), 2015, pp. 281–307.

Pennycook, Alistair: "Plurilithic Englishes: Towards a 3D model". In Murata, Kumiko/Jenkins, Jennifer (eds.), *Global Englishes in Asian contexts. Current and future debates*. Palgrave Macmillan: Basingstoke, UK, 2009, pp. 194–207.

Pennycook, Alistair: *Language as a local practice*. Routledge: London, 2010.

Pennycook, Alistair: "Pushing the ontological boundaries of English". In Hall, Christopher/Wicaksono, Rachel (eds.), *Ontologies of English. Conceptualising the language for learning, teaching, and assessment.* Cambridge University Press: Cambridge, 2020, pp. 355–367.

Piller, Ingrid: *Linguistic diversity and social justice. An introduction to applied sociolinguistics.* Oxford University Press: Oxford, 2016.

Pitzl, Marie-Luise: "Creativity meets convention: Idiom variation and remetaphorization in ELF". *Journal of English as a Lingua Franca*, 1(1), 2012, pp. 27–55.

Saraceni, Mario (ed.): *Bloomsbury world Englishes* (Volumes 1–3). London: Bloomsbury, 2021.

Schmid, Hans-Jörg/Mantlik, Annette: "Entrenchment in historical corpora? Reconstructing dead authors' minds from their usage profiles". *Anglia*, 133(4), 583–623, 2015.

Schwieter, John W.: *The handbook of the neuroscience of multilingualism.* Wiley: Chichester, 2019.

Seidlhofer, Barbara: *Understanding English as a Lingua Franca*: Oxford University Press: Oxford, 2011.

Snell, Julia: "Dialect, interaction and class positioning at school: From deficit to difference to repertoire". *Language and Education*, 27(2), 2013, pp. 110–128.

Snell, Julia: "Critical reflections on the role of the sociolinguist in UK language debates". *Language in Society*, 47(3), 2018, pp. 368–374.

Skehan, Peter: *A cognitive approach to language learning.* Oxford University Press: Oxford, 1998.

Stefanowitsch, Anatol/Flach, Susanne: "The corpus-based perspective on entrenchment". In Schmid, Hans-Jörg (ed.), *Entrenchment and the psychology of language learning: How we reorganize and adapt linguistic knowledge.* De Gruyter Mouton: Berlin, 2017, pp. 101–127.

Styler, Will: *The EnronSent corpus. Technical report 01–2011.* University of Colorado at Boulder Institute of Cognitive Science: Boulder, CO, 2011.

Tammelin-Laine, Taina/Martin, Maisa: "Negative constructions in nonliterate learners' spoken L2 Finnish". In Ortega, Lourdes/Tyler, Andrea/Park, Hae In/Uno, Mariko (eds.), *The usage-based study of language learning and multilingualism.* Georgetown University Press: Washington, DC, 2016, pp. 75–90.

Thorne, Steven L./Reinhardt, Jonathon: "'Bridging activities,' new media literacies, and advanced foreign language proficiency". *Calico Journal*, 25(3), 2008, 558–572.

Tomasello, Michael: *Constructing a language. A usage-based theory of language acquisition.* Harvard University Press: Cambridge, MA, 2003.

Ullman, Michael T.: "The declarative/procedural model. A neurobiologically motivated theory of first and second language". In VanPatten, Bill/Williams, Jessica (eds.), *Theories of second language acquisition: An introduction* (2nd edn). Routledge: London, 2015, pp. 135–158.

Verhagen, Arie: "Grammar and cooperative communication". In Dąbrowska, Ewa/Divjak, Dagmar (eds.), *Handbook of cognitive linguistics*. De Gruyter Mouton: Berlin, 2015, pp. 232–252.

Vetchinnikova, Svetlana: "Usage-based recycling or creative exploitation of the shared code? The case of phraseological patterning". *Journal of English as a Lingua Franca*, 4(2), 2015, pp. 223–252.

Vetchinnikova, Svetlana: "On the relationship between the cognitive and the communal: A complex systems perspective". In Filppula, Markku/Klemola, Juhani/Mauranen, Anna/Vetchinnikova, Svetlana (eds.), *Changing English: Global and local perspectives*. Mouton de Gruyter: Berlin, 2017.

Wicaksono, Rachel/Hall, Christopher J.: "Using ontologies of English". In Hall, Christopher/Wicaksono, Rachel (eds.), *Ontologies of English. Conceptualising the language for learning, teaching, and assessment*. Cambridge University Press: Cambridge, 2020, pp. 368–375.

Widdowson, Henry G.: "The ownership of English". *TESOL Quarterly*, 28, 1994, pp. 377–89.

Hanna S. Andersen

With Norwegian eyes: The verbalization of goal-oriented motion events in Norwegian

Abstract: Departing from Slobin's (1991, 1996) *thinking-for-speaking* framework, this paper investigates the Norwegian verbalization of goal-oriented motion events and provides a more detailed analysis of this kind of motion events in Norwegian than in previous studies. Previous research has shown that speakers without grammatical aspect in their L1 both verbalize more often and pay more attention to a possible endpoint in goal-oriented motion events than do speakers with grammatical aspect in their L1 (e.g., von Stutterheim & Nüse 2003; Schmiedtová, von Stutterheim & Carroll 2011). As Norwegian is considered a language without grammatical aspect, one would expect Norwegian L1 speakers, in line with e.g., German speakers, to mention the endpoints to a greater extent than speakers of an aspect language, such as English.

In this study, 30 Norwegian L1 speakers participated in an experiment where they had to give descriptions of short film clips online. The question is to what extent the participants mention inferable endpoints, and to what extent when compared to speakers of German and English. Furthermore, the question is what role the videoclips play in this regard.

The findings show that the Norwegian speakers as expected align with speakers of German when it comes to the mentioning of endpoints. However, the differences between Norwegian and German on one side, and English on the other, are linked to the type of scenes used in the experiment. The differences appear more clearly – not when the inferable goal is either large or small – but when the inferable goal is unclear. The participants' interpretation of whether the goal will actually be reached is also reflected in their choice of prepositions in the Norwegian verbalizations.

The question of whether speakers of Norwegian, based on the findings can be said to take a so-called holistic perspective on motion events is discussed, as well as the use of the notion *holistic* in this context.

Keywords: motion events, *thinking-for-speaking*, endpoints, conceptualization, Norwegian L1

1. Introduction

Based on studies of a number of different languages, e.g., German, Algerian Arabic, English and Russian, von Stutterheim and Nüse (2003) postulate that there is a connection between grammatical aspect and the conceptualization of events. In this context, conceptualization is defined as the cognitive planning processes that are activated immediately before the actual language production, or in other words, the segmentation, information selection and structuring of conceptual content that takes place just before speaking (e.g., Levelt 1989; von Stutterheim & Nüse 2003; Schmiedtová, von Stutterheim & Carroll 2011). This so-called preverbal phase has often been assumed to be language independent (see Levelt 1989). The hypothesis of a language-specific conceptualization, by contrast, assumes that the preverbal phase is influenced by grammatical structures in the L1 (Carroll, von Stutterheim & Nüse 2004; Schmiedtová et al. 2011; von Stutterheim & Nüse 2003; von Stutterheim, Andermann, Carroll, Flecken & Schmiedtová 2012). The research in this line of work investigates whether grammatical structures, such as grammaticized aspect, play a role, not only for how one expresses oneself in a given language, or what one chooses to report, but also for what is being noticed or given attention to – e.g., visually – in an event. For example, in the case of goal-oriented motion events with an inferable endpoint, studies show that L1 users of German both verbalize more event endpoints and direct more visual attention towards the endpoints as measured by eye-tracking, than do L1 speakers of English and Russian when describing the very same events (Schmiedtová et al. 2011). Inferable endpoints in this case would be the possible goals for the motion shown in the video clip. One example from the experiment could be two women walking along the road in the direction of a house. Though an inferable endpoint (the house) is visible, the arrival upon the goal is not shown in the video clip.

In the present study, the verbalization of goal-oriented motion events with inferable endpoints in Norwegian is described, and the question of whether speakers of Norwegian take a so-called holistic perspective on such events is discussed. According to von Stutterheim and Nüse (2003), a *holistic perspective* is a view which includes some kind of closure to an activity – points of completion or results of an event. For example, German speakers often mention the point of arrival when describing motion events, or the products of activities when describing actions where some object is affected or created. Hence, they can be said to conceptualize dynamic situations as entities with boundaries, and boundedness is a crucial notion within this perspective. By contrast, under the perspective of *phasal decomposition,* events are viewed as ongoing processes or actions. This would constitute the preferred option for speakers of English, who frequently parse the event sequences into smaller units than the German speakers do. Ongoingness and the progression of events is crucial within this perspective, and the endpoint or outcome of an action does not form a necessary component of each event. To discuss whether Norwegian aligns with a holistic or phasal perspective (or somewhere in between) in the present study, online descriptions of goal-oriented motion events from 30 L1 speakers of Norwegian were elicited. The results were compared to data from speakers of German and English. The question of whether speakers of Norwegian, in line with German speakers, take a so-called holistic perspective on motion events is discussed, as well as the use of the notion *holistic* in this context.

2. Theoretical framework and state of art

2.1. Thinking-for-speaking, seeing-for-speaking

The theoretical framework of the study is Slobin's (1991, 1996) *thinking-for-speaking* hypothesis and the hypothesis of language-specific conceptualization (von Stutterheim & Nüse 2003; see also Carroll et al. 2004; Schmiedtová et al. 2011; von Stutterheim et al. 2012). Slobin is interested in the mental processes that take place just before or during the formulation of a message. He is most concerned with the parts of the utterance that are required by the grammar of the language – grammaticalized structures – and only in the moment in which the thought is mobilized for communication, that is, in the moment of speaking (Slobin 1996, p. 76). According to Slobin, the features that are grammaticalized in a language, and thus compulsory, are more easily accessible than the lexical variants which can be chosen freely, and consequently are not automatized in the same way. These obligatory grammatical categories also direct our attention, and the *thinking-for-speaking* hypothesis can thus be described as a modern, more moderate version of the Sapir-Whorf hypothesis, in which Slobin claims that the language we learn shapes the way we perceive reality when talking about it: "Whatever else language may do in human thought and action, it surely directs us to attend – while speaking – to the dimensions of experience that are enshrined in grammatical categories" (Slobin 1996, p. 71).

In line with Slobin, several scholars have been concerned with the importance of grammatical form in language production at an early stage of cognitive processing, namely "that of preparing content for verbalization" (Carroll et al. 2004, pp. 2–3), in other words, before the actual verbalization of the message, often referred to as the preverbal phase (Levelt 1989). While the *thinking-for-speaking* hypothesis claims that the conceptualization as a component of language production is based on language-specific principles, the level of specificity of these principles remains an open question (von Stutterheim & Nüse 2003, p. 852). Is it, like Levelt (1989) argues, only at the microstructural or local level in the planning process, the *how* – how is content packaged for verbalization? Or is it earlier, at the macrostructural or global level, the *what* – what is included in the content of the message (von Stutterheim & Nüse 2003, p. 852)? The claim that grammaticized meanings are already relevant at the global (but also local) level of message generation is important for this line of argumentation. In other words, grammaticized conceptual categories in the L1 are thought to influence segmentation and information selection before the actual formulation of the utterance begins, and the grammar hence influences not only how one expresses oneself in a language, but also what one chooses to include in the utterance, how finely divided the event is and what one directs attention to (e.g., visually). These claims thus extend Slobin's hypothesis by including the macro level and are often referred to as the *seeing-for-speaking* hypothesis, or the hypothesis of language-specific perspectivation (Carroll et al. 2004; Schmiedtová et al. 2011; von Stutterheim & Nüse 2003; von Stutterheim et al. 2012).

2.2. Out walking or on the way to a house? Previous research

Several studies have been conducted within the *thinking-for-speaking* framework, mainly along two different lines of inquiry: One is following Talmy's (1985, 2000) theory of cognitive semantics, looking at how speakers of different languages attend to and express path and manner of motion. The other is the one dealing with conceptual structures that are represented more by the grammar than by lexical semantics (for an overview, see Bylund 2011b; Bylund & Jarvis 2011; Pavlenko 2014).

To find a way to explore the role of language in the process of conceptualization, von Stutterheim and Nüse (2003) chose *events* as one of the possible windows into this process. When reporting an event, the level of granularity, the components selected (bounded/unbounded) as well as the perspective under which the event is viewed, are all decisions that must be taken before the linguistic form is activated. In a study of film retellings and descriptions of short video clips with different types of events, von Stutterheim and Nüse (2003) found that English L1 speakers described more events – they segmented the same events into smaller units – than did the German L1 speakers when describing the same film. They also found that English speakers focused more on the development of an event than on the possible endpoints of the same event. When describing short film clips of motion events, the English participants more often described the ongoing motion only, as in *two women are walking*, while the German participants to a greater extent also added the possible goal or endpoint, as in *zwei Frauen laufen auf dem Weg Richtung eines Hauses* 'two women are walking on a road in the *direction of a house*'. Based on these findings, von Stutterheim and Nüse (2003) argue that speakers of English take a more fine-grained, so-called phasal perspective, while speakers of German, by including the event endpoints, take a holistic perspective when describing the same event (see also Carroll et al. 2004; Schmiedtová et al. 2011; von Stutterheim et al. 2012). Von Stutterheim and Nüse (2003) link the differences in perspective-taking to grammatical aspect, thus arguing that there is a connection between grammatical aspect and the construal of events: "In our case we postulate that the structural feature [+/- aspect] induces a specific pattern of event construal" (p. 870). This connection is explained by the obligatory marking of the progressive or imperfective form of the verb, which makes the speaker naturally focus on the ongoing action. Speakers of languages without grammatical aspect on the verb are not forced to focus on the ongoing moment in the same way, as the notional category of ongoingness simply is less salient and will naturally look for a closure of the event (von Stutterheim & Nüse 2003, p. 870; see also Carroll et al. 2004; Schmiedtová et al. 2011; von Stutterheim et al. 2012).

The relation between grammatical aspect and event construal has also been explored by Bylund and Jarvis (2011), who looked at bilingual Spanish-Swedish speakers and compared them to monolingual control groups. The participants described motion events in short video clips in Spanish and Swedish, and responded to a grammaticality judgment test with aspectual contrasts in Spanish. The study showed that the more errors the bilingual participants made related to aspectual distinctions in Spanish, the more likely they were to verbalize the endpoints of the motion events in Spanish, following the Swedish pattern. These findings support the hypothesis that grammatical aspect and the perspective on motion events are interrelated, as postulated by von Stutterheim and Nüse (2003). However, Bylund and Jarvis (2011) explain the theoretical relationship between endpoint encoding and grammatical aspectual distinctions in a slightly different way, by adopting Langacker's (1987, 2008) theory of cognitive grammar as their theoretical foundation. As Langacker deals directly with the relationship between grammatical aspect and event construal, they adhere to his description of construal and its components *scope* and *viewing frame*, which a person adopts when construing a situation. The notions restricted temporal scope versus the maximal temporal scope correspond to the phasal versus the holistic perspective (for more on these notions, see Bylund & Jarvis 2011; Langacker 2008). However, the two interpretations are seen as compatible explanations, which despite somewhat different emphases lead to essentially the same predictions (Bylund & Jarvis 2011, p. 51).

Several studies have been conducted within the aspect–non-aspect line of research, and among the languages explored we find Algerian Arabic, English, German, Spanish, (von Stutterheim & Nüse 2003), Czech, Russian (Schmiedtová & Sahonenko 2008; Schmiedtová 2011; Schmiedtová 2013), Dutch (Flecken

2010), Norwegian (Behrens & Ramm 2003; Carroll et al. 2004; von Stutterheim & Carroll 2006), Swedish (Bylund 2011a, 2011b), and Afrikaans (Bylund, Athanasopoulos & Oostendorp 2013); for an overview, see Bylund 2011b; Mertins 2018 or Pavlenko 2014. Although Norwegian L1 is listed above, a thorough description of the Norwegian results in the endpoint study is still lacking (see Section 2.4).

2.3. More than just linguistic data

Criticisms to the reported studies are primarily related to the *thinking* in Slobin's *thinking-for-speaking*-hypothesis. By studying language, one can document linguistic diversity, but not necessarily cognitive differences (e.g., Pourcel 2003). As Gullberg (2011) points out, it is difficult to show exactly how a person conceptualizes. In other words, one can examine what people choose to say, but not why they say it. Also, linguistic data does not necessarily demonstrate what people notice and remember (see also Athanasopoulos & Bylund 2013; Holum 2009; Mertins 2016). To gain a better understanding of the cognitive processes behind language production, Schmiedtová et al. (2011) used eye-tracking and memory tests, in addition to speech onset time (SOT), in their investigations of motion events. In these studies, they found that native speakers of non-aspect languages (e.g., German and Dutch) direct their visual attention differently than speakers of aspect languages, such as English, Russian and Spanish. For example, the German participants' gaze lingers significantly longer on the endpoints, and they also return to them more often than the Russian speakers. The German participants also waited longer to start speaking than the English and the Spanish. They fixated on the endpoints both before and after they started talking, while the English participants started speaking before looking towards the endpoints (Carroll et al. 2004). The German participants also remembered the endpoints in the relevant scenes better than the Russian participants for the same type of scene (von Stutterheim et al. 2012). These findings indicate that speakers of different languages have a different conceptualization of the same event, and the differences in conceptualization lead to differences in eye movements, verbalization, and memory. To be able to show linguistic effects on cognition, one must therefore combine language production data with other methodologies. Such methodologies could be eye-tracking, categorization and memory tasks, analysis of gestures, and so forth. (Gullberg 2011; Athanasopoulos & Bylund 2013; Mertins 2016, 2018).

2.4. Thinking for speaking in Norwegian

What do motion events look like from a Norwegian 'perspective'? There are already several studies of Norwegian within the *thinking-for-speaking* framework. However, most of the studies in a Norwegian context are so-called transfer studies, where the questions explored concern how different features are learned in Norwegian L2, and to what extent conceptual patterns from the L1 are transferred or can affect the L2 learning (e.g., Holum 2009; Johansen 2011; Malcher 2011; Nordanger 2009; Szmynska 2010; Vulchanova et al. 2012; for an overview of Norwegian transfer studies, see Golden et al. 2017; Gujord & Ragnhildstveit 2018; Mannsåker, Nistov & Nordanger 2020). Also, along with studies on the conceptualization of spatial expressions and the use of prepositions, most of these studies are based on Talmy's (2000) typological division of languages according to whether the verbs encode many elements of the action (so-called verb-framed languages) or whether meaning elements such as place, time and direction are added using satellites (satellite-framed languages). Holum (2009) studied boundary-crossing events in Norwegian L1 and Spanish learners of Norwegian L2, using video clips similar to the scenes used as control scenes in the current study (see methods section), and found that the Spanish learners of Norwegian L2 often kept the conceptualization patterns from their L1.

Following the hypothesis of language-specific conceptualization, to my knowledge, only Behrens and Ramm (2003) have looked at the relation between event conceptualization and grammatical aspect in Norwegian L1. In a first analysis of verbalizations of video scenes they found that the Norwegian L1 speakers express the endpoints on average just as often as the German L1 speakers they were compared to (38 % vs. 41 %, respectively), while the English L1 speakers score significantly lower (18 %), thus suggesting that the [+/ - grammatical aspect] influences the perspectivation taken on motion events. However, no information about the video clips or the differences between them is provided, and the results are described as preliminary findings by the authors (Behrens & Ramm 2003, pp. 129, 139). They also ask questions about information structure and the choice of thematically noteworthy objects, and comment that Norwegian only partially overlaps with German in this respect, placed just in between English and German, and that further analysis of Norwegian data and comparison with English and German will be fruitful for the project. Carroll et al. (2004) cluster Norwegian with Dutch and German, based on film retellings, where they found that the Norwegian L1 speakers based the temporal sequences on bounded events, in line with German, and in contrast to English, which anchor the events on a deictic point of reference (i.e., the 'now'). Furthermore, in a study of verbalization of single events, they found that Norwegian and German speakers tend to construe a possible endpoint in scenes where those could only be inferred, whereas speakers of English and Arabic were unlikely to do so, and they thus conclude that "(…) Norwegian and German speakers construe events under a holistic perspective" (Carroll et al. 2004, p. 20). As the Norwegian results were used to contrast to the aspectual languages, details of the Norwegian verbalizations were not analyzed in the study. Behrens, Flecken and Carroll (2013) also used single video clips on Norwegian L1 speakers, but they looked at the aspectual question from a different perspective: by discussing a possible grammaticalization of aspect in Norwegian, German, and Dutch. Based on the same video material as the current study, they investigated the activity scenes and not the motion events, due to the lack of aspectual constructions in motion events. The aim of the current study is thus for the first time to provide a more in-depth analysis of goal-oriented motion events where the endpoint is not reached (and no boundary crossed) in Norwegian L1. Furthermore, as already mentioned, the Norwegian results will be compared to results from English and German, to see whether Norwegian aligns with a holistic or phasal perspective (or somewhere in between). Also, the impact of the material used will be discussed.

2.4.1. Grammatical aspect or not?

While English must mark obligatory progressive aspect in the present tense (*be* + V-*ing*), this does not apply for German, in which explicit marking of verbal aspect is not obligatory in any context. *Grammatical aspect* is here defined as a grammatical marking of ongoingness, marked with verb morphology (see Mertins 2018; Schmiedtová 2011; von Stutterheim et al. 2012; see also Comrie 1976/2001). Like German, Norwegian does not have grammatical aspect in the present tense, but aspectual content can be expressed lexically (see Behrens et al. 2013; Tonne 2001). Tonne (1999, 2001) divides the available forms in Norwegian into two subgroups – the pseudo-coordinations, and the prospec group. The first consists of two inflected verbs coordinated with *og* 'and', as in 'en dame *sitter og strikker*' 'a lady is knitting', lit. 'a lady *sits and knits*'. And then there are the prospec-forms, which consist of inflected verbs with a preposition followed by an infinitive, as in *holder på å vaske* 'he is cleaning', lit. 'he holds on to clean'. There is an ongoing discussion as to whether Norwegian pseudo-coordinations may appear to be either partially, or in the process of being grammaticalized (e.g., Behrens et al. 2013; Kinn 2018, Lødrup 2017a, 2017b; Tonne 1999, 2001), but

Norwegian is commonly regarded as a non-aspect language in this context. Still, the quite frequent use of lexical forms to express aspectual content could lead to the assumption that Norwegian might, after all, differ from German in this respect, and hence, also when it comes to the frequency of expressing endpoints.

2.4.2. Research questions

The aim of the current study is to provide a more detailed description of the verbalization of motion events in Norwegian than previously done. The research questions are: To what extent do Norwegian L1 speakers mention the endpoints in goal-oriented motion events with inferable goals? How do the results from Norwegian L1 speakers compare to those from German and English L1 speakers? Since one could expect scenes with a larger goal to attract more endpoint designations than scenes with a smaller and more distant goal, will the results be influenced by the type of scene used in the experiment?

In the results, the expectation is to find support for the claim made in previous studies (Behrens & Ramm 2003; and Carroll et al. 2004) that Norwegian speakers mention the inferable endpoints in line with German speakers and to a larger degree than speakers of English. Still, as Norwegian has a more frequent use of lexicalized aspectual forms than German, as well as the fact that most Norwegians speak English relatively well (in fact, it is almost impossible to find Norwegian participants who do not speak English),[1] one might expect to find Norwegian somewhere in between the two. Finally, based on the analysis, the paper questions whether it would be correct to say that Norwegian takes a so-called holistic perspective on motion events (as defined by von Stutterheim & Nüse 2003), and provides some reflections on the notion 'holistic' in this context.

3. "With Norwegian eyes": Methods and materials

The data collection was part of a larger project, led by Christiane von Stutterheim and Barbara Schmiedtová (now Mertins), and the data was collected in Oslo in 2007/2008. Parts of the data were analyzed in connection with the above-mentioned study on progressive aspect in Norwegian, Dutch, and German (Behrens et al. 2013). While their focus was mainly on the activity scenes and the use of aspectual

1 Norwegian children learn English from 1st grade in school, and they get frequent exposure to English through e.g., TV, films, social media, gaming, and music. Norwegian learners of English generally perform well on European language tests measuring various aspects of grammatical competence (Johansen 2020).

expressions, the current study investigates the scenes showing motion events, and from a different perspective: that of endpoint naming in Norwegian.

3.1. Participants

Norwegian participants: The participants were the same as the participants in Behrens et al. 2013: a group of 30 students (17 f, 13 m) aged 18–29 years, from the University of Oslo. All participants had Norwegian as their L1 and spoke one or more foreign languages. Background information was collected in a short questionnaire where participants were asked what language(s) they spoke daily with family, siblings, or partner, what, if any, other foreign language(s) they knew and what level of competency they gauged themselves to be in these respective languages, and about their educational background. Participants were excluded if the questionnaire showed that they had lived for a long time abroad, and/or if they were functionally bilingual as children (i.e., growing up as bilinguals). *Comparison groups (English and German):* The participants from the German part of the project were 20 students (11 f, 9 m) aged 18–24 years, from the University of Heidelberg. The German participants spoke English to varying degrees. The 20 English participants (14 f, 6 m), aged 20–26 years, were from various English universities. No information about knowledge of foreign languages is provided for the English participants. The experiment was performed under the same conditions across countries, following the same experimental procedure.

3.2. Materials

The material consisted of 60 video clips, displaying everyday situations without any connection to each other.[2] Each clip lasted six seconds, followed by a white screen for eight seconds (for the participant to complete the description). Clips showing goal-oriented motion events with or without arrival at an endpoint were embedded among distracter scenes showing different activities. The critical scenes (n = 12) show goal-oriented motion events where the endpoint is not reached: A person, an animal or a vehicle is moving on or along a road or a path, as in Figure 1, left. The scene ends before the endpoint is reached, but a possible or inferable endpoint is visible in all cases (e.g., two ladies walking on a road, at the end of which there is a large house).

---

2 The videos were developed and shared by Barbara Mertins (copyright). All images (screen shots) from the data material are reproduced with permission from Barbara Mertins, TU Dortmund.

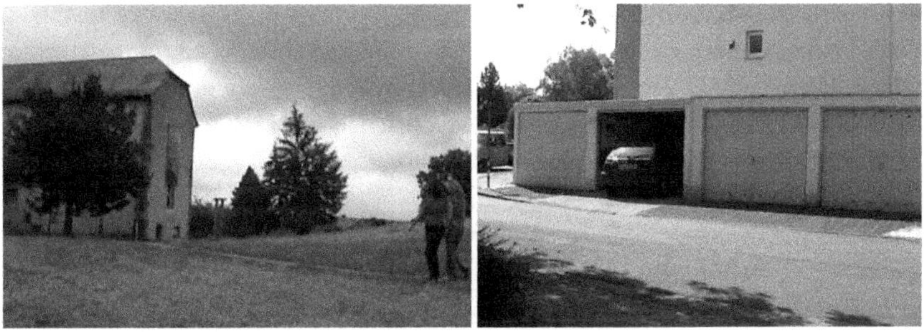

Figure 1: Screen shot of a critical scene (endpoint not reached). Two ladies are walking in the direction of a house, but the clip stops before they get there (left). Example of a control scene (endpoint reached). A car is driving into a garage (right).

In the control scenes (*n* = 12) the endpoint is reached (e.g., a man is walking through the door into a house). Because the action is completed (and a boundary crossed), the endpoints are expected to be mentioned to a greater degree than in the critical (and non-boundary-crossing) scenes.[3]

The distracter scenes (*n* = 36) consisted of various types of activities (e.g., a woman cleaning, drinking coffee, etc.), activities with the production of or change of an object (e.g., a man folding a paper airplane) and situations with little degree of change (e.g., a dog sitting still, a light burning, etc.). All the scenes were set up in a pseudo-randomized order, i.e., there were four different lists containing pairs of similar scenes, and the pairs were placed in a random order. The participants received one of four different lists (see Appendix 1 for an overview of critical and control items).

3.3. Procedure

The participants were shown the video clips on a PC screen. The task was to *"tell us what is happening"* (in Norwegian: *"Du skal bare fortelle hva som skjer"*). The participants were told to start talking as soon as they understood what was happening in the clip, only focusing on the event without any extra details. The speech was audio recorded from the first to the last video clip. After the experiment, the participants filled out a questionnaire on their linguistic and

3 See e.g., Holum (2009) for a description of boundary-crossing situations in Norwegian and a discussion of Norwegian as an S-language according to Talmy's (2000) division into S- and V-languages.

educational background, before receiving an unannounced memory test, used to test memory performance with respect to the (potential) endpoints from the videos. Unfortunately, though a comparison of the Norwegian memory tests to those of German and English could have enriched the discussion, the raw data for Norwegian were no longer available, making a reliable calculation difficult. There is also no eye-tracking data from the Norwegian part of the study. Half of the recordings were done at the University of Oslo in November 2007 and the rest in September 2008, under identical conditions and with the same procedure.

The audio recordings were transcribed and coded for [+/- endpoint (EP)]. In Norwegian, sentences where a possible or inferable endpoint was mentioned, mostly after a preposition, was counted as [+ EP]. For example, someone or something [motion verb] *to, towards, in the direction of a place, into a place* or *going somewhere*. The prepositions *i* 'in' and *på* 'on' were coded as [+ EP] if they were used in the sense of direction/intention of arrival at an endpoint, such as in regular expressions such as *gå i butikken* 'walking to the shop', *gå på lekeplassen* 'walking to the playground', etc.[4]

4. Results

The coding was done by three independent coders, with an interrater reliability (IRR) of Fleiss' kappa = 0.956 (360 scenes, 3 raters) for critical scenes and Fleiss' kappa = 0.955 (359 scenes, 3 raters) for the control scenes, in other words, a very high degree of reliability.[5]

4.1. Endpoint encoding in goal-oriented motion events in Norwegian L1

There were great individual differences among the participants when it comes to endpoint encoding in the critical scenes. Some participants mentioned many endpoints, while others mentioned few. The two who mentioned the most encoded 10 out of 12 possible endpoints, and the two who mentioned the least each mentioned 1 and 2 only, while the majority were somewhere in the middle, giving a mean value of the group of 0.503 (SD = 0.19), that is, 50 % endpoint designation. There was also a difference between the scenes as to the attraction of endpoint encoding. For example, 29 out of 30 participants mentioned the

4 The coding is based on the coding criteria in Schmiedtová (2013).

5 All the statistical analyses were performed by Bård Uri Jensen at Høyskolen i Innlandet/MultiLing.

playground as the endpoint in a scene where a little boy is walking alone towards a climbing frame. At the opposite end, in a scene with a car driving on a country road with a village in the distance, or a lady biking on a path with houses in the distance, only 1–4 of the participants mentioned the endpoints. Between these extremes was a large group of scenes with a relatively high or medium degree of endpoint naming. The scenes could be divided into three groups by proportion of endpoint designation, for a later discussion of what these scenes have in common: scenes with a high number of endpoints mentioned (20–30 out of 30 participants); scenes with an intermediate number of endpoints mentioned (10–20 of 30); and scenes with a low number of endpoints mentioned (fewer than 10 participants; for an overview, see Appendix 2).

In the control scenes, the endpoints as expected were mentioned to a high degree by all the participants, and consistently higher than in the critical scenes. Six of the Norwegian participants mentioned the endpoints in all the scenes (12 out of 12 possible). The four participants with the least endpoint designations each had seven or eight endpoint designations, and the rest of the participants mentioned ten to eleven each. The mean value of the group was 86 % ($SD = 0.12$). There was no obvious connection between how individuals scored in the control versus the critical scenes, but this may be related to the fact that everyone scored high in the control scenes.

4.2. The use of prepositions in the critical versus the control scenes

Before comparing the numbers of endpoints mentioned in Norwegian to the English and German results, one further finding is presented, namely the use of prepositions in the critical versus the control scenes. In the critical scenes, the preposition *mot* 'towards' is decidedly the one most frequently used. A typical example[6] could be the scene where a man is crossing the street, walking in the direction of a blue car:

1. En mann går *mot* en bil
   'A man is walking (lit. walks) *towards* a car'

The preposition *til* 'to' is also quite frequently used:

2. En mann som går *til* bilen sin
   'A man walking (lit. who walks) *to* his car'

6 All the examples are authentic utterances from the experiment.

There are only a few examples in which we find other prepositions, as *inn i* 'into' (lit. 'in in'), *inn på* 'into' (lit. 'in on') and *inn mot* 'into' (lit. 'in towards'). One example is the scene where a car is driving in the direction of a gas station:

3. En bil som kjører *inn på* en bensinstasjon
   'A car driving (lit. that drives) *into* (lit. in on) a gas station

The control scenes differ from the critical scenes both in the higher proportion of endpoint designations and in terms of the prepositions used. While in the critical scenes the prepositions *mot* 'towards' and *til* 'to' are used almost exclusively, only having a few exceptions with *inn* 'in' and *inn i* 'into', the control scenes display the opposite use: *inn i*, *inn på*, *inn til* 'into' are used almost exclusively, while *mot* 'towards' and *til* 'to' only as exceptions and/or in combination with *inn*. A good example is the scene where a man is walking up a flight of stairs, entering the door of a large building:

4. En gutt som går *inn i* et hus, bygning
   'A boy walking into (lit. who goes into) a house, building'

There are a few cases with *til* 'to' and *mot* 'towards', but mostly in combination with *inn* 'in', as in:

5. Jeg ser en hvit bil kjøre *inn mot* en gårdsplass
   'I see a white car driving *in towards* a courtyard'

While the use of prepositions in boundary-crossing situations in Norwegian is already described by Holum (2009), it is only briefly mentioned here for the later discussion, where it will be contrasted to the choice of prepositions in the critical scenes, as one might argue that by choice of preposition, the speaker takes a stance as to whether the mentioned endpoint will actually be reached or not.

4.3. Comparison between the languages

Let us now compare the verbalization of endpoints in the Norwegian data to the German and the English results.[7] In the critical scenes, the Norwegian and the German participants consistently mentioned more endpoints than did the English participants. There was a significant difference between, on the one hand, Norwegian (mean 50 %) and German (mean 55 %), and on the other hand, English (mean 38 %). There was no significant difference between German

---

7 Since individual data was not available for English and German, the scene is used as the observation unit in the comparison.

and Norwegian (measured with a paired Cohens d ≈ 0.16, 95 % CI [−0.33, 0.67]), while there was a significant difference between Norwegian and English (measured with a paired *t*-test, $t \approx 2.40$, $N = 12$, p ≈ 0.035, D ≈ 0.12, 95 % CI [0.010, 0.23], d ≈ 0.40, 95 % CI [0.041, 0.75]). The distributions for the critical scenes are illustrated in Box plot 1.

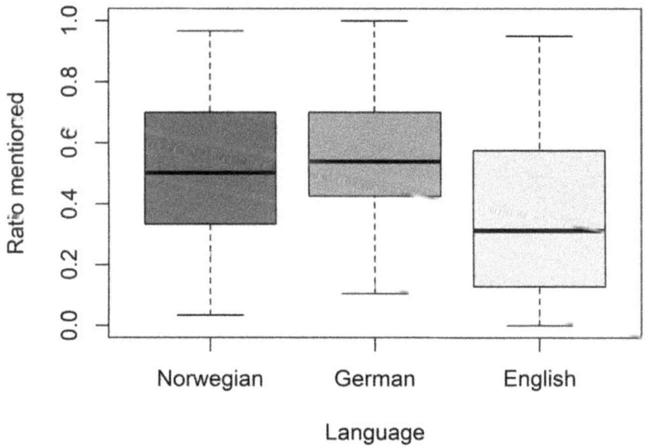

Figure 2: Proportion of endpoints mentioned, critical scenes, for Norwegian, German and English.

In the control scenes, as expected, the mentioning of endpoints was consistently higher than in the critical scenes in all three language es: For Norwegian, the mean value was 86 % ($SD = 0.14$), for German 89 % ($SD = 0.12$) and for English 86 % ($SD = 0.21$). There was no significant difference between Norwegian and English in the control scenes (measured with a paired Wilcoxon test, $V = 17.5$, $N = 12$, p ≈ 0.59; for key numbers, see Appendix 3). Let us now take a closer look at the differences between the scenes used in the experiment.

4.5. The differences between the type of scenes in the three languages

In the Norwegian L1 results, there was a lot of variation between the critical scenes when it comes to the endpoint attraction. In the control scenes, however, there was generally a high number of verbalized endpoints across all scenes. The verbalized endpoints are distributed differently across the 12 critical scenes in all the three languages (see Figure 3):

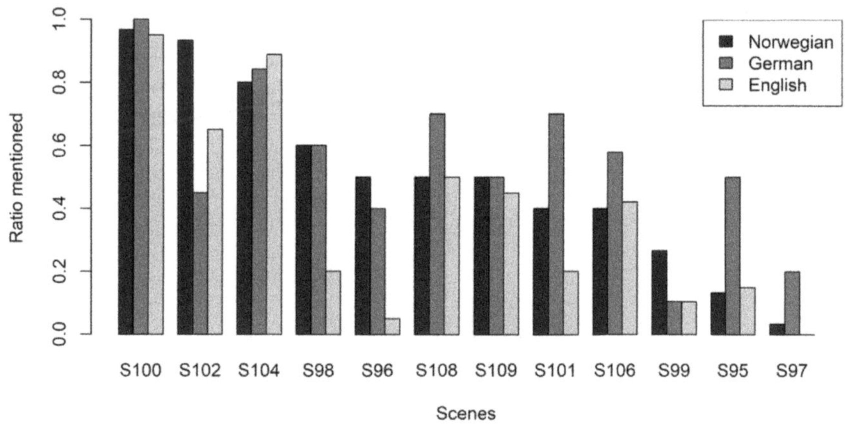

Figure 3: Key figures for the proportion of endpoints mentioned in the critical scenes for Norwegian, German and English. The S-numbers represent the name of the scene (for an overview, see Appendix 1).

For example, the scenes marked with S100 and S104 had high numbers of endpoint designation in all three languages, while the scenes S95, S97 and S99 had considerably less endpoint designations. In the middle of the bar plot, there is more variation (for a description of the scenes, see Appendix 1). Let us now turn to the discussion of the findings.

5. Discussion

In this section, the following questions will be discussed: (1) To what extent do Norwegian L1 speakers mention the endpoints in goal-oriented motion events, and how does Norwegian align compared to German and English? (2) What is the relation between endpoint designation and the salience of the goal? (3) What do the choice of prepositions tell us? And finally, (4) To what extent is it correct to call Norwegian a holistic language?

5.1. Differences between the three languages

While the difference in endpoint designation between Norwegian and German on the one side, and English on the other, can be linked to grammatical aspect as postulated by von Stutterheim and Nüse (2003), the fact that there is no significant difference in the production data between Norwegian and German might seem a bit surprising. This finding corresponds to the preliminary findings in Behrens and Ramm (2003), who also found no significant difference between Norwegian and German. But because Norwegian has many means to express aspectual content, as well as the discussion about a possible grammaticalization of the Norwegian pseudo-coordinations, one might have assumed that there would be a difference after all. However, as shown by Behrens et al. (2013), aspectual expressions are hardly used in motion events at all in Norwegian, giving less reason to expect a different outcome. More surprisingly perhaps, is that although all the participants speak English to a certain (mostly high) level, and although there is frequent language contact between Norwegian and English in daily life in Norway, this does not seem to have affected the results significantly in any direction. This contrasts to the findings of bidirectional transfer in the study of Spanish L1 learners of Swedish L2, where the participants had adopted the Swedish tendency of mentioning endpoints also when speaking Spanish, and showing less attentiveness towards aspectual contrasts when speaking Spanish than the monolingual control group (Bylund & Jarvis 2011). While the latter study shows traces of transfer from the L2 onto the L1, in our case, we do not see any (or at least not any obvious) effect of the English tendency of omitting endpoints in the Norwegian material as compared to the German.[8] This raises interesting questions for further inquiry as to when which traits will influence from the L2 back onto the L1 (e.g., why does the tendency for boundedness seem to work back from the L2 on the L1 in the case of the Spanish learners of Swedish, while the English tendency of omitting the endpoints, in our case, does not?). Here, of course, one explanation could be that our participants live in Norway, and despite the social prestige accorded to English in the Norwegian society, Norwegian is the dominant language, a factor of considerable significance (see e.g., Daller et al. 2011). All in all, based on the current study, there is no reason to believe that Norwegian L1 speakers take a very different perspectivation on goal-oriented motion events as compared to the German L1 speakers.

5.2. Qualitative differences in the video scenes

The variation in the results between the video clips in all three languages (as illustrated in Bar chart 1 above) can probably be partly explained by how obvious the (potential) goal of the motion is. Here, the concept of *salience* or *prominence* – how visible or in the foreground something is – can be useful (for a discussion of

8 It should be noted that this was not subject to inquiry in the current study (and the English proficiency of the participants not controlled for).

the concept, see Langacker 2000, pp. 6–8, 2008, p. 66). We can imagine that a large and eye-catching goal will attract more verbalizations of endpoints than one that is smaller and further away. In other words, the choice of method and material is crucial for this kind of study. Based on the actual number of endpoint designations in the Norwegian L1 material, the critical scenes can be divided into three groups, and the question is what the scenes in each group would have in common (for an exhaustive list of the grouped items, see Appendix 2). Group A: 20–30 designations out of a possible 30 (3 scenes), group B: 10–20 of 30 (6 scenes), and group C: 0–10 of 30 (3 scenes). Figure 4 (left) shows a screenshot of a prototypical example from group A, Figure 4 (right) is a prototypical example of group B, and Figure 5 (left) is a prototypical example of group C. The results correspond well with how salient or prominent the endpoint can be said to be in each scene. In group A – the scenes with the highest mentioning of endpoints – the car, the house and the playground are all large and relatively obvious goals for the motion. The scenes from group B, as will be shown in the discussion below, have a less clear goal. In group C, the two scenes with the least designations, the villages and the houses are at distance, and a third scene was cinematically not working well.[9] Let us take a closer look at a prototypical example from group A, depicting a scene with a prominent endpoint:

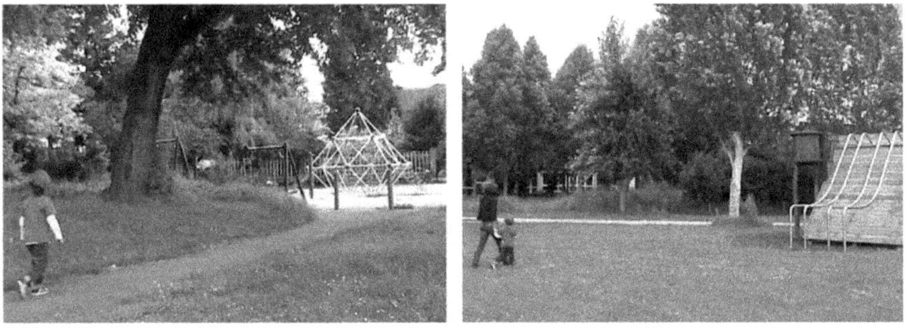

Figure 4: A little boy is walking towards a playground/large climbing frame, the scene stops just before the entrance (left). A lady and a child are walking in the park, in the direction of the climbing structure (right).

9 Scene 10: We first see an empty sidewalk cafe, then a lady comes along, crossing the square in the direction of some outdoor chairs or the corner of the house at the back. This scene is difficult to interpret (nothing happens at first), and most of the participants wait longer to start talking than with the other scenes. One can therefore discuss whether it should have been included at all, but it is included here for the sake of comparison, as it is included in the German and English material.

In this scene, a little boy is walking towards a large playground, but the clip ends just before he arrives there. Still, we are in no doubt about where he is going – it's simply not likely that he is going anywhere else. The fact that he is a child, walking alone, connects him more with the playground than just a walk in the park, for example. In fact, one could say that to a certain extent, the critical scenes with such a large and obvious goal resemble the control scenes; although a boundary is not being crossed in the video clip, it is likely that it will either be crossed or at least reached, and the endpoint is therefore mentioned to the same extent as in a control scene. The assumption that he is going to the playground is made by 29 out of 30 participants when seeing the clip (here by two of them):

6. En gutt som går *mot en lekeplass*, liten gutt
   (A boy walking *towards a playground,* small boy)

7. En gutt går *til lekeplassen*
   (A boy is walking *to the playground)*

For comparison, we can look at another and similar scene, but from group B, with a slightly less obvious goal (Figure 4, right): A mother and a small child are walking in a park in the direction of a climbing frame. Or are they just walking in the park? In this scene, only 15 out of 30 mention the climbing frame/play structure.

8. En dame og et barn går i en park *over plenen*
   (A lady and a child are walking in a park *across the lawn*)

9. En mor går med et barn *mot en lekeplass*
   (A mother is walking with a child *towards a playground*)

In group C, the goal is even further in the background. Admittedly, the car in the scene below must follow the road in the direction of the houses, but the endpoint is still less prominent and not necessarily the goal of the motion.

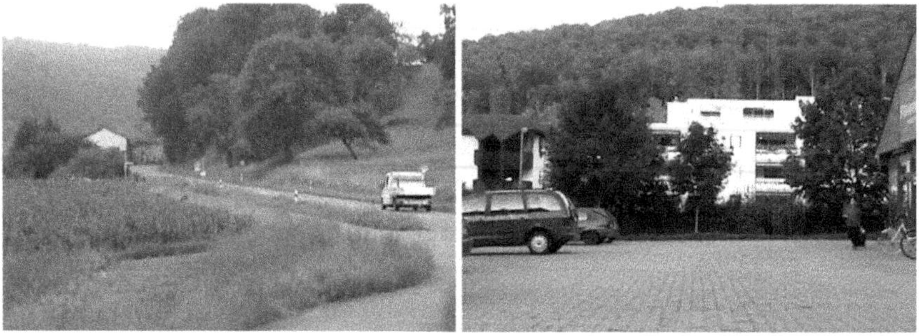

Figure 5: A van driving along a country road in the direction of a village / houses (left). A lady is walking from the shop and across the square in the direction of some cars (right).

In this clip, only 4 out of 30 participants mention the village or houses, while the others instead mention the road the car is driving *along* (17/30) or *on* (9/30):

10. En bil kjører *langs* en vei
    (A car is driving *along* a road)

11. En bil som kjører *på* en landsvei/bondevei
    (A car driving *on* a country road/farm road)

5.2.1. The scenes with an unclear goal

Let us take a closer look at the Norwegian participants' descriptions of the scenes in group B. These scenes are more complex, and it is not obvious where the agent is going, nor what the focus for information selection in the utterance should be. One example was described above, where a lady and a child are walking in a park – possibly towards a climbing structure (Figure 4). In another clip, a lady has just come out of a supermarket pulling a trolley bag behind her, walking across the square in the direction of some cars (Figure 6). In this scene, half of the participants (15 of 30) mentioned a potential endpoint (*the parking lot* or *a car*). But unlike the scenes described above, where the events are simple (e.g., the boy is walking towards the playground, the car is driving on a road), the Norwegian participants in this case describe more parts of the event: *out from the store*, and/or *across the square,* and/or *towards the car* (e.g., Examples 12 and 13 below).

12. En dame kommer *ut fra et kjøpesenter* og går *mot bilen sin*
    (A woman comes *out from a shopping center* and is walking *towards her car)*

13) Det er en dame som går - *med en trillekoffert* - *over en plass* - *mot noen biler*
(There is a lady walking - *with a trolley bag* - *across the square* - *towards some cars*)

Another scene with no obvious goal is illustrated in Figure 6. It starts off with a lady walking down a cobbled street in the direction of a barrier at the end. While it is unlikely that she's going to the barrier itself, one might imagine that she is going somewhere behind the barrier (e.g., the house) or turning to the street to the right or to the left. Yet, 18 out of 30 speakers mention the barrier in this scene:

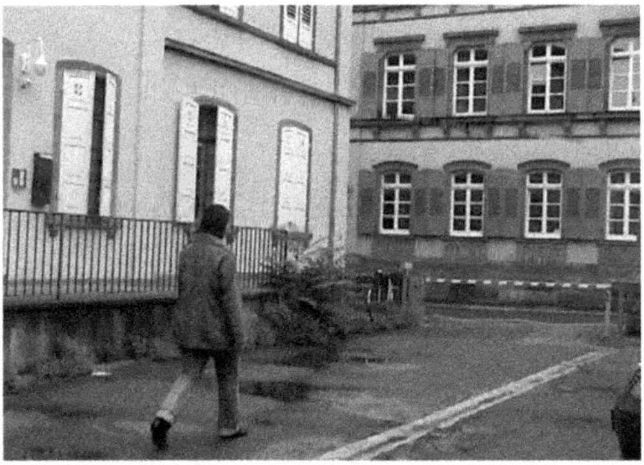

Figure 6: A girl is coming in from the left, walking in the direction of the barrier. The video clip ends when she is a few steps away from the barrier.

14. En person som går *mot en bom*
A person is walking *towards a barrier)*

15. En dame går nedover veien *mot en bom*
(A lady is walking down the road *towards a barrier*)

Although these are just a few examples, comparing the Norwegian results to the German and the English gives an interesting picture. In the scene with the barrier, 60 % (18 out of 30) of the Norwegian speakers and 60 % (12 out of 20) of the German mention the endpoint, versus only 20 % (4 of 20) of the English speakers. In the clip described earlier, in which a woman is walking from the supermarket towards the parking lot, we find a similar tendency: 50 % (15 out of 30) of the Norwegian speakers mention the endpoint, 40 % (8 of 20) of the German speakers, and only 5 % (1 of 20) of the English speakers. A similar pattern emerges in all the scenes from group B: the German and the Norwegian speakers mention more endpoints than the English. In other words, speakers of all the three languages seem to mention many endpoints when the goal is obvious, and few when the goal is in the distance. The difference between the aspect and non-aspect languages emerges most clearly in the scenes where the goal is less clear. When discussing whether a language is holistic, and when comparing across languages, it is therefore crucial that great caution is taken in the choice of material, and that the material used is identical across languages.

5.2.2. When the critical and control items resemble

By the crossing of a boundary, the control scenes can be described as having the highest level of goal-orientation possible. Although no boundary is crossed in the critical scenes, I argued above that some scenes resemble the control items since the goal is so obvious (and the boundary likely to be crossed), and these scenes have as many endpoint designations as the control scenes. Let us take a closer look at one critical (Figure 9, right) and one control scene (Figure 7, left) with similar content: a boy is walking on his own to the playground.

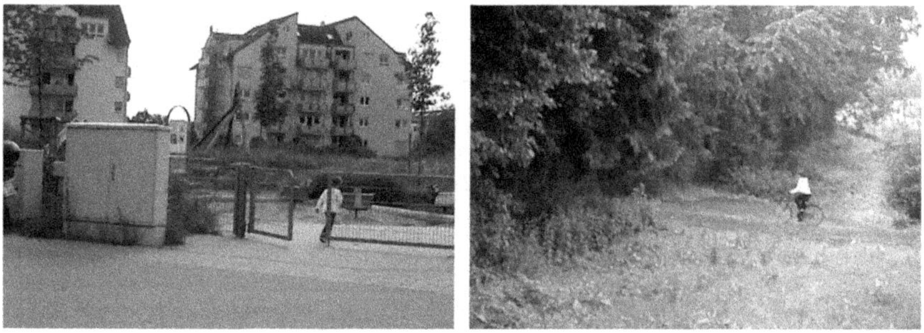

Figure 7: A boy is walking through the gate and into the playground (left). A lady is riding a bike. Is she on her way into the woods (or is she already there)? (right).

In the critical scene, the clip stops just before the boy would arrive at the playground, while in the control scene, the boy is walking into the playground through a gate (hence crossing a boundary). In the critical scene, 29 out of 30 participants mention the playground. In the control scene, also 29 of 30 participants mention the playground – in other words, a very high degree of endpoint designation in both cases. Yet there is a qualitative difference in the verbalizations between the two scenes in the choice of preposition. In the critical scene, the preferred prepositions are *mot* 'towards' (17) and *til* 'to' (10):

16. En gutt går *mot en lekeplass*
    (A boy is walking *towards a playground)*

17. En liten gutt *går til lekeplassen*
 (A little boy is walking *to the playground)*

In the control scene, the preferred prepositions are *inn på* and *inn til* 'into' (17 instances combined):

18. Et barn som går gjennom en port *inn på en lekeplass*
 (A child who is walking through a gate *into a playground*)

19. En gutt som går *inn til en lekeplass*
 (A boy who is walking *into a playground*)[10]

The differences in the choice of prepositions are further discussed in Section 5.3.

Whereas the control scenes in general have a high number of endpoint designations (22–30 of 30) in the Norwegian material, there is one control scene differing from the others by having a strikingly low number of endpoint designations (only 16). One could imagine that this scene has something in common with the critical scenes. A woman is riding a bike on a path in or into the forest (Figure 7, right). While the other control scenes mostly have an obvious endpoint (and a clear boundary-crossing), in this scene it is a question of interpretation whether the woman is on her way into the forest, or if she's already in the forest. Thus, this scene could be said to be less suitable as a control scene.

Interestingly in this context, when comparing the three languages, English still scores the lowest in this scene, with an endpoint mentioned in only 25 % of cases (5 of 20), while German and Norwegian have endpoints mentioned in 60 % (12 of 20) and 53 % (16 of 20) of cases, respectively. In other words, again we see that the endpoint designations drop and the difference between aspect and non-aspect languages emerges more clearly when the goal of the motion is unclear or becomes subject to interpretation.

5.3. The use of prepositions as a mark of reservation

As we have seen, even when the goal is large and obvious, there is a difference in the choice of prepositions, linked to whether a boundary is being crossed or not.

10 In this particular scene, in addition to *inn* 'in', there are a few examples of *mot* 'towards' and *til* 'to', and one could of course discuss further whether it is rather the gate that is the goal: the boy is going through the gate (crossing a boundary), and towards the playground. All the participants (29/30), however, mention the playground in their verbalizations (and 17 also mention the gate).

In the control scenes, the preposition *inn i* 'into' is preferred almost exclusively, while there is more variation in the critical scenes, mostly between *mot* 'towards', *til* 'to', and *inn til/mot* 'into/in towards'. This can be related to the uncertainty of the arrival at the (inferable) goal of the event. Let us take a closer look at meaning of the prepositions and a possible reservation of arrival at the endpoint.

Mot 'towards' – high degree of reservation: The word *mot* 'towards' means *i møte med* 'in the direction of; up to; (lit.) 'in meeting with' (Language Council of Norway & University of Bergen). In the critical scenes, it seems that the preposition *mot* is used precisely to express 'in the direction of' only, hence expressing reservation as to whether someone reaches the possible endpoint. In one example, we see a man crossing the street and walking in the direction of a blue car; but is he just crossing the street, or is he going to the car? And is the car necessarily his? These are questions that are answered more or less (in)directly in the participants' answers, both by mentioning (or not) the endpoint and by the choice of preposition, but also by the choice of pronouns. See the contrast between 20, 21, 22 and 23:

20. En mann går *mot en bil*
    (A man is walking *towards a car)*
21. En mann går *mot bilen sin*
    (A man is walking *towards his car*)

Another type of reservation could be linked to whether the car is his, or just a random car:

22. En type går *mot sin blå bil* / eller *det bør ikke være hans*
    (A guy is walking towards his blue car / or *it might not be his*)
23. Her er det en fyr som går *mot bilen sin* / eller *mot én bil*
    (Here's a guy walking *towards his car* / or *towards 'a' car*)

However, little reservation of this type is found in the material. In this scene, 28 out of 30 mention the car, and 10 of them with the phrase *bilen sin/sin bil* 'his car'. In the other scenes, the endpoints are also mentioned without much reservation other than what we may assume from the preposition *mot*.[11]

11 I mentioned that the preposition *mot* may be used to provide a reservation of arrival (i.e., uncertainty as to whether they will arrive at the goal). Tonne (2001, 2020) offers an alternative interpretation of the use of *mot*, that of a form of aspectual expression. Specifically, that the prepositions *til* and *mot* are associated with telicity and atelicity, respectively. Therefore, according to Tonne's interpretation, there would be a difference between *til lekeplassen* 'to the playground' (telic) and *mot lekeplassen* 'towards the playground' (atelic).

Til 'to' – medium degree of reservation: When using the preposition *til* 'to', we can assume that the participants consider the potential endpoint to be a probable goal of the motion, meaning *up to the goal*:

24. En person som går *til en bom*
    (A person walking *to a barrier*)

→ a person is going to the barrier, the motion ends here. The meaning changes when using the preposition *mot*:

25. En dame går nedover veien *mot en bom*
    (A lady is walking down the road *towards a barrier)*

→ a lady is walking in the direction of a barrier, but we don't know where she's actually heading. Again, we see that the preposition *mot* expresses another (and stronger) type of reservation than, for example, *til.*

Inn i 'into' – low/no degree of reservation: In one of the critical scenes, a car is driving along some tram tracks in the direction of a gas station. In this scene, only half of the participants (14/30) mention the gas station, and most of them express reservation as to whether the endpoint is reached, by using the prepositions *mot* or *til.* A couple of them, however, use the preposition *inn.* This can be said to be an expression of a strong assumption of the goal being reached, even if the clip stops before the car has driven into the station:

26. En hvit bil som kjører *inn på* en bensinstasjon
    (A white car driving *into* a gas station)

A similar, strong assumption can be found in the use of the word *hjem* 'home' in the critical scene where two women are walking along a road in the direction of a big house (Figure 1):

27. Her er det noen som går *hjem* fra en tur, to jenter som går *hjem* fra en tur
    (Here, there is someone going *home* from a walk, two girls going *home* from a walk)

In this case, the participant is assuming not only that the women are walking up to the house, but that they live there. These few examples are exceptions, though. Mostly, a reservation is expressed using *mot* 'towards', indicating that, although the endpoint is mentioned, the speaker does not assume that the endpoint will necessarily be reached.

5.6. A holistic perspective?

Would it be correct to say that Norwegian takes a holistic perspective on motion events, as defined by von Stutterheim and Nüse (2003)? Looking at the proportion of endpoint designations, Norwegian scores quite similarly to German, which in the literature is normally considered holistic. Norwegian also scores significantly higher than English, which is said to take a phasal perspective on the same events. Hence, these results seem to support the argument that Norwegian takes a holistic perspective in line with German. In Swedish, a language close Norwegian, there is also a preference for holistic event presentation (Bylund 2008).

Still, the term holistic could be debated. With a mean of 50 % endpoint designation, claiming that Norwegian in general takes a holistic perspective on motion events might be an overinterpretation of the data. In other contexts, it may be questionable to call 50 % a tendency. Also, in other studies, the numbers are even lower. For example, Behrens and Ramm (2003) reported a mean of endpoint designation of 38 % for Norwegian and 41 % for German, versus 18 % for English. Additionally, von Stutterheim and Nüse (2003) report that the numbers vary greatly: "If only 50 % of the speakers 'close' the event, English speakers do so even less frequently; and if 50 % of the English speakers mention the event in question, the amount of German speakers who do so is 90 %" (p. 862). In other words, rather than being either high or low, the numbers seem to be relative to each other. As we have seen, the proportion of endpoint designations also depends on the type of scene, which in turn underscores the significance of the choice of material. In other words, the languages can be more or less holistic, depending on the type of goal. In all three languages, scenes with a large and obvious endpoint attract many endpoint designations, whereas scenes with a distant endpoint attract fewer. The most interesting scenes in this respect are those which are more ambiguous (i.e., the scenes in group B, as discussed above), and this is where the difference between the aspect and non-aspect languages becomes most evident. Perhaps *semi-holistic* or *weakly holistic* would be more appropriate designations for Norwegian? Another way of putting it might be that Norwegian takes a *more* holistic perspective on motion events than languages with grammaticalized aspect.

Accordingly, dividing languages into distinct categories, like the holistic vs. the phasal perspective, is a bit rough, and it would be more fruitful to think of it in terms of a continuum, where some languages take a more holistic perspective, some a more phasal, and some possibly more in between. This will depend on the degree of the grammaticalization of the respective grammatical categories. Where English is less aspectual than, for example, Arabic, German is more holistic than Dutch (Mertins 2018). The differences we find in the scene types also reflect variation along a continuum to some degree. Interestingly, while we have described a 50 % verbalization of endpoints in the critical scenes, even when inferring an endpoint and including it in the utterance, the speaker takes a stance or certain reservation – marked by the choice of preposition – as to whether the endpoint will be reached or not. In other words, in Norwegian, it's not all-or-nothing, but a range of possibilities to express different kinds of goal-orientation. When thinking and speaking about languages and diversity, even the small nuances should be included for a better understanding of the phenomena in question.

6. Conclusion

So, what do motion events look like "with Norwegian eyes"? The aim of this article was to provide a more in-depth study of the verbalization of goal-oriented motion events in Norwegian than in earlier studies, and to discuss whether it is correct to say that Norwegian speakers take a holistic perspective on such events. In the investigated material, Norwegian L1 speakers mentioned the potential endpoints in on average 50 % of the cases in the critical scenes. In other words, mentioning endpoints is not mandatory in Norwegian, but the degree of endpoint naming depends on how large or obvious the possible goal of the motion is: scenes with a prominent and intermediate prominent goal impel higher rates of verbalization. The findings correspond roughly in line with the German results. The English L1 speakers, on the other hand, mention endpoints to a significantly lower degree in goal-oriented motion events with an inferable endpoint. The difference in endpoint designation between the languages is most visible in the scenes where the goal is moderately prominent or subject to interpretation. Based on these findings, Norwegian seems to follow the pattern proposed by von Stutterheim and Nüse (2003), that speakers of languages without grammatical aspect take a (more) holistic perspective on motion events than do speakers of aspect languages. But rather than claiming that Norwegian speakers in general take a holistic perspective on such events, I suggest moderating the use of the notion, depending on the situation, keeping in mind that a language might be more holistic relative to another – not necessarily excluding the unbounded option.

The linguistic data we have tells us something about how motion events are expressed in Norwegian. Compared with English, the results suggest that there is a difference between the two groups in the preverbal phase as to what is included in the utterance. Yet, to be able to say anything about the actual conceptualization process, a future study including other methodologies, such as e.g., eye-tracking and/or memory data, would be desired. An interesting question for further study is whether the preference for mentioning endpoints at large/medium-sized goals is expressed by Norwegian children to the same extent, and with the same choice of prepositions, as by adults. Another focus is to consider bilingual children growing up with two languages with competing perspectives on the same event: a more holistic endpoint-oriented perspective versus a more phasal perspective. These questions are currently being explored in an experimental eye-tracking study on monolingual Norwegian and simultaneously bilingual Norwegian-English children.

7. Acknowledgments

I want to thank the editors and anonymous reviewers for their valuable comments. Furthermore, I had the opportunity to discuss several aspects of the statistical analysis with Bård Uri Jensen. Thank you!

References

Athanasopoulos, P./Bylund, E. (2013). The 'thinking' in thinking-for-speaking. Where is it? *Language, Interaction and Acquisition, 4*(1), 91–100. John Benjamins Publishing Company. https://doi.org/10.1075/lia.4.1.05ath

Behrens, B., Flecken, M./Carroll, M. (2013). Progressive attraction: On the use and grammaticalization of progressive aspect in Dutch, Norwegian, and German. *Journal of Germanic Linguistics, 25*(2), 95–136. https://doi.org/10.1017/S1470542713000020

Behrens, B./Ramm, W. (2003). "Ser vi det samme eller styres vi av vår språklige kode?" Rapport fra det norske bidraget til det internasjonale språkprosjektet "Konseptualisering og språkspesifikk kunnskap". *NOA nr 24*, 109–142, ILN, UiO.

Bylund, E. (2008). Procesos de conceptualización de eventos en español y en sueco: Diferencias translingüísticas. *Revue Romane. Langue et littérature. International Journal of Romance Languages and Literatures, 43*, 1–24. Doi: https://doi-org.ezproxy.uio.no/10.1075/rro.43.1.02byl

Bylund, E. (2011a). Segmentation and temporal structuring of events in early Spanish-Swedish bilinguals. *International Journal of Bilingualism, 15*(1), 56–84.

Bylund, E. (2011b). Language-specific patterns in event conceptualization: Insights from bilinguals. In A. Pavlenko (Ed.), *Thinking and speaking in two languages* (pp. 108–142). Multilingual Matters.

Bylund, E./Athanasopoulos, P./Oostendorp, M. (2013). Motion event cognition and grammatical aspect. Evidence from Afrikaans. *Linguistics, 51*,929–955. Mouton de Gruyter. https://doi-org.ezproxy.uio.no/10.1515/ling-2013-0033

Bylund, E./Jarvis, S. (2011). L2 effects on L1 event conceptualization. *Bilingualism: Language and Cognition, 14*(1), 47–59. http://dx.doi.org/10.1017/S1366728910000180

Carroll, M./von Stutterheim, C./Nüse, R. (2004). The language and thought debate: A psycholinguistic approach. In C. Habel & T. Pechman (Eds.), *Approaches to language production* (pp. 183–218). Mouton de Gruyter.

Comrie, B. (2001). *Aspect*. Cambridge: Cambridge University Press (Original work published 1976).

Daller, M./Treffers-Daller, J./Furman, R. (2011). Transfer of conceptualization patterns in bilinguals: The construal of motion events in Turkish and German. *Bilingualism: Language and Cognition, 14*(1),95–119. Doi: https://doi.org/10.1017/S1366728910000106

Flecken, M. (2010). *Event conceptualization in language production of early bilinguals*. Proefschrift. Radboud Universiteit Nijmegen, Utrecht.

Golden, A./Jarvis, S./Tenfjord, K. (Eds.). (2017). *Crosslinguistic influence and distinctive patterns of language learning: Findings and insights from a learner corpus*. Multilingual Matters. ISBN 97s1-78309-876-7.

Gujord, A. K. H./Ragnhildstveit, S. (2018). Tverrspråkleg påverknad – Status og trendar i norsk andrespråksforsking. In A. K. H. Gujord & G. T. Randen (Eds.), *Norsk som andrespråk – Perspektiver på læring og utvikling* (pp. 133–163). Oslo: Cappelen Damm.

Gullberg, M. (2011). Thinking, speaking and gesturing about motion in more than one language. In A. Pavlenko (Ed.), *Thinking and speaking in two languages*. Bristol: Multilingual Matters.

Holum, L.-M. (2009). *Språkspesifikk konseptualisering og muntlig andrespråksproduksjon: En studie av uttrykk for bevegelsesmåte hos avanserte andrespråksinnlærere av norsk med spansk som førstespråk* [Master's thesis, University of Oslo]. DUO Research Archive. https://www.duo.uio.no/handle/10852/26826

Johansen, S. C. (2011). *Går på tur aldri sur: En korpusbasert studie av bevegelseshandlinger og morsmålstransfer i innlærertekster fra voksne informanter i norsk som andrespråk* [Master's thesis, University of Oslo]. DUO Research Archive. https://www.duo.uio.no/handle/10852/26696

Johansen, S. H. (2020). Hedging in spoken conversations by Norwegian learners of English. *Nordic Journal of Modern Language Methodology, 8*(2), 27–48. https://doi.org/10.46364/njmlm.v8i2.751

Kinn, T. (2018). Pseudocoordination in Norwegian: Degrees of grammaticalization and constructional variants. In E. Coussé, P. Andersson, & J. Olofsson (Eds.), *Grammaticalization meets constructional grammar. Constructional approaches to language 21*. John Benjamins Publishing Company, Amsterdam/ Philadelphia.

Langacker, R. W. (1987). *Foundations of cognitive grammar* (Vol. 1). Stanford: Stanford University Press.

Langacker, R. W. (2000). *Grammar and conceptualization*. Berlin: Mouton de Gruyter.

Langacker, R. W. (2008). *Cognitive grammar. A basic introduction*. Oxford: Oxford University Press.

Language Council of Norway/University of Bergen. (n.d.). Mot. In *Bokmålsordboka*. Retrieved May 10, 2022, from https://ordbokene.no/bm/39214/mot

Levelt, W. J. M. (1989). *Speaking. From intention to articulation*. Cambridge MA: MIT Press.

Lødrup, H. (2017a). Norwegian pseudocoordination with the verb drive 'carry on': Control, raising, grammaticalization. In M. Butt & T. H. King (Eds.), *Proceedings of the LFG'17 Conference* (pp. 264–284). CSLI Publications. https://web.stanford.edu/group/cslipublications/cslipublications/LFG/LFG-2017/abstr-loedrup.shtml

Lødrup, H. (2017b, September 29). *Sitte* og *arbeide* 'sit and work': Is Scandinavian pseudocoordination with posture verbs a grammaticalized progressive construction? [Institute seminar]. ILN, UiO.

Malcher, J. (2011). *Jeg liker å treffe folk i café. Man må nyter de fine tingene på verden!: preposisjoner og morsmålstransfer – En korpusbasert studie med i og på i fokus* [Master's thesis, University of Oslo]. DUO Research Archive. https://www.duo.uio.no/handle/10852/26695

Mannsåker, H./Nistov, I./Nordanger, M. (2020). Andrespråkslæring – Med vinkling fra kognitiv lingvistikk. In L. Kulbrandstad & G. B. Steien (Eds.), *Språkreiser. Festskrift til Anne Golden på 70-årsdagen 14. juli 2020* (p. 79–105). Novus, Oslo.

Mertins, B. (2016). The use of experimental methods in linguistic research: Advantages, problems and possible pitfalls. In T. Anstatt, C. Clasmeier, & A. Gattnar (Eds.), *Slavic languages in psycholinguistics. Chances and challenges for empirical and experimental research* (pp. 15–33). Tübingen: Narr Verlag.

Mertins, B. (2018). *Sprache und Kognition: Ereigniskonzeptualisierung im Deutschen und Tschechischen*. Berlin: Mouton de Gruyter.

Nordanger, M. (2009). *Keiserens nye klær? Lingvistisk og konseptuell transfer i markeringen av grammatikalisert definitt referanse i russiskspråklige og engelskspråkliges norske mellomspråk – En studie basert på ASK* [Master's thesis, University of Bergen]. Bergen Open Research Archive. https://bora.uib.no/bora-xmlui/bitstream/handle/1956/3620/63003650.pdf

Pavlenko, A. (2014). *The bilingual mind, and what it tells us about language and thought*. Cambridge: Cambridge University Press.

Pourcel, S. (2003). Rethinking 'Thinking for Speaking'. *Proceedings of the twenty-ninth annual meeting of the Berkeley Linguistics Society: General session and parasession on phonetic sources of phonological patterns: Synchronic and diachronic explanations*, vol. 29, pp. 349–358. http://journals.linguisticsociety.org/proceedings/index.php/BLS/article/viewFile/1007/788

Schmiedtová, B. (2011). Do L2 speakers think in the L1 when speaking in the L2? *Vigo International Journal Applied Linguistics, 8*(1), 139–179.

Schmiedtová, B. (2013). Traces of L1 patterns in the event construal of Czech advanced speakers of L2 English and L2 German. *International Review of Applied Linguistics in Language Teaching, 51*(2), 87–116. https://doi.org/10.1515/iral-2013-0005

Schmiedtová, B./Sahonenko, N. (2008). Die Rolle des grammatischen Aspekts in Ereignis-Enkodierung: Ein Vergleich zwischen Tschecnischen und Russischen Lernern des Deutschen. In P. Grommes & M. Walter (Eds.), *Fortgeschrittene Lernervarietäten: Korpuslinguistik und Zweitsparcherwerbs-forschung* (pp. 45–71). Niemeyer, Berlin: Niemyer Verlag.

Schmiedtová, B./von Stutterheim, C./Carroll, M. (2011). Language-specific patterns in event construal of advanced second language speakers. In A. Pavlenko (Ed.), *Thinking and speaking in two languages* (pp. 66–107). Bristol: Multilingual Matters.

Slobin, D. I. (1991). Learning to think for speaking: Native language, cognition, and rhetorical style. *Pragmatics, 1*(1), 7–25. https://doi.org/10.1075/prag.1.1.01slo

Slobin, D. I. (1996). From "thought and language" to "thinking for speaking". In J. J. Gumperz & S. C. Levinson (Eds.), *Rethinking linguistic relativity* (pp. 70–96). Cambridge: Cambridge University Press.

Szmynska, O. (2010). *Konseptualisering av rommet hos polske norskinnlærere – Utfordringer og diagnoser. En korpusbasert studie med i og på i fokus* [Doctoral dissertation, Adam Mickiewicza University]. Adam Mickiewicz University Repository. https://repozytorium.amu.edu.pl/bitstream/10593/1269/9/KONSEPTUALISERING%20AV%20ROMMET%20HOS%20POLSKE%20NORSKINNLARERE.pdf

Talmy, L. (1985). Lexicalization patterns: Semantic structure in lexical forms. In T. Shopen (Ed.), *Language typology and syntactic description, vol. III: Grammatical categories and the lexicon* (pp. 56–149). Cambridge: Cambridge University Press.

Talmy, L. (2000). *Toward a cognitive semantics.* MIT Press, Cambridge, Mass.

Tonne, I. (1999). A Norwegian progressive marker and the level of grammaticalization. *Languages in Contrast*, *2*, 131–159. https://doi.org/10.1075/lic.2.1.08ton

Tonne, I. (2001). *Progressives in Norwegian and the theory of aspectuality* [Doctoral dissertation, University of Oslo]. Unipub.

Tonne, I. (2020). «… noen ganger sitter vi og diskuterer om skolen…». Bruk av pseudokoordinering med positurverb i norsk som andrespråk. In L. Kulbrandstad & G. B. Steien (Eds.), *Språkreiser. Festskrift til Anne Golden på 70-årsdagen 14. juli 2020.* Novus, Oslo.

von Stutterheim, C./Andermann, M./Carroll, M./Flecken, M./Schmiedtová, B. (2012). How grammaticized concepts shape event conceptualization in language production: Insights from linguistic analysis, eye tracking data, and memory performance. *Linguistics*, *50*(4), 833–867. https://doi.org/10.1515/ling-2012-0026

von Stutterheim, C./Carroll, M. (2006). The impact of grammatical temporal categories on ultimate attainment in L2 learning. In H. Byrnes, H. D. Weger-Guntharp/K. Aprang (Eds.), *Educating for advanced foreign language capacities* (pp. 40–53). Washington D.C.: Georgetown University Press.

von Stutterheim, C./Nüse, R. (2003). Processes of conceptualization in language production: Language-specific perspectives and event construal. *Linguistics*, *41*(5), 831–881.

Vulchanova, M. D./Martínez, L./Eshuis, R./Listhaug, K. (2012). No evidence of L1 path encoding strategies in the L2 in advanced Bulgarian speakers of Norwegian. *Spatial Cognition & Computation*, *12*(4), 275–304. https://doi.org/10.1080/13875868.2012.658931

Appendices

Appendix 1

Overview of stimuli

Critical scenes (endpoint not reached)

1. **95_car.cornfield:** *a car driving along a country road in the direction of a small village*
2. **96_stepout.woman.supermarket**: *a woman is coming from a shopping mall, heading for the parking lot/cars*
3. **97_bicycle.village:** *a woman is biking on a country road, a village in the distance*
4. **98_walking.barrier**: *a woman is walking towards a barrier at the end of the street*
5. **99_walking.cafe**: a woman is walking in the direction of an empty sidewalk café
6. **100_walking.playground.one**: *a child is walking on a path towards a playground*
7. **101_climbing.ladder**: *a man is climbing a ladder upwards, towards a balcony*
8. **102_wal+5 king.car**: *a man is crossing the street, walking in the direction of a blue car*
9. **104_walking.house.two**: *to women are walking on a country road in the direction of a house*
10. **106_riding.barrier**: *a woman is riding a horse towards a barrier*
11. **108_walking.playground.two**: *a woman and a child are walking in a park in the direction of a climbing frame*
12. **109_gasstation.mpg**: *a car is driving through a crossroads in the direction of a petrol station*

Control scenes (endpoint reached)

1. **80_garage.long**: *a car is driving into a garage*
2. **81_trainstation**: *a woman is hurrying into a train station*
3. **82_van.gate**: *a van is driving through a gate into a courtyard*
4. **83_bicycle.gate**: *a man is biking into a gate (disappearing)*
5. **84_bicycle.forrest**: *a woman is biking in (into?) a forest*
6. **85_entering.shop**: *an elderly woman is entering a supermarket*
7. **87_running.dog.door**: *a dog is running through a doorway*
8. **88_walking.cat**: *a cat is walking from one room to another*

9. **89_walking.playground.oneP**: *a boy is walking through a gate into a playground*
10. **90_walking.churchdoor**: *a man is walking up a stairway and entering the door of a church*
11. **91_walking.horse.box:** *a horse is walking into its stable*
12. **93_train.tunnel**: *a train is driving into a tunnel*

Appendix 2: Scenes divided according to the number of endpoint designations in Norwegian L1

(A) Scenes with a high degree of endpoint designation (20–30 of 30N)

1. S100: A child is walking on a path towards a playground: 29/30
2. S102: A man is crossing the street, walking in the direction of a blue car: 28/30
3. S104: Two women are walking on a country road in the direction of a house: 24/30

(B) Scenes with an intermediate degree of endpoint designation (10–20 of 30N)

4. S98: A woman is walking towards a barrier at the end of the street: 18/30
5. S96: A woman is coming from a shopping mall, heading for the parking lot/cars: 15/30
6. S108: A woman and a child are walking in a park in the direction of a climbing frame: 15/30
7. S109: A car is driving through a crossroad in the direction of a petrol station: 14/30
8. S106: A woman is riding a horse towards a barrier: 12/30
9. S101: A man is climbing a ladder upwards, towards a balcony:12/30

(C) Scenes with a low degree of endpoint designation (below 10 of 30N)

10. S99: A woman is walking in the direction of an empty sidewalk café: 8/30
11. S95: A truck on a country road is driving towards a village: 4/30
12. S97: A woman is biking on a country road, a village in the distance: 1/30

Appendix 3: Key numbers for Norwegian, German and English – critical and control scenes.

Critical scenes (N12)					
Language	**Min**		*Mean value*	**Standard deviation**	**Max**
Norwegian (N30)	0.033		***0.50***	0.29	0.97
German (N20)	0.11		***0.55***	0.25	1
English (N20)	0 (n=1)		***0.38***	0.32	0.95
Control scenes (N12)					
Language	**Min**		***Mean value***	**Standard deviation**	**Max**
Norwegian (N30)	0.53		***0.86***	0.14	1 (n=3)
German (N20)	0.60		***0.89***	0.12	1 (n–4)
English (N20)	0.26		***0.86***	0.21	1 (n=5)

Katrin Odermann

Mehrsprachigkeit und Schriftspracherwerb: Vorteile von Mehrsprachigkeit durch früh entwickeltes metalinguistisches Bewusstsein

Abstract: Prejudices against multilingualism are partly generated by a misinterpretation of the results of the frequently quoted PISA studies: Poor school performance is seen as a consequence of an "immigrant background" that is then linked to poor skills in German language. However, the socioeconomic status is the variable that explains most of the variation found in such studies. The acquisition of written language is considered a key issue in the German education system. However, the foundations for successful acquisition of written language are not laid in elementary school, but already before in the family environment. As a result, children with parents of a low socioeconomic status are particularly disadvantaged as they have less contact with texts, books, libraries, and other relevant input sources. This preschool experience influences the emergence and development of metalinguistic awareness, which in turn is a prerequisite for the onset of literacy acquisition. Phonological awareness and its influence on written language acquisition have been subject of many previous studies and shown to be especially important for the first phase of written language acquisition. Less research has been done on other types (e.g., morphological or syntactic) of metalinguistic awareness. Multilingual children must constantly apply metalinguistic awareness because of the daily exposure to two or more languages that they have to learn to differentiate at all linguistic levels. Numerous studies have demonstrated the advantage of multilinguals in the development of executive functions such as attentional control which seem to be related to an earlier emergence of metalinguistic awareness. Despite these advantages of multilingualism, there are only deficit-oriented approaches in the field of literacy acquisition with respect to multilingualism. Future research on literacy acquisition, metalinguistic awareness, and multilingualism should be more benefit-oriented and also should investigate the aspects of metalinguistic awareness, preferably using experimental psycholinguistics methods in addition to behavioral studies.

Keywords: acquisition of written language, executive functions, metalinguistic awareness, multilingualism, bilingualism

1. Einleitung

Weltweit existieren etwa 6.900 Sprachen, die in etwa 200 Nationalstaaten gesprochen werden. Dies bedeutet, es gibt 30 mal so viele Sprachen wie Länder, sodass Mehrsprachigkeit aus globaler Sicht keineswegs als ein rares Phänomen bezeichnet werden kann (Romaine 1989). Allein in Europa werden zum Beispiel in Ländern wie Spanien, der Schweiz oder Belgien mehr als eine Sprache gesprochen. Auch in Deutschland ist Mehrsprachigkeit aufgrund der über 60 Jahre langen Einwanderungsgeschichte mittlerweile eher Normalität als Ausnahme: 26 % der Menschen in Deutschland haben einen Migrationshintergrund[1] (Statistisches Bundesamt 2021). Der Anteil liegt bei Schüler*innen sogar bei 33 % (Statistisches Bundesamt 2019) und es wird davon ausgegangen, dass der Anteil von Schüler*innen mit Migrationshintergrund in Großstädten bei ca. 50 % liegt (Jacob 2021). Wie viele der Menschen in Deutschland tatsächlich zwei- oder mehrsprachig sind, ist dennoch schwer zu berechnen, da hierzu nicht nur die Menschen mit Migrationshintergrund gehören, sondern auch weitere Personen, die aus verschiedenen Gründen täglich mehrere Sprachen nutzen. Somit dürfte der Anteil der Mehrsprachigen noch weit über dem der Menschen mit Migrationshintergrund liegen.

Ungeachtet der großen Zahl von Mehrsprachigen bestehen nicht nur aus der breiten Öffentlichkeit, sondern auch seitens der Bildungsinstitutionen immer noch hartnäckige Vorurteile gegenüber Mehrsprachigkeit und Bilingualismus. Eines dieser Vorurteile ist, dass Kinder, die zwei- oder mehrsprachig aufwachsen, keine der beiden Sprachen „richtig" sprechen (die sogenannte *doppelte Halbsprachigkeit*) (Delucchi Danhier & Mertins 2018) und die damit vermeintlich verbunden schlechten Deutschkenntnisse der Kinder in Folge zu schlechten Schulleistungen führen. Da die Kompetenzen in der deutschen Sprache als Hauptfaktor für den Bildungserfolg mehrsprachiger Kinder gesehen werden (Huschka et al. 2020), wird von Kinderärzt*innen, Erzieher*innen und Lehrer*innen oft eine exklusive Förderung der deutschen Sprache gefordert. Die deutsche Sprache zu fördern ist sicherlich ein richtiger Ansatz, wenn nicht ebenfalls gleichzeitig dazu geraten würde, die Herkunftssprachen zu vernachlässigen, aufzugeben oder gar zu verbieten.

1 Der Begriff *Migrationshintergrund* muss kritisch betrachtet werden, da er keine Aussage über die Mehrsprachigkeit der Personen gibt. Migrationshintergrund weist nur auf die Herkunft der Familie und Vorfahren hin. Eine Person hat auch dann Migrationshintergrund, wenn sie selbst keine Migrationserfahrungen gemacht hat.

Schlechtere Schulleistungen der Schüler*innen mit Migrationshintergrund in PISA-Studien, insbesondere schlechte Leseleistungen, werden als Konsequenz des Migrationshintergrunds und den damit einhergehenden schlechten Deutschkenntnissen interpretiert. Bei dieser Darstellung der Ergebnisse wird Migrationshintergrund mit Mehrsprachigkeit stillschweigend gleichgesetzt und diese Mehrsprachigkeit bezogen auf bestimmte Sprachen, nämlich Migrationssprachen wie z. B. Türkisch, Polnisch oder Arabisch. Mehrsprachigkeit durch Bildungssprachen wie z. B. Englisch, Französisch oder Spanisch werden dagegen in der Regel als positiv gewertet, obwohl es aus der Sicht der Linguistik keine Wertigkeit der Sprachen gibt. Auch der sozioökonomische Status der Kinder mit Migrationshintergrund als Erklärungsvariable wird zur Interpretation der PISA-Daten nicht systematisch herangezogen. Vielmehr wird eine Korrelation zwischen Migrationshintergrund, Mehrsprachigkeit mit bestimmten Sprachen und schlechten Schulleistungen angenommen, die für die Erklärung der identifizierten Varianz nicht zutrifft. Weder Migrationshintergrund noch Mehrsprachigkeit mit bestimmten Sprachen sind für die schlechten Schulleistungen der Kinder verantwortlich, sondern der sozioökonomische Status der Familien. Durch die Einbeziehung des sozioökonomischen Status in die Auswertung der Ergebnisse wird nämlich die Korrelation zwischen der Variable Migrationshintergrund und schlechteren Schulleistungen aufgehoben. In der Expertise des SVR-Forschungsbereichs (SVR-Forschungsbereich – Forschungsbereich beim Sachverständigenrat deutscher Stiftungen für Integration und Migration 2016) wurde in diesem Sinne herausgearbeitet, dass bei alleiniger Betrachtung des Migrationshintergrund zur Erklärung von Kompetenzen der Schüler*innen, dieser als statistisch bedeutsamer Faktor nur drei bis sechs Prozent der Unterschiede erklärt. Unter Einbeziehung der sozialen Herkunft verliert der Migrationshintergrund vollständig an statistischer Bedeutung. „Bei gleichem Bildungshintergrund der Eltern und gleicher sozioökonomischer Lage erzielen Jungen und Mädchen aus bestimmten Herkunftsgruppen (z. B. der spanischen oder vietnamesischen Herkunftsgruppe) sogar überdurchschnittlich gute Ergebnisse." (Mendt 2020). Dadurch wird deutlich, dass nicht der Migrationshintergrund *per se*, sondern die soziale Herkunft eine entscheidende Rolle beim Schulerfolg der Kinder spielt (Mendt 2020).

Der Schriftspracherwerb stellt dabei eine Schlüsselrolle für den Erfolg im deutschen Schulsystem dar (Huschka et al. 2020). Die Grundlagen des Schriftspracherwerbs, also die Vorstellungen von Schrift, die das Kind entwickelt, werden im Sinne von Bredel et al. (2011) bereits vor der Einschulung in der familiären Umgebung geschaffen, beispielsweise durch ein lesendes Umfeld. Zu diesen Grundlagen des Schriftspracherwerbs gehört auch die Entwicklung des metalinguistischen Bewusstseins, in dem Sinne, dass es dem Kind erlaubt, über Sprache als System nachzudenken und diese zu abstrahieren. Metalinguistisches Bewusstsein bezeichnet das Wissen über linguistische Strukturen und das Können, dieses Wissen gezielt abzurufen (Grosjean & Li 2012). Nur durch diese Fähigkeiten können Kinder die Bilateralität sprachlicher Zeichen verstehen, indem sie die graphische Bedeutung der Zeichen von der inhaltlichen Bedeutung trennen und ihre Arbitrarität verstehen.

Ziel dieses Beitrags ist es, die Schnittstelle zwischen Schriftspracherwerb, metalinguistischem Bewusstsein und Mehrsprachigkeit anhand theoretischer Grundlagen zu beleuchten, um aufzuzeigen, dass Mehrsprachigkeit keineswegs Nachteile, sondern vor allem Vorteile für den Schriftspracherwerb mit sich bringt. Der Artikel ist wie folgt strukturiert: Zunächst werden die Voraussetzungen für einen erfolgreichen Schriftspracherwerb dargestellt (Kapitel 2). Ein besonderes Augenmerk liegt dabei auf der Entwicklung des metalinguistischen Bewusstseins und dessen unterschiedlichen sprachlichen Ebenen als Prädiktor für die Lese- und Schreibfähigkeit. Kapitel 3 behandelt die Vorteile von Mehrsprachigkeit bezüglich der exekutiven Kontrolle und deren Einfluss auf die Entwicklung des metalinguistischen Bewusstseins. Des Weiteren wird anhand ausgewählter Studien der mehrsprachige Vorteil bei metalinguistischen Fähigkeiten aufgezeigt. Anschließend wird in Kapitel 4 das Thema Schriftspracherwerb in Bezug zur Mehrsprachigkeit gesetzt und die Hypothese, dass mehrsprachige Kinder durch ein früher entwickeltes metalinguistisches Bewusstsein, Vorteile beim Schriftspracherwerb haben, diskutiert.

2. Voraussetzungen für den Schriftspracherwerb: Familiäres Umfeld und metalinguistisches Bewusstsein

Schriftspracherwerb ist der Erwerb der Lese- und Schreibfähigkeit und beginnt in ausgewählten Bereichen bei Kindern bereits vor dem Eintritt in die Grundschule (Schneider 2017). So sind einige drei- bis vierjährige Kinder durchaus in der Lage, erste Einsichten in das orthografische Prinzip zu erwerben und im Alter von vier und fünf Jahren können bei manchen Kindern erste wichtige Entwicklungsstufen des Schriftspracherwerbs festgestellt werden (Bredel et al. 2011). Dementsprechend können Vorschulkinder beispielsweise bestimmte Logos von Supermärkten oder Tankstellen identifizieren und wiedererkennen. Dabei nehmen sie die Wörter ganzheitlich wahr, ohne die einzelnen Buchstaben unterscheiden zu können (Schneider 2017). Andere Kinder verfügen in diesem Alter zusätzlich über Buchstabenwissen und sind in der Lage, innerhalb eines Wortes einzelne Buchstaben zu identifizieren oder innerhalb eines

Satzes einzelne Wörter zu erkennen. Dies zeigt, dass Kinder mit dem Eintritt in die Grundschule unterschiedliche Vorkenntnisse im Bereich Schriftsprache aufweisen, sodass kaum von gleichen Ausgangsbedingungen für den Schriftspracherwerb ausgegangen werden kann (Schneider 2017). Besonders Kinder mit Eltern eines niedrigen sozioökonomischen Status scheinen hier benachteiligt zu sein, da der Erwerb der Schriftsprache von dem Input aus der Familie und der Gesellschaft direkt abhängig ist (Bredel et al. 2011). Im Gegensatz dazu haben Kinder, die durch ein bildungsnahes familiäres Umfeld mit Texten oder Büchern Kontakt zur Schriftsprache haben, über Gelesenes sprechen und häufiger Buchhandlungen oder Bibliotheken besuchen, nachweislich Vorteile beim Schriftspracherwerb (Hurrelmann 2009). Schulleistungsstudien wie IGLU stellen darüber hinaus fest, dass sich die Anzahl der vorhanden Bücher im Elternhaus als signifikante Einflussgröße auf die Lesefertigkeit auswirkt (Bos et al. 2003). Schründer-Lenzen (2006) weist ebenfalls darauf hin, dass bildungsnahe Familien einen höheren Wert auf Schriftsprache legen und diese positive Einstellung auf den Lerngegenstand Lesen übertragen werden kann.

Solche vorschulischen Erfahrungen, die die Kinder in der Familie oder auch im Kindergarten sammeln können, haben Auswirkungen auf die frühe Entwicklung des metalinguistischen Bewusstseins, welches als eine Grundvoraussetzung für den Beginn des Schriftspracherwerbs angesehen wird und auch im späteren Verlauf Schüler*innen dazu befähigt zu kompetenten Leser*innen und Schreiber.inen zu werden. Grosjean und Li (2012) fassen metalinguistisches Bewusstsein als das Wissen über linguistische Strukturen und das Können dieses Wissen intendiert abzurufen auf. Metalinguistische Fähigkeiten befähigen Kinder dazu, linguistische Strukturen zu analysieren und grammatische Regeln zu erkennen (Grosjean und Li 2012). Es ist eine Fähigkeit, die grundlegend und entscheidend für die Entwicklung komplexen Sprachgebrauchs (z. B. das Verständnis von Metaphern) und Schriftspracherwerb bei Kindern ist, da es ermöglicht, die Bedeutung eines Wortes von seiner Form zu trennen. Diese Trennung und die damit verbundene Einsicht in die Symbolhaftigkeit von Schrift zeichnet die erste der drei Phase des Schriftspracherwerbs nach Uta Frith (1986) aus. Diese sind: 1. logographemischen Phase, 2. Alphabetische Phase und 3. Orthographische Phase. Die Trennung von Wortbedeutung und graphischer Form in der logographemischen Phase gibt dem Kind Einsicht in die zwei Aspekte der Zeichen und wird als Bilateralität der Zeichen verstanden. Ursprünglich geht die Theorie der Bilateralität auf Ferdinand de Saussure (Saussure 2019) zurück und besagt, dass jedes Zeichen eine Ausdrucksseite (*signifiant*) und eine Inhaltseite *(signifié)* hat. Mit dem *signifiant* wird das Lautbild eines Wortes bezeichnet und mit dem *signifié* ist die Bedeutung gemeint. Um diese Einsicht in die Symbolhaftigkeit der Zeichen zu gewinnen und dessen Arbitrarität zu verstehen, müssen spezifische kognitive Fähigkeiten entwickelt sein, wie z. B. die Aufmerksamkeitskontrolle (exekutive Funktion). Nach Bialystok und Barac (2012) stellt besonders die Arbitrarität eine besonders hohe Anforderung an die Aufmerksamkeitskontrolle, weil es keine von außen nachvollziehbare Beziehung zwischen den Wörtern einer bestimmten Sprache und dem Konzept, das sie repräsentieren, gibt. Diese ist arbiträr und Kinder müssen zunächst lernen, die graphische Form eines Wortes von seiner Bedeutung zu trennen, um diese dann durch kontrollierte Aufmerksamkeit separat zu betrachten und auf allen sprachlichen Ebenen zu analysieren (Barac & Bialystok 2012).

Für den ganzen Prozess des Schriftspracherwerbs ist somit das metalinguistische Bewusstsein grundlegend, um beispielsweise beim Lesen aus Wörtern und Texten den Sinn des Gelesenen zu entnehmen. Besonders das schnelle und hochautomatisierte Abrufen der Wörter und ihrer Bedeutungen aus dem mentalen Lexikon zeichnen gute Leser aus (Schneider 2017). Längsschnittstudien belegen, dass eine Entwicklung des metalinguistischen Bewusstseins vor Schuleintritt positive Auswirkungen auf den Erwerb von Lese- und Schreibfähigkeiten in der Grundschule hat, z. B. durch schnellere Wortdekodierung oder der höheren Geschwindigkeit bei der Informationsverarbeitung (Schneider 2017).

Obwohl das metalinguistische Bewusstsein alle sprachlichen Ebenen umfasst, wurde im Zusammenhang mit dem Schriftspracherwerb bislang überwiegend das phonologische Bewusstsein untersucht. In der Forschung herrscht Konsens darüber, dass das phonologische Bewusstsein ausschlaggebend für den Schriftsprach- und Leseerwerb ist (Bredel et al. 2011; Bryant et al. 1990; Moll et al. 2012). Das phonologische Bewusstsein lässt sich als „[…] die Fähigkeit, ein lautliches Wort mit seiner Silben- und Betonungsstruktur in untergeordnete Einheiten – im engeren Sinn Laute, im weiteren Sinn Silben bzw. Silbenkonstituenten – zu gliedern." (Bredel et al. 2011, S. 91) definieren. Ein weiter entwickeltes phonologisches Bewusstsein befähigt Kinder beim Schriftspracherwerb dazu, sich auf die lautlichen Aspekte von Sprache zu konzentrieren und dabei die Wortbedeutung zu abstrahieren. Die Relevanz des phonologischen Bewusstseins für den Schriftspracherwerb belegt u.a. die Studie von Schneider und Näslund (1993), die im letzten Kindergarten Jahr verschiedene Prädikatoren, wie Intelligenz, Arbeitsgedächtnis und phonologisches Bewusstsein, für den Schriftspracherwerb bei den Proband*innen teste und nach den ersten zwei Grundschuljahren die Wortdekodierung , das Leseverstehen und die Rechtschreibung der Proband*innen prüfte. Die Studie zeigt, dass alle im Vorfeld getesteten Prädikatoren einen signifikanten Einfluss auf den Schriftspracherwerb hatten, wobei das phonologische Bewusstsein den stärksten direkten Einfluss auf die Lese- und Rechtschreibfähigkeit hatte (Schneider & Näslund 1993).

Schründer-Lenzen (2013) sieht das phonologische Bewusstsein sogar als zentrale Vorläuferfähigkeit des Schriftspracherwerbs an und Schneider (2017) bezeichnet die übergeordnete phonologische Informationsverarbeitung als eine relevante Voraussetzung für den Schriftspracherwerb. Diese Verarbeitung wird in das phonologische Bewusstsein, die Kapazität des Arbeitsgedächtnisses und die Benenngeschwindigkeit untergliedert. Das phonologische Bewusstsein zeigt sich bei Kindern durch das Erkennen von Reimen, das Identifizieren einzelner Wörter in Sätzen, die Gliederung von Silben in Wörtern und das Erkennen von unterschiedlichen Wortlängen. Besonders letzteres stellt für Vorschulkinder eine große Herausforderung dar, da sie in dem Alter nicht in der Lage sind, die Bedeutung des Wortes von der Struktur zu trennen. Schneider (2017) nennt an dieser Stelle das Beispiel „Bus vs. Kinderwagen". Vorschulkinder haben oft Schwierigkeiten, bei der Frage nach der Länge der beiden Wörter ihre Bedeutung zu unterdrücken und ziehen die Schlussfolgerung, dass „Bus", aufgrund seiner Größe in der realen Welt, das längere Wort sein müsse. Sie sind noch nicht in der Lage, sich auf die Buchstabenzahl zu fokussieren (Schneider 2017).

Neben dem phonologischen Bewusstsein wird auch die Rolle oder der Einfluss des semantischen Bewusstseins für die Lesefähigkeit erforscht. Frost (2001) zeigt, dass die phonologische Bewusstheit ebenfalls eine entscheidende Rolle für das Lesen spielt, allerdings begrenzt sich die Relevanz auf das Anfangsstadium des Lesenlernens, die logographemische Phase. Im weiteren Verlauf des Erwerbs von Lesefähigkeiten hat das semantische Bewusstsein im Sinne der Dekodierung auf Wortebene sowie übergeordneter semantischen Strategien eine wichtigere Bedeutung (Wolf & Katzir-Cohen 2001). Eine dieser Strategien ist die Ambiguitätserkennung. Diese ist als Teil des metalinguistischen Bewusstseins auf semantischer Ebene ausschlaggebend für die Dekodierung auf Wortebene, da Kinder bewusst Kontrolle über die zugrundeliegenden mentalen Prozesse ausüben müssen, um zu erkennen, dass Wörter und Sätze Doppelbedeutungen haben und sie in der Lage sein müssen, diese Bedeutungen neu zu verarbeiten (Zipke et al. 2009). Folglich ist das semantische Bewusstsein die zweite metalinguistische Ebene, die eine wichtige Voraussetzung für den Schriftspracherwerb darstellt.

Nur wenige Studien haben sich bislang mit dem semantischen Bewusstsein im Zusammenhang mit Schriftspracherwerb auseinandergesetzt. Eine dieser wenigen Studien ist die Langzeitstudie von Frost et al. (2005). In dieser

Studie wird die Beziehung zwischen vorschulischen semantischen Fähigkeiten (Wortschatz, Satzverständnis und Satzbau), phonologischem Bewusstsein und Leseverstehen bei Kindern und Jugendlichen in regelmäßigen Abständen vom dritten bis zum sechzehnten Lebensjahr untersucht. Es konnte gezeigt werden, dass das semantische Bewusstsein (Wortschatz, Sprachverständnis und Satzproduktion) im Alter von drei Jahren, Interesse für Bilderbücher im Alter von drei Jahren und phonologisches Bewusstsein im Alter von sechs Jahren, die Lesefähigkeit im Alter von 16 Jahren signifikant beeinflussen, indem die Leseleistungen der 16-Jährigen mit diesen Eigenschaften besser waren als die, der Jugendlichen ohne diese Eigenschaften.

Eine weitere Studie, die die Bedeutung des semantischen Bewusstseins für die Lesefähigkeit belegt, ist die Studie von Browne Rego & Bryant (1993). Diese zeigt, dass syntaktische und semantische Fähigkeiten dem Kind dazu verhelfen, mehrsilbige Wörter und Fremdwörter zu verstehen und zu lesen. In dieser Langzeitstudie wurden Kinder im Alter von fünf bis sechs Jahren über den Zeitraum des ersten Schuljahres untersucht. Im ersten Teil der Studie wurden drei Tests zum syntaktischen und semantischen Bewusstsein durchgeführt Der zweite Teil der Studie wurde fünf Monate später durchgeführt. Es wurde ein Lesetest durchgeführt, bei dem die Kinder zunächst einzelne Wörter kontextlos lasen und später Wörter, die in einen Kontext eingebettet waren. Kinder, die im ersten Teil der Studie eine höhere Punktzahl bei den syntaktischen und semantischen Aufgaben erreichten, konnten im zweiten Teil der Studie mehr im Kontext eingebettete Wörter lesen als Kinder mit einer niedrigeren Punktzahl im ersten Teil der Studie. Die Autoren schlussfolgern, dass Kinder die sensibel für semantische und syntaktische Kategorien sind, diese Kategorien erfolgreich als Hinweise beim Lesen einsetzen können.

Neben den Studien, die sich mit den einzelnen Ebenen des metalinguistischen Bewusstseins und dessen Auswirkungen auf den Schriftspracherwerb befassen, gibt es auch Studien, die einen möglichen Einfluss von Training auf die Entwicklung von metalinguistischem Bewusstseins zum Forschungsgegenstand machen. Besonders unter Einbezug von Mehrsprachigkeit sind diese Studien interessant, da Mehrsprachigkeit als eine Art regelmäßige Übung für das metalinguistische Bewusstsein, durch die konstante Auseinandersetzung mit zwei oder mehreren Sprachen, gesehen werden kann. Dieser Aspekt des Trainings wird in der Studie von Schneider et al. (1994) erforscht. Diese Studie belegt, dass metalinguistisches Bewusstsein – hier insbesondere das phonologische Bewusstsein – durch bewusstes Training gefördert werden kann. In der Studie wird allerdings nicht zwischen einsprachigen und mehrsprachigen Kindern unterschieden und auch der sozioökonomische Status der Eltern wird nicht berücksichtigt. Kinder der Trainingsgruppe nahmen an einem Förderprogramm teil, das aus 15-minütigen Trainingseinheiten (Sprachspiele) bestand und über 6 Monate täglich im Kindergarten durchgeführt wurde. Die Kontrollgruppe absolvierte den normalen Kindergartenalltag. Zu Beginn des ersten Schuljahres wurde mit den Kindern ein metalinguistischer Transfertest durchgeführt und Ende des ersten Schuljahres ein Lesetest. Die Studie belegt, dass Trainingseffekte sowohl bei dem metalinguistischen Transfertest als auch bei den Lesetests nachzuweisen sind und die Leseleistungen sich verbesserten, wenn das phonologisches Bewusstsein der Kinder gezielt gefördert wurde.

Die Studie von Zipke et al. (2009) kommt zu vergleichbaren Ergebnissen. Kinder im Durchschnittsalter von acht Jahren aus Familien mit niedrigem sozioökonomischem Status nahmen an der Studie teil. Der Fokus lag auf der Erkennung von Ambiguität von Wörtern und auf der Forschungsfrage, ob das Leseverstehen bei Kindern aus Familien mit niedrigem sozioökonomischem Status durch Training der Ambiguitätserkennung verbessert werden kann. Die Ergebnisse zeigen sowohl, dass die Instruktionen zur metalinguistischen Ambiguität effektiv waren und dieses Training das Leseverständnis der Schüler*innen verbesserte als auch, dass das Erkennen von mehrdeutigen Wörtern und Verarbeitung dieser einen positiven Einfluss auf den Schriftspracherwerb – insbesondere das Lesen – haben. Über die Nachhaltigkeit der Effekte, die für die Argumentation der Studie von großer Relevanz wäre, wurden jedoch keine Aussage gemacht.

Zusammenfassend kann man festhalten, dass die vorgestellte Forschung positive Auswirkungen eines gut entwickelten metalinguistischen Bewusstseins bei Kindern vor dem Schuleintritt auf den Erwerb des Schriftspracherwerbs in der Schule belegt. Zudem sind die unterschiedlichen Ebenen des metalinguistischen Bewusstseins zu unterschiedlichen Phasen des Schriftspracherwerbs von Bedeutung. Das phonologische Bewusstsein, das am meisten untersucht wurde, ist besonders zu Beginn des Schriftspracherwerbs wichtig, während das weniger erforschte semantische Bewusstsein eine ebenfalls wichtige Rolle und zwar in allen weiteren Erwerbsphasen spielt. Außerdem zeigen die vorgestellten Studien, die das phonologische Bewusstsein im Zusammenhang mit Schriftsprachleistungen untersucht haben, dass das metalinguistische Bewusstsein durch Übungen trainiert werden kann. Aufgrund dieser Ergebnisse lässt sich die Hypothese aufstellen, dass mehrsprachige Kinder durch den früheren Erwerb des metalinguistischen Bewusstseins schneller die Schriftsprache beim Schuleintritt erwerben und bessere Leistungen beim Lesen in den ersten Grundschuljahren erreichen könnten. Es ist aber zu beachten, dass bis dato vor allem metalinguistisches Bewusstsein von Kindern auf der phonologischen Ebene und dessen Beitrag zum Schriftspracherwerb untersucht wurde (Ibrahim et al. 2007). Folglich ist der Einfluss des phonologischen Bewusstseins auf das Lesenlernen weit anerkannt (Zipke et al. 2009). Es gibt kaum aber Studien, die sich mit dem semantischen Bewusstsein und deren Einfluss auf den Schriftspracherwerb beschäftigen. Das semantische Bewusstsein muss in Zusammenhang mit Mehrsprachigkeit weiter erforscht werden, da mehrsprachige Kinder beispielsweise an die Doppelbedeutung von Wörtern gewöhnt sind und dadurch eventuell bessere Leistungen in der Sinnentnahme von Sätzen und Texten erbringen könnten als monolinguale Kinder.

3. Vorteile von Mehrsprachigkeit: Exekutive Kontrolle und metalinguistisches Bewusstsein

Ergebnisse der Mehrsprachigkeitsforschung belegen, dass mehrsprachige Personen kognitive Vorteile gegenüber monolingualen Personen haben. Diese Vorteile leiten sich von ihrer Fähigkeit zwei oder mehr Sprachen zu gebrauchen und zu managen ab (Bialystok et al. 2004; Bialystok 2017; Grosjean & Li 2012; Hilchey & Klein 2011). Diese Vorteile wurden ausgiebig für die Organisation des Wortschatzes und das Abrufen der Bedeutung der Wörter aus dem mentalen Lexikon bei Mehrsprachigen untersucht. Besonders sogenannte Priming[2] Experimente eignen sich gut, um das mentale Lexikon zu erforschen. Beispielsweise zeigt Amengual (2016), dass bei bilingualen Personen beide Sprachen stets aktiv sind und bei mehrsprachigen Sprecher*innen somit ständig Wörter beider Sprachen koaktiviert werden. Diese Koaktivierung verlangt für die Sprachverarbeitung eine besondere Aufmerksamkeitskontrolle bei der Auswahl der intendierten Sprache und Unterdrückung der nicht geforderten Sprache oder Sprachen. Die dauerhafte und intensive Aufmerksamkeitskontrolle, der eine monolinguale Person nicht ständig ausgesetzt ist (Bialystok et al. 2009; Bialystok 2017), bringt mehrsprachigen Sprecher*innen Vorteile nicht nur für die Bewältigung von verbalen Aufgaben, sondern auch von nicht verbalen Aufgaben, die in Bezug zu den exekutiven Funktionen stehen wie z. B. die Aufmerksamkeitskontrolle (Bialystok 2017; Prior & MacWhinney 2010). Best und Miller (2010) sowie Blair (2016) verstehen unter exekutiven Funktionen kognitive Prozesse, die der adaptiven und zielgerichteten Kontrolle von Gedanken,

2 Beim Priming findet „durch einen vorausgegangenen Reiz eine Voraktivierung bzw. neuronale Bahnung im Gehirn statt [...], die die nachfolgende Verarbeitung (z.B. die nachfolgenden Reize) beeinflusst." Delucchi Danhier und Mertins (2018).

Verhalten und Gefühlen unterliegen. Miyake et al. (2000) gehen davon aus, dass die exekutiven Funktionen aus drei Hauptdomänen bestehen: Veränderung, Unterdrückung und Aktualisierung. Dementsprechend ist das konstante Aufmerksamkeitsmanagement, dem mehrsprachige Personen ständig ausgesetzt sind, eine mentale Übung für das exekutive System (Hilchey & Klein 2011).

Diese Fähigkeit mehrsprachiger Sprecher*innen, die Aufmerksamkeit auf einen bestimmten Aspekt und dessen Lösung schneller und präziser zu fokussieren, belegt Bialystok in einer Studie, in der sie anhand von Tests zum grammatischen Urteilsvermögen zeigte, dass bilinguale Kinder bei linguistischen Aufgaben ihre Aufmerksamkeit besser auf die relevante sprachliche Information fokussieren und für die Aufgabe unwichtige Informationen unterdrücken konnten als monolinguale Kinder desselben Alters (Bialystok 1992). Diese Ergebnisse weisen auf die weiter entwickelten exekutiven Funktionen der Aufmerksamkeitskontrolle und besser entwickelten Inhibitionsmechanismen bei bilingualen Kindern hin. Wie im vorigen Kapitel erläutert wurde, sind gerade diese Fähigkeiten beim Erwerb der Schriftsprache von zentraler Bedeutung, da die Unterdrückung irrelevanter Informationen es Kindern erlauben, ihre Aufmerksamkeit gezielt so zu steuern, dass sie die graphische Form eines Wortes und dessen Bedeutung getrennt voneinander betrachten und analysieren können.

Wie in Kapitel 2 dargestellt, müssen spezifische exekutive Funktionen, wie die Aufmerksamkeitskontrolle und die Unterdrückung, vorhanden sein, damit sich metalinguistisches Bewusstsein überhaupt entwickeln kann. Bereits Vygotsky (1964) stellte in seinem Buch „Thought and Language" erstmals die Vermutung auf, dass Bilingualismus die metalinguistischen Fähigkeiten von Kindern beeinflusst, da bilinguale Kinder stärker an die Willkürlichkeit der Wort-Bedeutung Verbindung gewöhnt sind und es einfacher für sie ist, diese zu kontrollieren. Auch Bialystok (1986) zeigt, dass bilinguale Kinder früher als monolinguale über ein metalinguistisches Bewusstsein auf grammatischer Ebene verfügen. Ihre Studie belegte, dass bilinguale Kinder grammatisch korrekte Sätze als richtig identifizierten, auch wenn der Satz semantisch keinen Sinn ergab. Monolinguale Kinder bezeichneten diese Sätze hingegen als grammatisch falsch. Dies zeigt, dass sie die semantischen Informationen schlechter oder gar nicht unterdrücken.

Die Metaanalyse von Adesope et al. (2010) von 63 Studien bestätigt die früheren Ergebnisse von Bialystok, dass Bilingualismus das metalinguistische Bewusstsein stärkt und eine Schlüsselkomponente dieses bilingualen Vorteils die Aufmerksamkeitskontrolle ist, die es den bilingualen Personen erlaubt, schneller relevante Merkmale zu beachten und irreführende auszublenden.

In dieser Metaanalyse wird jedoch nicht zwischen den verschiedenen Ebenen des metalinguistischen Bewusstseins unterschieden. Eine solche Unterscheidung ist jedoch notwendig, da sie unterschiedliche Phasen des Schriftspracherwerbs betreffen. So ist besonders das phonologische Bewusstsein zu Beginn des Schriftspracherwerbs, in der logographemischen Phase, von größter Bedeutung, während das syntaktische und semantische Bewusstsein in allen weiteren Phasen an Bedeutung gewinnt. Diese Unterscheideidung nehmen Reder et.al. (2013) in ihrer Studie zu bilingualen Vorteilen bezüglich des metalinguistischen Bewusstseins vor. Sie fanden heraus, dass französisch-deutsch bilinguale Kinder bessere Leistungen bei morphologischen und syntaktischen Bewusstseinsaufgaben zeigten als monolinguale französische Kinder und bestätigten damit ebenfalls frühere Ergebnisse von Bialystok (1986). Bei den Aufgaben zum phonologischen Bewusstsein fand die Studie hingegen keine Unterschiede zwischen den monolingualen und bilingualen Kindern. Dies lässt die Hypothese zu, dass mehrsprachige Kinder zu Beginn des Schriftspracherwerbs, in der das phonologische Bewusstsein eine zentrale Rolle spielt, sich nicht von monolingualen Kindern unterscheiden, jedoch in späteren Phasen des Schriftspracherwerbs Vorteile im Bereich des semantischen Bewusstseins gegenüber monolingualen Kindern entwickeln.

Es gibt auch Studien, die die zuvor dargestellten bilingualen Vorteile nicht identifiziert haben. Zum Beispiel untersuchten Rosenblum und Pinker (1983) die Word-Objekt Beziehung, dessen Verständnis Rückschlüsse auf die Entwicklung des metalinguistischen Bewusstseins zulässt. Sie stellten keine Unterschiede zwischen monolingualen und bilingualen Kindern fest, obwohl sie Alter, Geschlecht, nichtsprachliche Intelligenz und den sozioökonomischen Status der Eltern konstant hielten. Kritisch ist hier aber anzumerken, dass die Stichprobe nur aus 12 Proband*innen pro Gruppe bestand und somit die Ergebnisse nicht als repräsentativ gelten können. Außerdem sehen die Autoren als möglichen Grund für die abweichenden Ergebnisse zu anderen Studien, dass alle Eltern der Kinder Akademiker waren und die Kinder eventuell aufgrund der familiären Bildungsnähe weiterentwickelt waren, als für ihr Alter üblich. Auch die Studie von Altman et al. (2018) konnte keinen bilingualen Vorteil feststellen. Hier wurde die Rolle der Sprachdominanz in Beziehung zu metalinguistischem Bewusstsein auf morphologischer und lexikalischer Ebene untersucht. Die Proband*innen wurden in drei Gruppen eingeteilt: Monolinguale Kinder, bilinguale Kinder, dominant in der Herkunftssprache und bilinguale Kinder mit Dominanz in der Umgebungssprache. Die Ergebnisse zeigen keine Unterschiede zwischen den Gruppen der monolingualen und bilingualen Kinder, die in der Umgebungssprache dominant waren. Jedoch erbrachten die monolingualen Kinder bessere Leistungen als die Kinder mit Sprachdominanz in der Herkunftssprache, was auf einen geringeren Wortschatz in der Umgebungssprache zurückgeführt wurde. Altman et al. begründen diesen Befund damit, dass das metalinguistische Bewusstsein auf Spracherfahrungen und Sprachkenntnisse aufbaut. Metalinguistisches Bewusstsein kann somit in den verschiedenen Sprachen der Kinder unterschiedlich weit entwickelt sein. Um Ergebnisse zu erhalten, aufgrund derer die bilingualen Vorteile entkräftet werden könnten, müsste das metalinguistische Bewusstsein für jede Sprache des Kindes einzeln untersucht werden.

Obgleich Paap (2019) in seinem Artikel zum bilingualen Vorteil die Ansicht vertritt, dass zwar viele Studien den geschilderten Vorteil in den exekutiven Funktionen bestätigen, betont er dennoch, dass die Ergebnisse der Studien nicht aussagekräftig seien, da die bilingualen Vorteile auf sehr spezielle Fälle beschränkt seien und nicht für alle bilingualen Sprecher*innen übertragbar seien. Beispielsweise könnten sich Vorteile bei einer Gruppe von bilingualen Kindern zeigen, die in beiden Sprachen ausgeglichenen Input erhalten und balanciert bilingual sind. Bei einer anderen Gruppe bilingualer Kinder, die andere Voraussetzungen mitbringen, müssen diese Vorteile nicht unbedingt immer vorhanden sein bzw. identifiziert werden können. Diese Argumentation lässt sich aber entkräften, da die Ergebnisse zu den Vorteilen des Bilingualismus die breite Spanne individueller bilingualer Facetten widerspiegeln und die Diversität der Gruppe der Bilingualen kein Nachteil ist, sondern ein besonderes Merkmal der Bilingualen, welches bei der Auswertung der Ergebnisse beachtet werden muss. Im gleichen Sinne argumentieren auch (Barac & Bialystok 2012) und heben dabei hervor, dass die unterschiedlichen Gruppen bi- und mehrsprachiger Personen nicht unbedingt vergleichbare Ergebnisse bei linguistischen und metalinguistischen Aufgaben zeigen müssen, dennoch aber für die jeweilige Gruppe als repräsentativ gelten. Bei der Betrachtung der vermeintlich widersprüchlichen Datenlage sollten die Stichprobengröße, die Methoden sowie die Kriterien für die Zusammenstellung der Probanden*innen (Bilingualität vs. Monolingualität) immer in Betracht gezogen werden. Jede bilinguale Gruppe besteht immer aus einer relativ heterogenen Sprecher*innengruppe, die sich sowohl in ihren Sprachen als auch in den individuellen Spracherfahrungen unterscheidet. Um diese Varianz aufzufangen, müssen Faktoren wie Sprachdominanz, Input, sozioökonomische Faktoren sowie Spracheinstellungen der Familie und Gesellschaft bei der Auswertung unbedingt berücksichtigt werden. Eine gut funktionierende Methode, diese Faktoren konstant zu halten, sind standardisierte Elternfragebögen, die bei jeder Studie mitdurchgeführt werden sollten. Durch die Kombination verschiedener methodischer

Zugänge und unter Berücksichtigung aller Faktoren, die Bilingualität beeinflussen können, besteht dann mehr Hoffnung, dass Studien vergleichbare und valide Ergebnisse liefern werden.

Aus diesen Gründen macht die Gruppeneinteilung in mehrsprachige und einsprachige Kinder sowie der Vergleich dieser beiden Gruppen keinen Sinn. Diese Einteilung führt zu einem Vergleich zwischen zwei Gruppen, die sich in sich systematisch weiterhin durch andere Merkmale unterscheiden, die wiederum Auswirkungen auf die exekutiven Funktionen haben könnten und die Ergebnisse verfälschen würden (Paap 2019). Eines dieser Merkmale ist der Einfluss des sozioökonomischen Status der Eltern. Studien zeigen, dass ein geringer sozioökonomischer Status der Eltern Einfluss auf eine Reihe von kognitiven Systemen und das Hirnvolumen haben kann (Noble et al. 2012). Kinder, deren Eltern einen hohen sozioökonomischen Status haben, weisen dagegen bessere kognitive Leistungen auf und steigen mit besseren Voraussetzungen in die Schullaufbahn ein (Niklas & Schneider 2015). Der sozioökonomische Status der Eltern muss folglich in jeder Studie mit mehrsprachigen Kindern mit erhoben werden, um dessen Einfluss auf die Ergebnisse zu kontrollieren. Infolgedessen können Studien, die dem Vorteil von Mehrsprachigkeit widersprechen und den sozioökonomischen Staus nicht mit erheben, nicht ernst genommen werden.

Die Vorteile von Mehrsprachigkeit in Frage zu stellen, ist aufgrund der unterschiedlichen Zusammensetzung der Stichproben und Methoden, wie oben beschrieben, nicht nachvollziehbar. Wenn sämtliche Merkmale der bilingualen und monolingualen Gruppe, wie beispielsweise Alter, Geschlecht, Intelligenz, sozioökonomischer Status, Geschwisterkonstellation, Sprachinput und Sprachbalance konstant gehalten würden, könnte man nachweisen, dass die Mehrheit der Studien zur Untersuchung der exekutiven Funktionen und des metalinguistischen Bewusstseins von Kindern einen mehrsprachigen Vorteil zeigen. Der Vergleich unterschiedlicher Gruppen von Mehrsprachigen, mit den unterschiedlichen Ausprägungen der Mehrsprachigkeit führt selbstverständlich auch zu unterschiedlichen Ergebnissen, die dementsprechend interpretiert werden müssen.

Kurzum hat Mehrsprachigkeit *per se* das Potential, das Gehirn und die kognitiven Systeme zu modifizieren (Bialystok 2017) und fördert durch die ständige Sprachauswahl besonders die exekutiven Funktionen der Unterdrückung und Aufmerksamkeitskontrolle, basierend auf der Annahme, dass die Nicht-Zielsprache unterdrückt wird, um Interferenzen zu vermeiden (Bialystok 2017). Die exekutiven Funktionen stehen wiederum in Verbindung mit der Entwicklung des metalinguistischen Bewusstseins, welches folglich bei Mehrsprachigen früher entwickelt wird und Vorteile für den Schriftspracherwerb zur Folge hat.

4. Mehrsprachigkeit und Schriftspracherwerb

Wie bereits oben dargestellt, spielt die exekutive Kontrolle und das metalinguistische Bewusstsein eine wesentliche Rolle für einen erfolgreichen Schriftspracherwerb. In Anlehnung an frühere Studien wird hier die Hypothese aufgestellt, dass mehrsprachige Kinder schneller und früher die Schriftsprache erwerben könnten als monolinguale Kinder. Trotz der vielen Vorteile, die für andere Bereiche bereits belegt sind, gibt es im Bereich Schriftspracherwerb bei mehrsprachigen Kindern nur defizitorientierte Ansätze. Studien aus den Erziehungswissenschaften oder der Deutschdidaktik z. B. Schrüner-Lenzen (2004), untersuchen überwiegend die Beziehung zwischen verschiedenen didaktischen Methoden des Schriftspracherwerbs und den Leistungen im Lesen und Schreiben von Kindern mit Migrationshintergrund. Bei diesen Studien werden weder die Vorläuferkompetenzen des Schriftspracherwerbs noch der sozioökonomische Status der Eltern in die Analyse miteinbezogen, sodass keine Aussagen über die möglichen Vorteile von Mehrsprachigkeit und den Einfluss des sozioökonomischen Status auf den Schriftspracherwerb gemacht werden können. Deswegen sind die Ergebnisse dieser Studien für die Mehrsprachigkeitsforschung unbedeutend.

Gerade die Vorläuferkompetenzen des Schriftspracherwerbs sind aber ausschlaggebend für den späteren erfolgreichen Erwerb der Schriftsprache. Diese Kompetenzen sind bei ein- und mehrsprachigen Kindern – aufgrund der oben benannten Vorteile Mehrsprachiger in den exekutiven Funktionen und der Entwicklung des metalinguistischem Bewusstseins – unterschiedlich gut ausgeprägt. Jedoch befassen sich nur wenige Studien mit diesen Unterschieden und mit dessen Einfluss auf den Verlauf des Schriftspracherwerbs. So wird in der Studie von Huschka et al.(2020), ebenfalls defizitär orientiert, untersucht, ob die vorschulischen Prädikationsmuster für die Vorhersage von Lese- und Rechtschreibkompetenzen bei monolingualen deutschen Kindern und mehrsprachigen Kindern vergleichbar sind. Sowohl der sozioökonomische Status der Eltern als auch die kognitive Leistungsfähigkeit der Kinder wurden kontrolliert. In der Studie wurde die phonologische Bewusstheit, die phonologische Schleife,[3] die Benenngeschwindigkeit[4] und die behaviorale Selbstregulation[5]

3 Temporäres Speichern von Phoneminformationen im Kurzzeitgedächtnis (Huschka et al. 2020, S. 194).

4 Misst das Rekodieren von Phoneminformationen aus dem Langzeitgedächtnis (Huschka et al. 2020, S194).

5 Steuerung der eigenen Aufmerksamkeit, Folgen von Anweisungen und Unterlassen unangemessener Handlungen (Huschka et al. 2020, S. 194).

im letzten Jahr vor der Einschulung getestet. Zum Ende des ersten Schuljahres wurde die Lesegeschwindigkeit (anhand des Lesens von Pseudowörtern), das Leseverständnis (Satz- und Textverständnis) und die Rechtschreibung (Lückendiktate) untersucht. Die Befunde bestätigen die Ergebnisse der Studien zum phonologischen Bewusstsein bei monolingualen Kindern. So hat auch in dieser Studie das phonologische Bewusstsein bei monolingualen Kindern eine große Bedeutung für den Beginn des Schriftspracherwerbs und Auswirkungen auf die drei getesteten Bereiche: Lesegeschwindigkeit, Leseverständnis und Rechtschreibung. Die Ergebnisse zeigen aber auch, dass es unterschiedliche Prädiktoren für monolinguale und multilinguale Kinder im Hinblick auf den Schriftspracherwerb gibt. Für Mehrsprachige wirkt sich das phonologische Bewusstsein nur auf die Bereiche des Leseverstehens und der Rechtschreibung aus. Das bedeutet, dass ein gut entwickeltes phonologisches Bewusstsein im letzten Kindergartenjahr bei Mehrsprachigen bessere Lese- und Rechtsschreibleistungen zum Ende des ersten Schuljahres (wie auch bei einsprachigen Kindern) bewirkt. Für die Lesegeschwindigkeit hat das phonologische Bewusstsein jedoch bei Mehrsprachigen keine Bedeutung. Mehrsprachige, mit weniger gut entwickeltem phonologischem Bewusstsein erbrachten trotzdem eine hohe Lesegeschwindigkeit. Dies könnte damit zusammenhängen, dass die Lesegeschwindigkeit anhand des Lesens von Pseudowörtern gemessen wurde, bei denen Mehrsprachige ihre Vorteile der exekutiven Funktionen (Unterdrückung irrelevanter Informationen und Aufmerksamkeitskontrolle) zu Gute kommen könnten. Für die Mehrsprachigkeitsforschung ist die Tatsache, dass für monolinguale und bilinguale Kinder andere Ebenen des metalinguistischen Bewusstseins unterschiedliche Einflüsse auf die Bereiche des Schriftspracherwerbs haben, von großer Bedeutung. Weitere Studien sind notwendig, die die einzelnen Ebenen des metalinguistischen Bewusstseins untersuchen und deren Bedeutung für den Schriftspracherwerb bei bilingualen Kindern herausarbeiten.

Die Frage nach der Bedeutung anderer Ebenen des metalinguistischen Bewusstseins beim Schriftspracherwerb mehrsprachiger Kinder untersucht die Studie von Jasińska & Petitto (2018), deren Schwerpunkt im Gegensatz zu Huschka et al. (2020) nicht auf dem phonologischen Bewusstsein, sondern auf dem semantischen Bewusstsein liegt. Die Studie vergleicht die Lesekompetenzen von ein- und mehrsprachigen Kindern mit unterschiedlichem Erwerbsalter der weiteren Sprache. Zum Zeitpunkt der Studie waren die Kinder zwischen sechs und zehn Jahren alt. Die Autoren fokussieren auf das semantische Bewusstsein mit der Begründung, dass dieses ab dem Zeitpunkt, an dem Kinder zu erfahrenen Lesern werden, wichtiger als das phonologische Bewusstsein ist. Dies lässt sich dadurch begründen, dass die Konzentration auf die Bedeutung des Wortes effektiver und schneller ist, als die Fokussierung auf die Orthographie und das mühevolle Dekodieren der Wörter (Berends & Reitsma 2006). Die Ergebnisse der Studie belegen, dass Mehrsprachigkeit und das Alter des Erwerbsbeginns der zweiten Sprache (je früher desto besser) das Lesen und die Sprache von Kindern positiv beeinflussen. Dies zeigt sich daran, dass mehrsprachige Kinder monolinguale Kinder im Passagenverständnis übertrafen, indem sie mehr fehlende Wörter in den vorgegebenen Sätzen einsetzen konnten und ebenfalls bessere Ergebnisse beim Lesen von Pseudowörtern erbrachten, indem sie mehr unbekannte Wörter, bei denen die Graphem-Phonem Regeln der Zielsprache verletzt wurden, lesen konnten. Beim Lesen von zielsprachig korrekten Wörtern konnte kein Unterschied gefunden werden.

Grundsätzlich bietet der mehrsprachige Spracherwerb Kindern spezifische Sprachvorteile. Beispielsweise haben mehrsprachige Kinder in jeder ihrer Sprachen ein Wort für ein Objekt, sodass sie zwei oder mehr Bedeutungen für dasselbe Objekt haben. Dadurch haben sie ein frühes Verständnis für die willkürliche Beziehung zwischen realen Objekten und ihren linguistischen Ausprägungen. Dieses Verständnis hilft den Kindern bei der Trennung von graphischer Form und Bedeutung eines Wortes und ist eine Voraussetzung für den Beginn des Schriftspracherwerbs, wie in Kapitel 2 bereits erläutert. Diese spezifischen Sprachvorteile zeigen ebenfalls Huschka et al. (2020) sowie Jasińska & Petitto (2018) in ihrer Forschung. Sie untersuchten die Bedeutung verschiedener Teilaspekte oder Komponenten des metalinguistischen Bewusstseins für den Schriftspracherwerb, insbesondere für die Lesefähigkeit. Mehrsprachige Kinder können ihre Aufmerksamkeit besser auf die graphische Form der Wörter lenken und gleichzeitig die Bedeutung der Wörter unterdrücken. Somit erlangten Bilinguale in beiden Studien bessere Ergebnisse durch eine höhere Anzahl gelesener Wörter. Durch den Fokus auf den Vergleich von mehr- und einsprachigen Kindern konnte bewiesen werden, dass es unter Kontrolle des sozioökonomischen Status keine Defizite bei den mehrsprachigen Kindern gibt, sondern mehrsprachige Kinder sogar Vorteile beim Leseverstehen vorweisen, die sich in der Lesegeschwindigkeit und dem Leseverstehen niederschlagen.

Es fehlen in der Forschung bislang Studien, die den Effekt der Mehrsprachigkeit auf die verschiedenen Bereiche des metalinguistischen Bewusstseins und dessen Entwicklung im Zusammenhang mit dem Schriftspracherwerb systematisch untersuchen und sich nicht ausschließlich auf das phonologische Bewusstsein fokussieren. Inwieweit das semantische Bewusstsein ebenfalls eine Vorläuferkompetenz des Schriftspracherwerbs ist, wurde zwar bei monolingualen Kindern erforscht und belegt, stellt aber bei mehrsprachigen Kindern eine klare Forschungslücke dar. Zudem wurde keine Studie durchgeführt, die den Zusammenhang von Mehrsprachigkeit, Schriftspracherwerb und sozialer Herkunft systematisch untersucht.

5. Methodischer Zugang

Die hier vorgestellten Studien zum Schriftspracherwerb sind zum größten Teil Verhaltensstudien mit monolingualen Proband*innen. Der Fokus der Studien liegt darauf, Prädiktoren für einen erfolgreichen Schriftspracherwerb im Kindergartenalter zu identifizieren. Dabei wird insbesondere das phonologische Bewusstsein als der wichtigste Faktor untersucht und in den ersten beiden Grundschuljahren im Zusammenhang mit den Leistungen im Leseverständnis, Lesegeschwindigkeit sowie der Rechtschreibung weiter erforscht. Problematisch bei diesen Studien ist allerdings, dass sie kaum Elternfragebögen zur Erarbeitung der individuellen Faktoren (sozioökonomischer Hintergrund der Familie, lesendes Umgebung, sprachlicher Input usw.) einsetzen und somit keine Aussagen über das Zusammenspiel dieser Faktoren und den Prädiktoren für den Schriftspracherwerb machen können. Darüber hinaus werden die unterschiedlichen Ebenen des metalinguistischen Bewusstseins in der Regel zusammen und nicht einzeln untersucht. Somit können keine, auf die Teilaspekte des metalinguistischen Bewusstseins bezogenen Aussagen gemacht werden. Es gibt außerdem kaum einschlägige Forschung, die sich systematisch dem Schriftspracherwerb bei mehrsprachigen Kindern widmen würde. Die wenigen Studien sind defizitär orientiert und ziehen stets Vergleiche zwischen mehr- und einsprachigen Kindern, statt Bilinguale untereinander zu vergleichen. Dabei wird weiterhin von der monolingualen Norm ausgegangen und die Besonderheiten von Mehrsprachigen nicht berücksichtigt. Zukünftige Forschung zum Thema Schriftspracherwerb, Mehrsprachigkeit und metalinguistisches Bewusstsein sollte daher sowohl den sozioökonomischen Status, den Input in den jeweiligen Sprachen als auch die unterschiedliche Entwicklung des metalinguistischen Bewusstseins mehr- und einsprachiger Kinder untersuchen. Außerdem muss der Zusammenhang von Mehrsprachigkeit, metalinguistischem Bewusstsein und Schriftspracherwerb aus Sicht der Psycholinguistik näher untersucht werden und experimentelle Methoden wie Eye-Tracking oder EEG (Elektroenzephalografie) eingesetzt werden, um einen unmittelbaren Zugriff auf hochautomatisierte, kognitive sowie neuronale Prozesse, die mit den Prozessen der exekutiven Kontrolle einhergehen, zu ermöglichen. Der Vorteil des Zugangs durch psycholinguistische Methoden im Gegensatz zu behavioralen Methoden besteht darin, dass dieser keiner sozialen Erwünschtheit unterlegen ist und die Kombination beider Methoden die immer noch vor allem in der Gesellschaft bestehenden Mythen und Vorurteile gegenüber Mehrsprachigkeit weiter entkräften und hoffentlich auch endgültig ausgeräumt werden könnten. Dies könnte anhand folgender Forschungsfragen geschehen: Unterscheiden sich bilinguale von monolingualen Vorschulkindern im Zeitpunkt der Entwicklung ihres semantischen metalinguistischen Bewusstseins? Haben Vorschulkinder aus Familien mit einem niedrigeren sozioökonomischen Status ein weniger gut entwickeltes semantisches metalinguistisches Bewusstsein als Kinder aus Familien mit einem höheren soziökonomischen Status? Erwerben balancierte[6] bilinguale Kinder früher ein metalinguistisches Bewusstsein als nicht-balancierte bilinguale Kinder: Beginnen Kinder, die bereits vor Schuleintritt über ein semantisches metalinguistisches Bewusstsein verfügen früher zu lesen? Ist ein früh entwickeltes semantisches metalinguistisches Bewusstsein ein Prädiktor für einen erfolgreichen Schriftspracherwerb?

6. Fazit und Ausblick

Studien belegen eindeutig, dass es Zusammenhänge zwischen den Voraussetzungen für einen erfolgreichen Schriftspracherwerb und den Vorteilen von Mehrsprachigkeit gibt. Neben verschiedenen Vorläuferkompetenzen, die für einen erfolgreichen Schriftspracherwerb vorhanden sein müssen, spielt besonders ein früh entwickeltes metalinguistisches Bewusstsein eine entscheidende Rolle für den Schriftspracherwerb (Bredel et al. 2011). Für die Entwicklung des metalinguistischen Bewusstseins müssen bestimmte exekutive Funktionen – wie die Aufmerksamkeitskontrolle und Unterdrückung irrelevanter Informationen – vorhanden sein (Grosjean & Li 2012). Genau diese exekutiven Funktionen sind bei mehrsprachigen Kindern besser entwickelt als bei einsprachigen Kindern, da Mehrsprachige durch die Koaktivierung beider Sprachen einer dauerhaften und intensiven Aufmerksamkeitskontrolle ausgesetzt sind (Bialystok et al. 2009; Bialystok 2017). Dadurch haben mehrsprachige Kinder einen Vorteil, der sich darin äußert, dass das metalinguistischen Bewusstseins bei mehrsprachigen Kindern früher entwickelt ist als bei einsprachigen Kindern (Bialystok 1986, 2017; Reder et al. 2013). Des Weiteren zeigen Studien (Zipke et al. 2009), dass metalinguistisches Bewusstsein durch sprachliche Übungen, wie z. B. Reime erkennen, doppeldeutige Wörter zu Bildern zuordnen oder Silbentrennen, trainiert werden kann. Mehrsprachige Kinder haben

6 Sprecher*innen, die in beiden Sprachen ein vergleichbares Leistungsniveau haben.

täglich auf natürliche Weise diese sprachlichen Aufgaben zu meistern und sind somit im Vorteil, da Mehrsprachigkeit eine ständige mentale Übung für das exekutive System (Hilchey und Klein 2011) und das metalinguistische Bewusstsein ist. Das Management der Unterdrückung der nicht relevanten Sprache ist bei Mehrsprachigen voll automatisiert und erfolgt später sogar ganz ohne kognitiven Aufwand (Costa & Santesteban 2004).

Bisherige Studien zum metalinguistischen Bewusstsein und Schriftspracherwerb beruhen ausschließlich auf Verhaltensdaten, die zum größten Teil aus den Bildungs- und Erziehungswissenschaften stammen. Weitere Forschungen sollten die Schnittstelle Schriftspracherwerb, metalinguistisches Bewusstsein und Mehrsprachigkeit unter Einbezug des sozioökonomischen Status und der Nutzung der psycholinguistischen Methoden untersuchen und unterschiedliche experimentelle methodische Zugänge nutzen, um anhand neuer Daten, die unabhängig von sozialer Erwünschtheit sind, zu zeigen, dass Migrationshintergrund und/oder Mehrsprachigkeit keinen negativen Einfluss auf Schulerfolg haben, sondern Vorteile beim Erwerb der Schriftsprache mit sich bringen, wenn bestimmte Bedingungen erfüllt werden, wie z. B. ausreichender Input in beiden Sprachen. Die Bedeutung der verschiedenen Ebenen des metalinguistischen Bewusstseins (phonologische, morphosyntaktische, semantische und pragmatische) sollten dabei einzeln untersucht werden, um genaue Einblicke in ihren Einfluss auf den Schriftspracherwerb zu erlangen.

7. English summary: Multilingualism and literary acquisition

Multilingualism and Literacy Acquisition: Benefits of Multilingualism through early metalinguistic awareness

Since there are worldwide about 30 times more languages than countries, multilingualism is not a special case. Even though Germany has been an immigration country for more than 60 years, there are still many prejudices against multilingualism. These are partly generated by misinterpreting the data from large-scale assessment studies, such as the PISA study: Poor school performance is explained in terms of "immigrant background" and then linked to poor skills in German language. Certainly, low linguistic skills in German lead to poor school performance. However, the socioeconomic status is a variable that can explain poor school performance much better. Tacitly equating "migration background" with multilingualism is a mistake. The acquisition of written language is considered a key issue in the German education system. However, the foundations for a successful acquisition of written language are not laid in elementary school, but already before school enrollment, in the family environment. As a result, children with parents with a low socioeconomic status are particularly disadvantaged as they have less or no exposure to texts, books, and libraries. In contrast, families with a higher socioeconomic status place more emphasis on written language and transfer a positive attitude towards reading and learning to read. This preschool experience shapes the emergences and development of metalinguistic awareness, which in turn constitutes a prerequisite for the onset of literacy acquisition. Metalinguistic awareness is the knowledge about linguistic structures and the ability to retrieve them intentionally. It enables children to separate the meaning of a word from its form. This separation and the associated insight into the symbolic nature of writing characterizes the beginning of literacy acquisition. To gain insights into this separation, particular cognitive abilities (e.g., attentional control) must be at hand. Phonological awareness and its influence on written language acquisition have been subject of many previous studies and shown to be especially important for the first phase of written language acquisition. Less research has been done on the other aspects of metalinguistic awareness, such as semantic or morphological awareness. The few studies that have been conducted on these aspects show that semantic awareness is crucial for word decoding in the later stages of written language acquisition. It has been demonstrated that by selectively directing attention, children can, for example, detect word ambiguity. In addition, it has been shown that metalinguistic awareness can be trained and that an improvement in reading comprehension can be achieved through such training. Multilingual children must constantly apply metalinguistic awareness because of the daily exposure to two or more languages that they have to learn to differentiate at all linguistic levels. The use of attentional control and the suppression of irrelevant information are central for these processes. Numerous studies have provided evidence for advantages in multilinguals in the development of executive functions as well as metalinguistic awareness. Despite these findings, the deficit-oriented approaches are still predominant in the field of literacy acquisition in relation to multilingualism. Relevant studies examine, among other things, the relationship of different didactic methods of literacy acquisition with reading and writing achievement of children with "migration background". These studies do not include variables such as specific precursors of literacy acquisition, socioeconomic status, or the degree of multilingualism. As a result, this research does not add any significant value to the multilingualism discourse. Future research on literacy acquisition, metalinguistic awareness, and multilingualism should be more benefit-oriented and should also investigate all aspects of metalinguistic awareness, preferably using experimental psycholinguistics methods in combination with behavioral studies.

Literaturverzeichnis

Adesope, O. O./Lavin, T./Thompson, T./Ungerleider, C. (2010). A systematic review and meta-analysis of the cognitive correlates of bilingualism. *Review of Educational Research, 80*(2), 207–245. https://doi.org/10.3102/0034654310368803

Altman, C./Goldstein, T./Armon-Lotem, S. (2018). Vocabulary, metalinguistic awareness and language dominance among bilingual preschool children. *Frontiers in Psychology, 9*, 1953. https://doi.org/10.3389/fpsyg.2018.01953

Amengual, M. (2016). The perception of language-specific phonetic categories does not guarantee accurate phonological representations in the lexicon of early bilinguals. *Applied Psycholinguistics, 37*(5), 1221–1251.

Barac, R./Bialystok, E. (2012). Bilingual effects on cognitive and linguistic development: Role of language, cultural background, and education. *Child Development, 83*(2), 413–422. https://doi.org/10.1111/j.1467-8624.2011.01707.x

Berends, I. E./Reitsma, P. (2006). Addressing semantics promotes the development of reading fluency. *Applied Psycholinguistics, 27*(2), 247–265.

Best, J. R./Miller, P. H. (2010). A developmental perspective on executive function. *Child Development, 81*(6), 1641–1660. https://doi.org/10.1111/j.1467-8624.2010.01499.x

Bialystok, E. (1986). Factors in the growth of linguistic awareness. *Child Development, 57*(2), 498–510. https://doi.org/10.2307/1130604

Bialystok, E. (1992). Attentional control in children's metalinguistic performance and measures of field independence. *Developmental Psychology, 28*(4), 654–664. https://doi.org/10.1037/0012-1649.28.4.654

Bialystok, E. (2017). The bilingual adaptation: How minds accommodate experience. *Psychological Bulletin, 143*(3), 233–262. https://doi.org/10.1037/bul0000099

Bialystok, E./Craik, F. I. M./Klein, R./Viswanathan, M. (2004). Bilingualism, aging, and cognitive control: evidence from the Simon task. *Psychology and aging, 19*(2), 290–303. https://doi.org/10.1037/0882-7974.19.2.290

Bialystok, E./Craik, F. I./Green, D. W./Gollan, T. H. (2009). Bilingual minds. *Psychological Science in the Public Interest, 10*(3), 89–129.

Blair, C. (2016). Developmental science and executive function. *Current Directions in Psychological Science*, *25*(1), 3–7. https://doi.org/10.1177/0963721415622634

Bos, W./Lankes, E. M./Prenzel, M./Schwippert, K./Walther, G./Valtin, R./Voss, A. (2003). Welche Fragen können aus einer gemeinsamen Interpretation der Befunde aus PISA und IGLU fundiert beantwortet werden? *Zeitschrift für Pädagogik*, *49*(2), 198–212.

Bredel, U./Fuhrhop, N./Noack, C. (2011). *Wie Kinder lesen und schreiben lernen*. Tübingen: Francke Verlag.

Browne Rego, L. L./Bryant, P. E. (1993). The connection between phonological, syntactic and semantic skills and children's reading and spelling. *European Journal of Psychology of Education*, *8*(3), 235–246.

Bryant, P. E./MacLean, M./Bradley, L. L./Crossland, J. (1990). Rhyme and alliteration, phoneme detection, and learning to read. *Developmental Psychology*, *26*(3), 429–438. https://doi.org/10.1037/0012-1649.26.3.429

Costa, A./Santesteban, M. (2004). Lexical access in bilingual speech production: Evidence from language switching in highly proficient bilinguals and L2 learners. *Journal of Memory and Language*, *50*(4), 491–511. https://doi.org/10.1016/j.jml.2004.02.002

Delucchi Danhier, R., & Mertins, B. (2018). Psycholinguistische Grundlagen der Inklusion: Schwerpunkt Bilingualismus. In S. Hußmann & B. Welzel (Hrsg.), *DoProfiL – Das Dortmunder Profil für inklusionsorientierte Lehrerinnen- und Lehrerbildung* (S.161–178). Münster: Waxmann.

Frith, U. (1986). Psychologische Aspekte des orthographischen Wissens: Entwicklung und Entwicklungsstörung. In G. Augst, *New trends in graphemics and orthography*. Berlin: Mouton der Gruyter.

Frost, J. (2001). Differences in reading development among Danish beginning-readers with high versus low phonemic awareness on entering grade one. *Reading and Writing*, *14*(7/8), 615–642. https://doi.org/10.1023/A:1012041804933

Frost, J./Madsbjerg, S./Niedersøe, J./Olofsson, Å./Sørensen, P. M. (2005). Semantic and phonological skills in predicting reading development: From 3–16 years of age. *Dyslexia*, *11*(2), 79–92.

Grosjean, F./Li, P. (2012). *The psycholinguistics of bilingualism* (1. Aufl.). Chichester: Wiley-Blackwell.

Hilchey, M. D./Klein, R. M. (2011). Are there bilingual advantages on nonlinguistic interference tasks? Implications for the plasticity of executive control processes. *Psychonomic Bulletin & Review*, *18*(4), 625–658. https://doi.org/10.3758/s13423-011-0116-7

Hurrelmann, B. (2009). Sozialhistorische Rahmenbedingungen von Lesekompetenz sowie soziale und personale Einflussfaktoren. In N. Groeben/B. Hurrelmann (Hrsg.), *Lesekompetenz. Bedingungen, Dimensionen, Funktionen* (S. 123–149).

Huschka, S. S./Emde, K. R./Brandenburg, J. (2020). Zur Vorhersage der Schriftsprache durch vorschulische Kompetenzen. *Frühe Bildung*, *9*(4), 193–202. https://doi.org/10.1026/2191-9186/a000496

Ibrahim, R./Eviatar, Z./Aharon-Peretz, J. (2007). Metalinguistic awareness and reading performance: A cross language comparison. *Journal of Psycholinguistic Research*, *36*(4), 297–317. https://doi.org/10.1007/s10936-006-9046-3

Jacob, L. (2021). Mehrsprachigkeit als Forschungsgegenstand. In *Englischlernen unter den Voraussetzungen lebensweltlicher Mehrsprachigkeit* (S. 1–50). Wiesbaden: Springer VS. https://doi.org/10.1007/978-3-658-31918-2_1

Jasińska, K. K./Petitto, L. A. (2018). Age of bilingual exposure is related to the contribution of phonological and semantic knowledge to successful reading development. *Child Development*, *89*(1), 310–331.

Mendt, A. (2020). Kurz und Bündig Bildung final. Sachverständigenrat für Integration und Migration, abgerufen am 05.01.2023 unter: https://www.svr-migration.de/wp-content/uploads/2019/03/2020_Kurz_und_Buendig_Bildung_final.pdf

Miyake, A./Friedman, N. P./Emerson, M. J./Witzki, A. H./Howerter, A./Wager, T. D. (2000). The unity and diversity of executive functions and their contributions to complex "Frontal Lobe" tasks: a latent variable analysis. *Cognitive psychology*, *41*(1), 49–100. https://doi.org/10.1006/cogp.1999.0734

Moll, K./Wallner, R./Landerl, K. (2012). Kognitive Korrelate der Lese-, Leserechtschreib- und der Rechtschreibstörung. *Lernen und Lernstörungen*, *1*(1), 7–19. https://doi.org/10.1024/2235-0977/a000002

Niklas, F./Schneider, W. (2015). With a little help: Improving kindergarten children's vocabulary by enhancing the home literacy environment. *Reading and Writing*, *28*(4), 491–508. https://doi.org/10.1007/s11145-014-9534-z

Noble, K. G./Houston, S. M./Kan, E./ Sowell, E. R. (2012). Neural correlates of socioeconomic status in the developing human brain. *Developmental Science*, *15*(4), 516–527. https://doi.org/10.1111/j.1467-7687.2012.01147.x

Paap, K. R. (2019). The bilingual advantage debate: Quantity and quality of the evidence. Schwieter, J.W./Paradis, M. (Ed.). *The handbook of the neuroscience of multilingualism*, (S. 701–735). Hoboken NJ: Wiley-Blackwell.

Palmer, M. B. (1972). Effects of categorization, degree of bilingualism and language upon recall of select monolinguals and bilinguals. *Journal of Educational Psychology*, *63*(2), 160–164. https://doi.org/10.1037/h0032443

Prior, A./MacWhinney, B. (2010). A bilingual advantage in task switching. *Bilingualism: Language and Cognition*, *13*(2), 253–262.

Reder, F./Marec-Breton, N./Gombert, J.-E./Demont, E. (2013). Second-language learners' advantage in metalinguistic awareness: A question of languages' characteristics. *The British journal of educational psychology*, *83*(Pt 4), 686–702. https://doi.org/10.1111/bjep.12003

Romaine, S. (1989). *Bilingualism*. Oxford: Blackwell.

Rosenblum, T./Pinker, S. A. (1983). Word magic revisited: Monolingual and bilingual children's understanding of the word-object relationship. *Child Development*, *54*(3), 773–780.

Schneider, W. (2017). *Lesen und Schreiben lernen: Wie erobern Kinder die Schriftsprache?* (1. Aufl.). *Kritisch hinterfragt*. Berlin/Heidelberg. Springer Verlag.

Schneider, W./Näslund, J. C. (1993). The impact of early metalinguistic competencies and memory capacity on reading and spelling in elementary school: Results of the Munich Longitudinal Study on the Genesis of Individual Competencies (LOGIC). *European Journal of Psychology of Education*, *8*(3), 273–287. https://doi.org/10.1007/BF03174082

Schneider, W./Visé, M./Reimers, P./Blaesser, B. (1994). *Auswirkungen eines Trainings der sprachlichen Bewusstheit auf den Schriftspracherwerb in der Schule*. Universitätsbibliothek Würzburg, abgerufen am 05.01.2023 unter: https://opus.bibliothek.uni-wuerzburg.de/opus4-wuerzburg/frontdoor/deliver/index/docId/7020/file/Schneider_W_OPUS_7020.pdf

Schründer-Lenzen, A. (Hrsg.). (2006). *Risikofaktoren kindlicher Entwicklung: Migration, Leistungsangst und Schulübergang* (1. Aufl.). Wiesbaden: Verlag für Sozialwissenschaften.

Statistisches Bundesamt. (2019, 9. April). *33% der Schülerinnen und Schüler mit Migrationshintergrund*. Statistisches Bundesamt, abgerufen am 05.01.2023 unter: https://www.destatis.de/DE/Presse/Pressemitteilungen/Zahl-der-Woche/2017/PD17_006_p002.html

Statistisches Bundesamt (2021). Bevölkerung mit Migrationshintergrund – Ergebnisse des Mikrozensus 2021 – Fachserie 1 Reihe 2.2 – 2021 (Erstergebnisse). Statistisches Bundesamt, abgerufen am 05.01.2023 unter: https://www.destatis.de/DE/Themen/Gesellschaft-Umwelt/Bevoelkerung/Migration-Integration/Publikationen/Downloads-Migration/migrationshintergrund-2010220217004.pdf?__blob=publicationFile

SVR-Forschungsbereich – Forschungsbereich beim Sachverständigenrat deutscher Stiftungen für Integration und Migration (Hrsg.). (2016). *Doppelt benachteiligt? Kinder und Jugendliche mit Migrationshintergrund im deutschen Bildungssystem.*

Vygotsky, L. S. (1964). Thought and language. *Bulletin of the Orton Society, 14*(1), 97–98. https://doi.org/10.1007/BF02928399

Wolf, M./Katzir-Cohen, T. (2001). Reading fluency and its intervention. *Scientific Studies of Reading, 5*(3), 211–239. https://doi.org/10.1207/S1532799XSSR0503_2

Zipke, M./Ehri, L. C./Cairns, H. S. (2009). Using semantic ambiguity instruction to improve third graders' metalinguistic awareness and reading comprehension: An experimental study. *Reading Research Quarterly, 44*(3), 300–321.

Hendrik Trescher

Leichte Sprache – Anlass zur Diskussion

Abstract: Easy Language is finding its way into pedagogical practice as well as into scientific debates. It primarily intends to contribute to the empowerment of people with learning difficulties and is often included in demands for accessibility, participation, and inclusion of people who usually understand written and verbal language only to a limited extent. While Easy Language is becoming an important practical tool for this group of people, there is a risk that can be often seen as a 'panacea' and a kind of 'guarantee of inclusion'. The ambivalences that inevitably go hand in hand with the use of Easy Language are not reflected and discussed enough, although they raise many questions. This article discusses a number of controversies and issues connected to Easy language and its use, for example the supposed linguistic 'simplifications' of Easy Language or the role of the translator.

Keywords: Easy language, ambivalence, learning disability, disability, participation

1. Einleitung

Mittels Leichter Sprache sollen in erster Linie die Teilhabemöglichkeiten an Praxen der Mehrheitsgesellschaft von Menschen mit Lernschwierigkeiten erweitert werden. Demnach wird Leichte Sprache auch vielfach in Forderungen nach Teilhabe, Barrierefreiheit und Inklusion von Menschen, die Schrift- und Verbalsprache nur eingeschränkt verstehen, aufgegriffen. Leichte Sprache soll einen Zugang zur ‚schwierigen' – also der üblichen – Schrift- bzw. Verbalsprache (er)öffnen, indem diese vereinfacht und der Inhalt somit einem erweiterten Personenkreis zur Verfügung gestellt wird.[1]

Leichte Sprache entstand Ende der neunziger Jahre, Anfang des 21. Jahrhunderts in Selbstvertretungskreisen von Menschen mit Lernschwierigkeiten

1 In dem hier vorliegenden Beitrag wird sich nicht mit einer genuin linguistischen Fragestellung Leichter Sprache auseinandergesetzt. Es geht hier viel mehr um eine edukatorisch-gesellschaftliche Perspektive mittels derer auf Leichte Sprache geblickt wird. Demnach sind hierbei auch linguistische Kennzeichen sowie die technische Bedeutung (Leichter) Sprache nicht von Relevanz, sondern vielmehr die gesellschaftliche und edukatorische Bedeutung und Funktion einer ‚Sondersprache' allgemein – unabhängig davon, wie diese sich gestaltet.

und ist dort sowie in großen Teilen der dazugehörigen Handlungspraxis sowie der jeweiligen Bezugswissenschaften mittlerweile weitestgehend als Werkzeug des ‚barrierefreien' Informationszugangs anerkannt, aus dem Teilhabemöglichkeiten erwachsen können (u.a. Kaczmarzik 2019; Lange & Bock 2016; Seitz 2014; Bock 2014; Jekat et al. 2014). Dieser Anspruch und dieses Versprechen werden von unterschiedlicher Seite problematisiert. Ein Grund dafür ist, dass „Texte, die sich selbst als ‚Leichte Sprache' ausweisen, [...] keineswegs einheitlich" (Bock et al. 2017, S. 12 f) sind, wodurch diese in gewisser Weise beliebig erscheint. Außerdem fehlt es bei der Beschäftigung mit Leichter Sprache an einer pädagogischen Rahmung, anhand derer reflektiert werden kann, welche Rolle Leichte Sprache im Kontext pädagogischen Handelns einnimmt bzw. einnehmen kann. Als Kernproblematik kristallisiert sich jedoch eine mangelnde theoretische Fundierung Leichter Sprache heraus. Es liegt demnach ein hoher Forschungsbedarf vor, der von unterschiedlicher Seite angeführt wird (u.a. Poncelas & Murphy 2007; Kupke & Schlummer 2010; Sutherland & Isherwood 2016; Bergelt et al. 2016; Kaczmarzik 2018; Schuppener et al. 2018; Bredel et al. 2016; Bock 2014; Trescher 2021, 2020).

Während Leichte Sprache vermehrt Anklang in der (sonder-)pädagogischen Praxis sowie in wissenschaftlichen Diskursen der Linguistik und Sonderpädagogik findet, wird sich mit den Ambivalenzen Leichter Sprache bisher eher unzureichend befasst. Zur Verdeutlichung der Ambivalenzen werden in diesem Beitrag (noch) offene Fragen bezüglich Leichter Sprache gestellt und diskutiert. Zunächst wird ein kurzer Überblick gegeben, was unter Leichter Sprache verstanden wird, wer die Adressat*innen und was die Ziele Leichter Sprache sind sowie in welchen Bereichen sie verwendet wird.

2. Leichte Sprache

2.1 Was ist Leichte Sprache?

Im Gegensatz zur ‚schwierigen' Sprache, welche in Abgrenzung zur Leichten Sprache alle Facetten der Alltagssprache einschließt, zeichnet sich Leichte Sprache formell meist „unter anderem durch kurze Hauptsätze [...], [dem] weitgehenden Verzicht auf Nebensätze, die Verwendung von bekannten Wörtern" (Kellermann 2014, S. 7) sowie einem optisch ‚vereinfachten' Erscheinungsbild im Sinne eines bspw. übersichtlichen, großen Schriftbilds und der visuellen Unterstützung mittels Piktogramme und Bilder aus. Das, was insgesamt unter Leichter Sprache verstanden wird, unterscheidet sich ein Stück weit abhängig davon, aus welcher Perspektive auf dieses Phänomen geblickt wird. Während sonderpädagogische, oftmals eher handlungsorientierte Perspektiven, Leichte Sprache vor allem im Lichte einer Ermächtigungspraxis und als Werkzeug zu barrierefreier Teilhabe verstehen (u. a. Aichele 2014), wenden sich sprachwissenschaftlich orientierte Zugänge primär den sprachlichen Gegebenheiten zu und verstehen Leichte Sprache überwiegend als „eine künstlich geschaffene Varietät, deren Kodifizierung und Normierung sich noch in einem Stadium der Aushandlung befindet" (Linz 2017, S. 148; siehe auch Bock 2014). An dieser Stelle zeichnen sich bereits erste Ambivalenzen, Widersprüche und Brüche in der Beschäftigung mit Leichter Sprache ab, die mit Blick auf ihre handlungspraktische, pädagogische Umsetzung noch deutlicher werden.

2.2 Wer sind die Adressat*innen Leichter Sprache?

Als Adressat*innen Leichter Sprache werden in den jeweils bezugsrelevanten wissenschaftlichen Diskursen Menschen mit ‚Lernschwierigkeiten', ‚kognitiven Beeinträchtigungen' oder ‚geistiger Behinderung' angeführt (u.a. Poncelas & Murphy 2007; Kupke & Schlummer 2010; Bergelt 2018; Karreman et al. 2007; Bock & Lange 2017). Teilweise wird darauf aufmerksam gemacht, dass Leichte Sprache auch für Personen sinnvoll sein kann, denen das Lesen und Verstehen ‚schwieriger' Schriftsprache schwerfällt, wie es teils auf Sprachanfänger*innen, Nicht-Muttersprachler*innen oder Analphabet*innen zutreffen kann (Köhler 2016). Einige Autor*innen fassen das Zielgruppenspektrum noch weiter (siehe bspw. Stefanowitsch 2014; Maaß et al. 2014; Aichele 2014). Köhler schreibt, dass die Adressat*innen Leichter Sprache so vielfältig sind, „wie die Gründe, warum Menschen Lese-, Schreib- und Verständnisschwierigkeiten haben" (ebd. 2016, S. 134). Die Heterogenität der Adressat*innengruppe stellt Produzent*innen von Texten in Leichter Sprache vor die Schwierigkeit, dass nicht sichergestellt werden kann, dass dies alle Rezipient*innen verstehen (siehe Maaß et al. 2014). Diese Problematik lässt Stefanowitsch zu folgender Überlegung kommen: „Es ist fraglich, ob es für eine derart heterogene Zielgruppe eine einheitliche Lösung geben kann oder sollte" (ebd. 2014, S. 11 f). Reaktionen auf Überlegungen solcher Art spiegeln sich in den Entwicklungen verschiedener vereinfachter Varietäten der deutschen Sprache wider, wie bspw. Leichte Sprache und Einfache Sprache , welche im alltäglichen Sprachgebraucht teils synonym verwendet werden, sich jedoch u.a. darin unterscheiden, dass Einfache Sprache durch einen komplexeren Sprachstil sowie einer meist nicht (stark) optisch vereinfachten Schrift gekennzeichnet ist (siehe u.a. Kellermann 2014; Köhler 2016; Lange & Bock 2016; für den englisch- und polnischsprachigen Diskurs problematisiert dies Przybyla-Wilkin 2016). Auch ‚Leichte Sprache

Plus', eine Art Kombination Leichter und Einfacher Sprache (siehe Maaß 2020), stellt eine vereinfachte Variation deutscher Sprache dar.

Es wird deutlich, dass hinsichtlich der Frage, welche Merkmale der jeweiligen ‚Sprache' zuzuordnen sind, unterschiedliche Ansichten bestehen. Letztendlich muss bei der Betrachtung der Adressat*innengruppe stets bedacht werden, dass ein Großteil der als Adressat*innen eingestuften Personen gar nicht lesen kann. Für diese Personen bleiben folglich Barrieren bestehen (Kurzenberger et al. 2012).

2.3 Was sind Kontexte und Ziele Leichter Sprache?

Leichte Sprache soll im Alltag dem Abbau sprachlicher Barrieren dienen, sodass Teilhabemöglichkeiten der Adressat*innengruppe am gesellschaftlichen Leben erweitert werden (Schuppener et al. 2019). Die Bereiche, in denen Leichte Sprache Teilhabechancen erweitern soll, sind weit und umfassen u.a. Arbeitsleben (Bergelt et al. 2016; Schuppener et al. 2018), Erwachsenenbildung (Kupke & Schlummer 2010), kulturelle Angebote (Rüstow & Volkmann 2013), (inklusiven) Unterricht (Köhler 2016; Fajardo et al. 2014), Gesundheitsinformationen (Chinn 2017; Hurtado et al. 2014), Finanzverwaltung (Kahl & Pöld-Krämer 2014) oder auch juristische Fachtexte (Rink 2016). Leichte Sprache zielt in dieser Hinsicht also auf die Förderung des eigenständigen Handelns der Adressat*innen sowie der Mitbestimmung und -gestaltung gesellschaftlicher Prozesse ab (Kahl & Pöld-Krämer 2014; Sutherland & Isherwood 2016; Antener et al. 2018). Dabei darf nicht außer Acht gelassen werden, dass Leichte Sprache oftmals aus Gründen der Legitimation eines Gegenstandes oder einer Institution und aus einem äußeren Inklusionsdruck heraus angewendet wird (Reichstein 2016), wodurch ihre Akzeptanz bei Pädagog*innen, Adressat*innen und Mehrheitsgesellschaft womöglich geschmälert wird. Leichte Sprache wird außerdem von nicht zu unterschätzenden „ökonomischen und machtpolitischen Faktoren (mit)bestimmt" (Bock et al. 2017, S. 14) und ist somit auch ein (lukratives) Geschäftsmodell (Zurstrassen 2015), das Gefahr läuft, ihr eigentliches Ziel – Teilhabe für Menschen mit Lernschwierigkeiten ermöglichen – zu untergraben (siehe zur Ökonomisierung von Sprache bspw. Bourdieu (2005)).

3. Anlass zur Diskussion

Wie oben bereits angeführt, ist Leichte Sprache und der Umgang mit ihr sehr ambivalent. Um das Ausmaß der Ambivalenzen erkennen und verstehen zu können, müssen einige Punkte bezüglich Leichter Sprache diskutiert werden.

Dabei lassen sich diese grob in drei verschiedene – (1) gesellschaftliche, (2) technische und (3) pädagogische – Aspekte einteilen. Aufgrund ihrer Ambivalenz sind die folgenden Diskussionspunkte und damit einhergehenden Fragen nicht endgültig zu beantworten, dienen jedoch dazu die (möglichen) Problematiken mit Fokus auf die pädagogische Relevanz Leichter Sprache aufzudecken und zu reflektieren sowie eine Diskussion bzgl. dieser anzuregen.

3.1 Gesellschaftliche Aspekte

3.1.1 Gesonderte Sprache im Kontext einer inklusiven Gesellschaft

Auf der einen Seite gelingt es durch Leichte Sprache Teilhabebarrieren abzubauen und einen (erweiterten) Zugang für Menschen, welche routinemäßig nur eingeschränkt Schrift- und Verbalsprache verstehen, an den Praxen der Mehrheitsgesellschaft zu ermöglichen. Auf der anderen Seite stellt sich jedoch gleichzeitig die Frage: Ist es hinnehmbar, dass im Kontext von Forderungen nach einer inklusiven Gesellschaft eine gesonderte Sprache für bestimmte Menschen die Lösung sein soll? Mit der Forderung einer gesonderten Sprache werden die Adressat*innen gleichzeitig als ‚besonders', (kognitiv) beeinträchtigt' oder ‚behindert' hervorgebracht. „Leichte Sprache, das wird hier deutlich, sorgt somit einerseits für Teilhabe, geht aber mit der Zuschreibung an das Gegenüber einher, auf Leichte Sprache angewiesen zu sein und unterstellt damit ein Defizit" (Seitz 2014, S. 4). Leichte Sprache wird demnach nicht nur als inklusive Praxis, sondern auch als behindernde Praxis wirksam.

3.1.2 Hervorbringung einer ‚behinderten Identität'

Mit der Etablierung einer Sprache, die eigene Regeln, Ausdrucks- und Gestaltungsformen besitzt und von einer bestimmten Gruppe von Menschen verwendet wird – wie beispielsweise die Gebärdensprache –, geht auch immer eine gewisse Identitätsstiftung einher. Während im Zuge bspw. der Gebärdensprache diese von den Adressat*innen sowohl rezipiert als auch produziert wird, ist im Kontext von Leichter Sprache bisher nicht geklärt, ob jene Adressat*innen diese nicht nur rezipieren, sondern auch produzieren sollten, welches die Entstehung einer Sprachcommunity stärkt. Denn die Zugehörigkeit zu einer bestimmten Sprachgemeinschaft produziert kulturelle Identität und kann zudem zu einer Art Solidarisierung und Vergemeinschaftung untereinander beitragen. Problematisch ist jedoch, dass Leichte Sprache meist von einer homogenen Adressat*innenschaft ausgeht, welche jedoch so nicht existiert (Köhler 2016). Dabei stellt sich die Frage: Bringt Leichte Sprache eine undifferenzierte

,behinderte Identität' hervor? Die Gruppe der Menschen, die routinemäßig nur eingeschränkt Schrift- und Verbalsprache verstehen und nicht (ausreichend) lesen können, ist sehr heterogen und umfasst Menschen mit unterschiedlichstem Unterstützungsbedarf. Leichte Sprache schafft eine Art Sondergruppe, die – unabhängig ihres Unterstützungsbedarfs – (lediglich) nicht an der ,schwierigen' Sprache der Mehrheitsgesellschaft teilnehmen kann, aufgrund sprachlicher Exklusivität jedoch allgemeingültigen Ausschluss erfährt.

*3.1.3 Produktion von Inklusionsverlierer*innen*

Leichte Sprache wird derzeit vor allem in der Schriftsprache verwendet. Die meisten Menschen mit Lernschwierigkeiten oder geistiger Behinderung können jedoch nicht (ausreichend) lesen. Leichte Sprache kann in diesem Fall „ebenso eine Barriere darstellen […] wie schwere Sprache" (Kurzenberger et al. 2012, S. 122). Es wird demnach (lediglich) die Grenze derjenigen verschoben, die weiterhin umfassend an Barrieren stoßen, dadurch umfänglich Ausschluss erfahren und Gefahr laufen in gewisser Weise zu „Inklusionsverlierer*innen" (Becker 2016, S. 33; siehe auch Trescher 2018b) zu werden. Es stellt sich hierbei die Frage: In welchem Ausmaß werden Inklusionsverlierer*innen produziert? Für Menschen, die nicht (ausreichend) lesen können, wird trotz Leichter Sprache Ausschluss fortgeführt. Denn selbst mit technischer Unterstützung wie bspw. Vorlesesoftwares, wodurch jedoch auch ein weiteres Hilfsmittel dazukäme, ist nicht garantiert, dass Leichte Sprache so beim Empfänger ankommt, wie vom Sender ursprünglich intendiert. Im Einzelfall können damit ggf. noch Schwierigkeiten beim Lesen umgangen werden, aber gerade, wenn es um die Kombination von Schriftsprache und Piktogrammen bzw. Bilder geht – wie im Zuge von Leichter Sprache üblich – muss die Person das Dargestellte lesen und verstehen können. In gewisser Weise wird durch Leichte Sprache eine Gruppe von Menschen gebildet, die (sogar) trotz Leichter Sprache keine erweiterten Teilhabemöglichkeiten erfahren können.[2]

2 An dieser Stelle soll jedoch auch noch einmal darauf hingewiesen werden, dass es in diesem Beitrag nicht um die ,Verteuflung' Leichter Sprache geht, sondern lediglich darauf aufmerksam gemacht werden soll, dass die bereits aufgeführten (und noch kommenden) Diskussionspunkte bei der Konstruktion von Leichter Sprache bedacht werden müssen.

3.2 Technische Aspekte

3.2.1 Regeln der Schriftsprache

In grundschuldidaktischen Auseinandersetzungen wurde in der Vergangenheit immer wieder mehrperspektivisch diskutiert, inwiefern es sinnvoll wäre, die Regeln der Schriftsprache zu lockern, um ihre Verwendung zu erleichtern.[3] So könnten beispielsweise die orthographischen Regeln – entlang der Logik der Leichten Sprache – gelockert werden, wodurch sich die ‚schwierige' Schriftsprache zu einer ‚leicht(er)en' Schriftsprache entwickeln könnte. Dabei stellt sich jedoch die Frage: Nach welchen Regeln sollte Sprache schriftlich festgelegt werden, sodass diese für alle verständlich und nachvollziehbar ist? In diesem Zusammenhang stellt sich zudem die Frage: Wer ist ‚alle'? „Es ist fraglich, ob es für eine derart heterogene Zielgruppe eine einheitliche Lösung geben kann oder sollte" (Stefanowitsch 2014, S. 11 f).

3.2.2 Neue Lingua Franca

Wie bereits oben verdeutlicht, gehen mit dem Stellenwert einer Sondersprache auch Herausforderungen einher. Gleichzeitig nimmt das Phänomen der Sondersprache zu – so gibt es immer mehr (virtuelle) Räume, in denen nur noch in einer Sprache kommuniziert wird, die allen Diskursbeteiligten bekannt ist. Bei sogenannten ‚Massively Multiplayer Online Role-Playing Games' (MMORPG) – ein Computerspielformat, in dem mehrere Spieler gleichzeitig spielen und im Spiel direkt oder indirekt miteinander interagieren und kommunizieren können – kommunizieren die Spieler*innen weltweit beispielsweise überwiegend mit (englischsprachigen) Abkürzungen und Ausdrücken (Stertkamp 2017). Auch die Verwendung von Emojis (bspw. im Kontext von Chat-Kommunikation, Tweets oder Posts) kann zu den Phänomenen der Sondersprache gezählt werden. Hierbei wird vor allem der schnelle Wandel sowie die immerzu neuen Praxen solcher Sondersprachen deutlich. Der Unterschied hierbei – im Vergleich zur Leichten Sprache – ist jedoch, dass die Diskursbeteiligten sich selbst für die Teilnahme dieses spezifischen Diskurses entschieden haben, auch wenn jene Diskurse gewisse Kenntnisse dieser Sondersprache

3 Da bereits viel Forschung diesbezüglich vorangetrieben und weiterhin ausgeführt wird, wird an dieser Stelle nicht weiter im Detail auf die Überlegungen zur Lockerung der Schriftsprache eingegangen. Wie bereits oben dargelegt, geht es in diesem Beitrag ausschließlich um eine edukatorisch-gesellschaftliche Perspektive auf Leichte Sprache.

bereits voraussetzen und man sich diesem Diskurs zu einem bestimmten Grad unterwerfen muss. Es findet in diesen Fällen allerdings nicht aufgrund sprachlicher Barrieren eine Ausgrenzung von dem Gesamtdiskurs der ‚schwierigen' Sprache statt. Der sprachliche Stellenwert von Leichter Sprache, in die ‚schwierige' Sprache übersetzt wird, sollte diskutiert werden. Wäre es möglich, Leichte Sprache als eine Art ‚Lingua Franca' zu etablieren, die von allen (deutschsprachigen) Menschen verstanden, geschrieben und gesprochen wird? Auch hier könnten weiter Barrieren und Ausschluss entstehen, wenn bspw. die gesamte Kommunikation auf Englisch geführt wird. Dabei würde es sich dann jedoch um Sonderdiskurse und keine Alltagsdiskurse, welche für alle zugänglich sein sollten, handeln. Im Zuge dieser Diskussion stellt sich zudem die Frage: Sollte Leichte Sprache anstatt als eine ‚eigene Sprache' nicht eher als eine „Varietät" (Bock et al. 2017, S. 12) des Deutschen verstanden werden? Mit Blick auf die oben angeführten Sondersprachen (bspw. Emojis) wird jedoch auch deutlich, dass man die Etablierung einer bestimmten ‚Lingua Franca' bzw. ‚Sprachvarietät' nur bedingt vorschreiben kann. So lässt sich diese (meist) in der offiziellen Kommunikation (wie bspw. Informationsbroschüren oder Internetauftritten) sowie im öffentlichen Leben (z. B. in Supermärkten oder Bahnhöfen) umsetzen. Spätestens in privaten Kommunikationsformen (wie Alltagskommunikation aber auch Chats, Tweets, Posts etc.) kann darauf jedoch kein Einfluss genommen werden, da damit eine umfangreiche Überwachung des Privaten einhergehen würde, diese wäre aus diversen Gründen kaum zu rechtfertigen.

3.2.3 Anglizismen, Jugendsprache und anderen adaptiven (An-) Forderungen an Sprache

Im Laufe der Zeit hat sich Englisch als „die Verkehrssprache schlechthin" (Leitner 2009, S. 8) entwickelt. Sie gilt als eine der Sprachen, die global die meisten Menschen zumindest ansatzweise sprechen und verstehen und mittels dieser zumindest ein einfacher Informationsaustausch möglich ist. Dabei fließt die englische Sprache – im Sinne von Anglizismen – immer mehr in die (deutsche) ‚Lingua franca' ein und verändert (teils) das deutsche Sprachbild. Auch die sogenannte Jugendsprache beeinflusst – zumindest in bestimmten Diskursen wie bspw. den jeweiligen Peer-Groups – das deutsche Sprachbild. Dazu kommen andere (An-) Forderungen an Sprache wie beispielsweise gendergerechte Formulierungen. Die Änderungen des (deutschen) Sprachbilds sind Ergebnisse kultureller Einflüsse und Veränderungen. Demnach vollzieht sich in der Integration von englischer Sprache, Anglizismen, Jugendsprache und anderer (An-) Forderungen ein Stück weit auch (diskursspezifisch) kulturelle Teilhabe. Eine schlichte ‚Übersetzung' dieser wäre folglich gleichbedeutend mit kulturellem Ausschluss. Es stellt sich daher die Frage: Wie gehen wir mit Anglizismen, Jugendsprache und anderen adaptiven (An-)Forderungen an Sprache um? Um eine (kulturelle) Teilhabe zu ermöglichen, müssten diese in der Übersetzung in Leichte Sprache berücksichtigt und nicht einfach übersetzt bzw. darauf verzichtet werden. Vor allem auf die (umfassend) ‚gendergerechte' Sprache und diverse Formulierungen bzw. Adressierungen wird (umfassend) verzichtet. Dabei gibt es bereits ausgearbeitete Vorschläge, wie auch in Leichter Sprache gendergerecht formuliert werden kann (siehe hierzu bspw. Rocktäschel 2020). Diese Übersetzungspraxis wirft die Frage auf: Welche Änderungen an routinemäßiger Sprache sind (moralisch) ‚wertvoller'?

3.2.4 Vereinfachung des Inhalts

Mit der technischen bzw. formellen Vereinfachung geht meist zwangsläufig auch eine inhaltliche Vereinfachung einher. Bei der ‚Übersetzung' von ‚schwieriger' Sprache in Leichte Sprache kommt es zu inhaltlichen Auswahl- und Deutungsprozessen (Zurstrassen 2015; Bock 2014), weshalb komplexe Inhalte nicht immer vollständig und uneingeschränkt transportiert werden können (Kupke & Schlummer 2010). Mit einer Um- bzw. Neuformulierung in Leichte Sprache gehen auch immer inhaltliche Verluste einher. Neben der Ambivalenz der Selektion ist mit der ‚Übersetzung' in Leichte Sprache auch die Ambivalenz der Interpretation verbunden. Da der Inhalt immer aus Perspektive der übersetzenden Person wieder- und weitergegeben wird, findet dabei prinzipiell eine gewisse Interpretation des Inhalts statt.

Ein Beispiel hierfür ist ein Lexikon-Eintrag auf der Homepage der Bundeszentrale für politische Bildung zum Stichwort ‚Bundesland'.[4] Dort heißt es in ‚schwieriger Sprache':

> *„B. bezeichnet eine politisch-territoriale Einheit (Gliedstaat) und die zweite staatliche Ebene eines Bundesstaates, wobei die Benennung variieren kann (in AUT und DEU: Länder; in CHE: Kantone; in Australien und USA: states = Bundesstaaten; in CAN: provinces = Provinzen). Die B. verfügen über eigene legislative, exekutive und judikative Organe mit eigenen (in den Bundesverfassungen unterschiedlich festgelegten) Zuständigkeitsbereichen." (Schubert & Klein 2020, o.S.)*

---

4 Es sei hier darauf hingewiesen, dass es neben dem Eintrag zum Stichwort „Bundesland" auch noch weitere, ausführlichere Einträge zum Stichwort „Bundesländer" gibt.

Der Eintrag zum Stichwort ‚Bundesland' in Leichter Sprache[5] lautet auf der Homepage der Bundeszentrale für politische Bildung:

> *„Ein Bundesland ist ein Teil eines Bundesstaates. Bundesländer haben eigene Parlamente und eigene Regierungen. Mehrere Bundesländer zusammen bilden einen Bundesstaat. Deutschland ist ein Bundesstaat. Zu Deutschland gehören diese 16 Bundesländer: Baden-Württemberg, Bayern, Berlin, Brandenburg, Bremen, Hamburg, Hessen, Mecklenburg-Vorpommern, Niedersachsen, Nordrhein-Westfalen, Rheinland-Pfalz, Saarland, Sachsen, Sachsen-Anhalt, Schleswig-Holstein, Thüringen. Jedes Bundesland hat ein eigenes Parlament. Das Parlament eines Bundeslandes nennt man meistens Landtag. Jedes Bundesland hat eine eigene Regierung: Die Landesregierung. Für manche Dinge gibt es in den Bundesländern auch eigene Gesetze. Diese Gesetze gelten nur in dem Bundesland. Zum Beispiel werden die Gesetze für Schulen in den Bundesländern gemacht." (Bundeszentrale für politische Bildung 2022, o.S.)*

Eine Selektion ist hier zunächst darin zu erkennen, dass in ‚schwieriger' Sprache – im Gegensatz zur Leichten Sprache – mehrere, ausführlichere Einträge zum Stichwort ‚Bundesland' bzw. ‚Bundesländer' vorliegen. Das Problem der Interpretation wird zudem darin deutlich, dass Inhalte, wie bspw. der Verweis auf eigene exekutive und judikative Organe, herausgenommen werden. Durch das Weglassen von Informationen wird eine Dichotomie zwischen Personen, welche ‚schwierige' Sprache mit komplexen oder vorausgesetzten Inhalten verstehen, und Personen, die dies nicht tun, gefestigt.

Mit Blick auf die zwei Ambivalenzen, welche bei der ‚Übersetzung' auftreten, stellt sich die Frage: Wie sollte mit der Vereinfachung des Inhalts umgegangen werden? Zum einen muss beachtet werden, dass mit der Reduktion von Komplexität und Inhalt die adressierten Personen als ‚weniger wissend' hervorgebracht werden. Zum anderen ist zur Vermittlung komplexer Inhalte eine Komplexitätsreduktion manchmal sogar notwendig (siehe bspw. Schiewe 2017). Demnach ist die Vereinfachung des Inhalts im Kontext Leichter Sprache und die damit einhergehende Selektion und Komplexitätsreduktion unbedingt mehrperspektivisch zu betrachten.

3.2.5 Vereinfachung von Sprache – im Sinne einer kulturellen Praxis

Sprache wird von „politischen und institutionellen Rahmungen ebenso wie von sozialen, ethischen und ökonomischen Regelhaftigkeiten und Interessen beeinflusst" (Holly 2013, S. 58) und ist demnach eine kulturelle Praxis. Es stellt

---

5 Es sei hier darauf hingewiesen, dass es in Leichte Sprache nur einen Eintrag zum Stichwort „Bundesland" und keinen weiteren Eintrag zum Stichwort „Bundesländer" gibt.

sich die Frage: Ist es überhaupt möglich, Sprache – im Sinne einer kulturellen Praxis – zu vereinfachen? Insbesondere im literarischen Sinne – Literatur, Dichtung, Liedtext und vieles mehr – ist Sprache selbst der Gegenstand. Müssen/sollten bestimmte Diskurse ihr (begründet) elaboriertes Sprachsystem, Einzelsprache und das Sprechen selbst ändern? Vor allem im literarischen Sinne transportiert Sprache Emotionen und ruft diese hervor – sie wird emotional wahrgenommen. Sie hat demnach eine Erlebnisebene, die getrennt von der bloßen Weitergabe von Information betrachtet werden muss. Mit Blick auf die (inhaltliche) Komplexitätsreduktion im Zuge der ‚Übersetzung' in Leicht Sprache muss folgende Frage gestellt werden: Kann Leichte Sprache die Erlebnisebene (von Emotionen) gleichermaßen transportieren wie ‚schwierige Sprache'?

3.2.6 Abhängigkeit von ‚Übersetzenden'

Wie mit der Frage bzgl. der inhaltlichen Vereinfachung bereits deutlich wurde, befindet sich die Person, welche in Leichte Sprache ‚übersetzt', in einer überaus bedeutsamen Position. Sie hat die Aufgabe inne, relevante und unverzichtbare Inhalte von weniger relevanten Inhalten zu unterscheiden und zu abstrahieren. Zudem entscheidet sie, welche Texte und Informationen überhaupt in Leichter Sprache zur Verfügung gestellt werden. Menschen, die routinemäßig nur eingeschränkt Schrift- und Verbalsprache verstehen, sind demnach stark von den ‚Übersetzenden' abhängig. Wie sollte mit der Abhängigkeit von ‚Übersetzenden' umgegangen werden? Durch die (alleinige) Auswahl, Interpretation und Verschriftlichung der Inhalte von Menschen ohne eingeschränkte Schrift- und Verbalsprache für Menschen mit eingeschränkter Schrift- und Verbalsprache findet eine deutliche Fremdsteuerung statt.

Auch wenn Übersetzungsbüros sogenannte Kontrollgruppen aus Menschen mit routinemäßig eingeschränkter Schrift- und Verbalsprache einsetzen, kann dieses Problem nicht ausreichend gelöst werden. Es bestehen zwar bereits viele Ideen der Standardisierung und es wird weiterhin viel Forschung diesbezüglich betrieben, letzten Endes ist jedoch, wie oben erwähnt, aufgrund des komplexen und heterogenen Adressatenkreises keine vollkommene Vereinheitlichung möglich, zumindest dann nicht, wenn niemand mehr von dem ‚System Leichte Sprache' ausgeschlossen werden soll. In Bezug auf das Prüfen Leichter Sprache stellt sich zudem die Frage nach unabhängiger Kontrolle und ‚Objektivität' (Trescher 2021).

Aufgrund der bereits oben dargestellten Ambivalenzen der Selektion und Interpretation sowie der Abhängigkeit von ‚Übersetzenden' variieren die

Übersetzungspraxen in Leichte Sprache teils deutlich. Darüber hinaus gibt es bezüglich der ‚Übersetzung' in Leichte Sprache kein Prüfkriterienkatalog (Baumert 2016; Bredel et al. 2016). Inwiefern sind unterschiedliche Übersetzungsvarianten beliebig und wie sollte mit dieser Beliebigkeit verfahren werden?

Zwar existieren Regeln für die Übertragung von Texten in Leichte Sprache, da Leichte Sprache jedoch kein geschützter Begriff ist, variieren diese teils (stark) – nicht zuletzt, da diese von unterschiedlichen Seiten bereitgestellt werden. „Texte, die sich selbst als ‚Leichte Sprache' ausweisen, sind keineswegs einheitlich und auch nicht durchgängig regelkonform gestaltet" (Bock et al. 2017, S. 12 f). Texte in Leichter Sprache werden primär von sogenannten Übersetzungsbüros für Leichte Sprache erstellt, die mittlerweile deutschlandweit entstanden sind. Problematisch ist dabei, dass zwar Übersetzungen vorgenommen werden und/oder Texten teils ein sogenanntes Prüfsiegel verliehen wird (z. B. von der Lebenshilfe Bremen[6]), dass jedoch, wie hervorgehoben, keine einheitlichen Regeln zur ‚Übersetzung' bestehen, denn es gibt bislang „kein elaboriertes, wissenschaftlich überprüftes und evaluiertes einheitliches Konzept für ‚Leichte Sprache'" (Zurstrassen 2017, S. 55; siehe auch Maaß et al. 2014; Ledergerber 2019). Demnach stellt sich die Frage: Welche (Übersetzungs-) Regeln gelten wann? Die uneinheitlichen und nicht allgemeingültigen Regeln, über die viel diskutiert wird und welche bis heute mittels verschiedener (experimenteller) Forschung versucht werden aufzustellen, verstärken die bereits dargelegte Abhängigkeit sowie Beliebigkeit von Leichter Sprache. Zudem wird dadurch die Identifizierung und Kontrolle der teils verschiedenen Interessen der unterschiedlichen Aktuer*innen im Kontext Leichter Sprache erschwert. Die Übersetzungstätigkeiten im Zuge Leichter Sprache sowie Leichte Sprache im Allgemeinen können sich nämlich auch als ein lukratives Geschäftsmodell eigenen (Zurstrassen 2015; siehe auch Bock et al. 2017). Vor allem die handlungspraktische Auseinandersetzung mit Leichter Sprache ist wiederholt „von ökonomischen und machtpolitischen Faktoren (mit)bestimmt" (Bock et al. 2017, S. 13 f). So sind bspw. Übersetzungsbüros sehr teuer und es ist nicht immer einfach auszuhandeln, wer wann wie was übersetzt. Auch ist der Zugang zu sowie die Besetzung von sogenannten Prüfgruppen nicht transparent (Trescher 2021). Im Zuge dessen stellt sich die Frage: Wer profitiert letzten Endes (wie und letztlich auch am meisten) von Leichter Sprache?

6 Das Büro für Leichte Sprache der Lebenshilfe Bremen (zuletzt am 30.03.2022).

3.3 Pädagogische Aspekte

3.3.1 Infantilisierungseffekt

Menschen mit Lernschwierigkeiten gelten als primäre Adressat*innen Leichter Sprache (siehe u.a. Poncelas & Murphy 2007; Kupke & Schlummer 2010; Bergelt 2018; Karreman et al. 2007; Bock & Lange 2017). Diese beschreiben immer wieder, dass Leichte Sprache – nicht zuletzt aufgrund der oftmals verwendeten Piktogramme – eine infantilisierende Wirkung auf sie haben kann bzw. hat (Trescher 2018b).

Durch die infantilisierende Wirkung Leichter Sprache werden die Adressat*innen als kindlich und in gewisser Weise als ‚behindert' hervorgebracht (Trescher 2018b), wodurch Leichte Sprache zur Behinderungspraxis wird. (Wie) ist es möglich, den Infantilisierungseffekt, welcher häufig mit dem Gebraucht von Leichter Sprache einhergeht, zu umgehen? Die Problematisierung der Infantilisierungserfahrungen findet sich auch in der Fachliteratur wieder, wobei diese dort teils negiert werden, was mit Blick auf die geschilderten Erfahrungen für die Menschen, welche diese Art von Infantilisierung wahrgenommen haben, problematisch ist (siehe u.a. Kupke & Schlummer 2010; Rüstow & Volkmann 2013). Es wird erneut deutlich, dass mit Leichter Sprache zwar Teilhabemöglichkeiten eröffnet werden, gleichzeitig jedoch auch Ausschluss reproduziert wird. Die zentrale Frage ist letztlich: Was bedeutet dies als pädagogische Herausforderung, bzw. wie ist damit umzugehen, dass das Verwenden Leichter Sprache in pädagogischen Settings erstmal auch eine ungewollte ‚Nebenwirkung' hat? Vielmehr muss diskutiert werden, wie mit dem infantilisierenden Charakter Leichter Sprache pädagogisch umzugehen ist. Vor allem mit Blick auf die Bestrebungen im Sinne von ‚weg von einer paternalistischen Fürsorgehaltung hin zu einer Idee von Assistenz als Unterstützungsleistung', welche nicht erst seit dem Inklusionsparadigma (nicht nur) in der Sonderpädagogik Einzug erhalten haben, gilt es Leichte Sprache kritisch zu reflektieren – denn gerade durch Leichte Sprache wird eine Statusungleichheit und eine deutliche Abhängigkeit der betreuten Personen (re-)produziert.

3.3.2 Pädagogischer Umgang mit dem Label Leichte Sprache

Wie bereits oben diskutiert, können mit Leichter Sprache Infantilisierungseffekte einhergehen. Zudem kann mit dem Einsatz der Leichten Sprache als Sondersprache ein defizitärer Blick auf die AdressatInnen verfestigt werden. Pädagog*innen müssen sich daher bei der Auseinandersetzung mit Leichter Sprache folgende Fragen stellen: Wie ist mit dem Label Leichte Sprache pädagogisch umzugehen? Wie wird damit umgegangen, dass Leichte Sprache ein Vermittler ist, der gleichzeitig in gewisser Weise ‚statuserniedrigt'?

Auch müssen mit Blick auf die (zukünftigen) Lesekompetenzen der Adressat*innen mögliche negative Auswirkungen diskutiert werden. Was bedeutet es für den pädagogischen Auftrag, wenn ein ‚niedriger Standard' realisiert wird? Im Zuge dessen sollte thematisiert werden, „ob Leichte Sprache mit ihrem eigenen Regelwerk nicht sogar die Ausgrenzung von Menschen mit Lernschwierigkeiten fördern kann, wenn diese auf den zunehmend normierten Schreib- und Sprachstil der ‚Leichten Sprache' hin sozialisiert werden" (Zurstrassen 2015, S. 130). Es besteht das Risiko, dass mit zunehmender Fokussierung auf Leichte Sprache pädagogisches Handeln eingeschränkt wird, indem Schreib-, Lese- und Verstehenskompetenzen nur zu einem gewissen Grad gefördert werden. Darüber hinaus müssen die zugeschriebenen Kompetenzen nicht den tatsächlichen Fähigkeiten der adressierten Personen von Leichter Sprache entsprechen. Gerade in institutionalisierten Wohnformen – im Sinne ambulant bzw. stationär betreuten Wohnens –, in denen Menschen mit Lernschwierigkeiten oftmals leben, wird Gefahr gelaufen, dass durch den Gebrauch von Leichter Sprache, welche (wie oben dargestellt) meist von einer homogenen Adressat*innenschaft ausgeht, allen Personen die gleichen Verstehenskompetenzen zugesprochen und -zugänge geboten werden. Dadurch kann der Horizont Einzelner begrenzt und eine behindernde Praxis implementiert werden.

4. Fazit und Ausblick

Leichte Sprache sieht sich zahlreichen Herausforderungen (in Form von Ambivalenzen) ausgesetzt, von denen einige zuvor bereits problematisiert wurden. Diese sind u.a. die Zugrundelegung uneinheitlicher beziehungsweise nichtevaluierter Regeln, der Ausschluss der Adressat*innen von Fachdiskursen, inhaltliche Vereinfachungen, die Heterogenität der Adressat*innengruppe, die Gefahr der Infantilisierung der Adressat*innen sowie die Negierung ebendieser Problematik.

Diskursteilhabe vollzieht sich entscheidend über Sprache. Dies ist u.a. darin begründet, dass Gesellschaft in „der kulturellen Praxis der Sprache und des Sprechens" (Dietrich 2014, S. 475) konstituiert wird (siehe auch Foucault 2003b; Villa 2012; Bourdieu 2005; Bertau 2015; Stefanowitsch 2014). Sprache, in der Systemtheorie ‚Kommunikation' genannt, ist also ein kulturelles Werkzeug – eine Praxis –, anhand dessen sich Teilhabe vollzieht und anhand dessen das Subjekt in je bestimmter Art und Weise hervorgebracht wird. Sprache ist insofern „selbst produktiv, konstituiert ihre eigene Realität" (Krasmann 1995,

S. 252) und ist somit als performativer Akt zu verstehen, der sich (in foucaultscher Hinsicht) machtvoll vollzieht (Butler 1993; Villa 2012; Dietrich 2014). Sprache ist „weder unschuldig (also frei von Ideologie oder Geschichte) noch ist sie frei von Macht: Diskurse sind produktiv, das heißt, dass sie etwas hervorbringen, also etwas erschaffen" (Villa 2012, S. 20). Sprache als machtvolle Praxis vollzieht sich also in Diskursen und (re-)produziert somit (bestimmte) Subjektivitäten (Trescher 2015; siehe Foucault 1976, 1978, 2003a, 2005). Wird demnach Sprache, auf welche Weise auch immer, eingeschränkt, so entstehen Barrieren, die die Teilhabe an der Konstitution von Welt behindern (Dietrich 2014; siehe dazu auch Humboldt 2019) und die das Subjekt in gewisser Weise als ‚behindert' hervorbringen. Eine Subjektivierung als ‚sprachbehindert' ist unmittelbar gleichbedeutend mit Ausschluss von (je bestimmten) Diskursen. „Wem es gelingt, sprachliche Räume zu besetzen, der hat innerhalb des Diskurses eine Machtposition inne, von der aus er den Diskurs lenken und beeinflussen kann" (Böttinger 2019, S. 155). Spracherwerb und -nutzung ist folglich unmittelbar verknüpft mit der „Übernahme der in der sprachlichen Ordnung enthaltenen gesellschaftlichen Ordnung" (Dietrich 2014, S. 482; siehe auch Bourdieu 2005). Dadurch wird Teilhabe an einer Sprachgemeinschaft respektive eines bestimmten Diskurses reguliert. Diese/r „entspricht der Ordnung der sprachlichen Tätigkeit, der die Teilnehmenden angehören, sie entsteht aus allen spezifischen Sprachpraktiken aller Sprecher dieser Gemeinschaft" (Bertau 2015, S. 102). Sprache kann insofern als Medium verstanden werden, als „ein notwendiger Vermittler, der die Subjekte einander vermittelt *als* aufeinander bezogene Subjekte" (Bertau 2015, S. 96 f; siehe auch Krasmann 1995). Teilhabe an der Sprachgemeinschaft ist dabei gleichbedeutend mit kultureller Teilhabe – bringt Sprache den Menschen doch, in mancher Hinsicht, erst als „kulturfähig" (Brinkmann 1981, S. 31) hervor. In der Konsequenz geht mit dem Ausschluss von Sprache respektive der jeweiligen Sprachgemeinschaft der Ausschluss von Kultur einher – kulturelle Teilhabe wird behindert. Teilnehmende eines je bestimmten Diskurses erkennen sich dadurch (an), dass jede/r Einzelne „mit bestimmten sprachlichen Formen spricht und bestimmte sprachliche Formen annimmt und nicht zurückweist" (Bertau 2015, S. 99). Ausschluss vollzieht sich folglich, wenn die Sprechenden nicht gehört werden, da sie bspw. die Sprache des (je bestimmten) Diskurses nicht vollumfänglich beherrschen und somit in gewisser Weise als ‚sprachlos' hervorgebracht werden (Trescher & Hauck 2020; Trescher & Klocke 2014; siehe auch Brinkmann 1981). „Die Validierung des Gesprochenen ist Ratifizierung durch die Zuhörerschaft" (Bertau 2015, S. 100). Wird dies im Kontext Leichter Sprache gedacht, so muss eine weitere Frage diskutiert werden: Inwiefern wird durch Leichte Sprache zwar Teilhabe an der sprachlichen Konstitution von Gesellschaft möglich, erfolgt dadurch allerdings auch eine ‚leichte', das heißt ggf. eingeschränkte, zumindest aber veränderte Form der Teilhabe? Leichte Sprache ist insofern ambivalent, da sie sich zwischen Teilhabeermöglichung und Behinderungspraxis bewegt: Sie eröffnet Teilhabemöglichkeiten, „geht aber mit der Zuschreibung an das Gegenüber einher, auf Leichte Sprache angewiesen zu sein und unterstellt damit ein Defizit" (Seitz 2014, S. 4). Leichte Sprache manifestiert einen Sonderstatus derjenigen, die damit adressiert werden, und subjektiviert sie in dieser Hinsicht als ‚behindert'. Es bleibt letztlich auch eine politische Entscheidung, wie in Zukunft mit Leichter Sprache umgegangen wird und wer mit ihr wie adressiert wird. Eines ist jedoch klar, ein ‚Allheilmittel' gegen Ausschluss bestimmter Personen, ist sie sicherlich nicht.

5. English summary: Easy language – cause for discussion

Easy language - cause for discussion

Easy language is finding its way into (pedagogical) practice as well as into scientific debates. It (primarily) intends to contribute to the empowerment of people with learning difficulties and is often included in demands for accessibility, participation and inclusion of people who usually understand written and verbal language only to a limited extent. While Easy Language is becoming an important practical tool, there is a high risk that this type of language could be interpreted and handled as a 'panacea' or a kind of 'guarantee of inclusion'. Such contradictions that inevitably go hand in hand with the use of Easy Language are not part of the current discourse on inclusion (cf. Poncelas & Murphy 2007; Kupke & Schlummer 2010; Sutherland & Isherwood 2016; Bergelt et al. 2016; Kaczmarzik 2018). They, nevertheless, raise many questions.

One of the main problems is that despite the fact that Easy language can open up opportunities for participation, it can also limit access to participation since it can act as a kind of barrier itself. Some questions regarding the use of Easy Language need to be posed and answered:

- Is not kind of ironic that within the discourse about inclusive society we demand a special language for people with learning disabilities?
- Easy language is mainly used as written language – most of the people with learning difficulties cannot read (sufficiently). To what extent does Easy Language continue to exclude people who cannot read sufficiently? Are these

people at risk of becoming "losers of the process of inclusion" (Becker 2016, p. 33; Trescher 2018b)?

- Should Easy Language be further seen and used as a special type of language into which 'difficult' language is translated, or is it feasible to establish Easy Language as a kind of "lingua franca"?
- Further issues emerge in relation technical and linguistic simplifications of Easy Language, which are connected to simplifications of content (Zurstrassen 2015; Bock 2014; Kupke & Schlummer 2010). Do for example certain scientific discourses have to change their (reasonably elaborated) language? How do we deal with borrowings from English, youth language, or gender speech? In general terms, is it at all possible to simplify language (seen as an expression of culture) (Trescher 2018)?
- Easy Language translations are always created from the perspective of the translator. However, there are no standardized rules for the translations. How should this problem be tackled? How do deal with different translation variants?
- Some people with learning difficulties find it discriminating using a 'special (needs)' language. Is it possible to counteract the infantilizing effect related to the use of Easy Language?
- What does it mean for an educational approach if a 'lower standard' is to be realized? Will this possibly generate another disability practice?

The present paper is dedicated to the critical discussion of Easy Language by illustrating and reflecting these questions in detail.

Literaturverzeichnis

Aichele, Valentin: „Leichte Sprache – Ein Schlüssel zu „Enthinderung" und Inklusion". In: *Aus Politik und Zeitgeschichte* 64 (9–11), 2014, S. 19–25.

Antener, Gabriela /Girard-Groeber, Simone/Lichtenauer, Annette: Empowerment durch Leichte Sprache. „Das Projekt «Einfach leicht verständlich» als Beitrag zur Ermächtigung von Menschen mit kognitiver Beeinträchtigung". In: *Schweizerische Zeitschrift für Heilpädagogik* 24 (7–8), 2018, S. 44–50.

Baumert, Andreas: *Leichte Sprache – Einfache Sprache. Literaturrecherche – Interpretation – Entwicklung*. Bibliothek der Hochschule Hannover: Hannover, 2016.

Becker, Uwe: *Die Inklusionslüge. Behinderung im flexiblen Kapitalismus*. Transcript: Bielefeld, 2016.

Bergelt, Daniel: „Wie wird Leichte Sprache geprüft? Abbildung der gegenwärtigen Prüfpraxis“. In: *Teilhabe* 57 (4), 2018, S. 168–173.

Bergelt, Daniel/Goldbach, Anne/Seidel, Anja: „Leichte Sprache im Arbeitsleben. Analyse der derzeitigen Nutzung von Texten in Leichter Sprache im beruflichen Kontext von Menschen mit Lernschwierigkeiten“. In: *Teilhabe* 55 (3), 2016, S. 106–113.

Bertau, Marie-Cécile: „Sprache: öffentliche Praxis im Medium des Dritten“. In: Alkemeyer, Thomas/Schürmann, Volker/Volbers, Jörg (Hg.): *Praxis denken. Konzepte und Kritik*. Springer VS: Wiesbaden, 2015, S. 81–107.

Bock, Bettina M.: „„Leichte Sprache“: Abgrenzung, Beschreibung und Problemstellungen aus Sicht der Linguistik“. In: Jekat, Susanne J./Jüngst, Heike Elisabeth/Schubert, Klaus/Villiger, Claudia (Hg.): *Sprache barrierefrei gestalten. Perspektiven aus der Angewandten Linguistik*. Frank & Timme: Berlin, 2014, S. 17–51.

Bock, Bettina M./Lange, Daisy: „Empirische Untersuchungen zu Satz- und Textverstehen bei Menschen mit geistiger Behinderung und funktionalen Analphabeten“. In: Bock, Bettina M./Fix, Ulla/Lange, Daisy (Hg.): *„Leichte Sprache“ im Spiegel theoretischer und angewandter Forschung*. Frank & Timme: Berlin, 2017, S. 253–274.

Bock, Bettina M./Lange, Daisy/Fix, Ulla: „Das Phänomen „Leichte Sprache“ im Spiegel aktueller Forschung. Tendenzen, Fragestellungen und Herangehensweisen“. “. In: Bock, Bettina M./Fix, Ulla/Lange, Daisy (Hg.): *„Leichte Sprache“ im Spiegel theoretischer und angewandter Forschung*. Frank & Timme: Berlin, 2017, S. 11–31.

Böttinger, Traugott: „Zur Notwendigkeit einer pädagogischen Sprache – Ringen um Deutungsmacht im theoretischen Diskurs“. In: Dederich, Markus/Ellinger, Stephan/Laubenstein, Désirée (Hg.): *Sonderpädagogik als Erfahrungs- und Praxiswissenschaft. Geistes-, sozial- und kulturwissenschaftliche Perspektiven*. Verlag Barbara Budrich: Opladen, 2019, S. 155–176.

Bourdieu, Pierre: „Die verborgenen Mechanismen der Macht enthüllen“. In: Bourdieu, Pierre: *Die verborgenen Mechanismen der Macht*. Hg. v. Margareta Steinrücke. VSA: Hamburg, 2005.

Bredel, Ursula/ Lang, Katrin/ Maaß, Christiane: „Zur empirischen Überprüfbarkeit von Leichte-Sprache-Regeln am Beispiel der Negation“. In: Mälzer, Nathalie (Hg.): *Barrierefreie Kommunikation – Perspektiven aus Theorie und Praxis*. Frank & Timme: 2016, S. 95–115.

Brinkmann, Hennig: *Sprache als Teilhabe. Aufsätze zur Sprachwissenschaft*. Pädagogischer Verlag Schwann (Sprache der Gegenwart, 14): Düsseldorf, 1981.

Bundeszentrale für politische Bildung/bpb (Hrsg.): *einfach POLITIK: Lexikon.* Autor/inn/en: Meyer, D./Schüller-Ruhl, T./Vock u.a., R./ Redaktion (verantw.): Wolfram Hilpert (bpb). Bonn: 2022. https://www.bpb.de/kurz-knapp/lexika/lexikon-in-einfacher-sprache/ [30.06.2022]

Butler, Judith: „Für ein sorgfältiges Lesen". In: Benhabib, Seyla/Butler, Judith/Cornell, Drucilla/Fraser Nancy (Hg.): *Der Streit um Differenz. Feminismus und Postmoderne in der Gegenwart.* Fischer: Frankfurt am Main, 1993, S. 122–132.

Chinn, Deborah: „Learning how to be (a) patient: visual analysis of accessible health information leaflets for people with intellectual disabilities". In: *Disability & Society* 32 (10), 2017, S. 1485–1509.

Dietrich, Cornelie: „Sprache". In: Wulf, Christoph/Zirfas, Jörg (Hg.): *Handbuch Pädagogische Anthropologie.* VS: Wiesbaden, 2014, S. 475–484.

Fajardo, Inmaculada/Ávila, Vicenta/Ferrer, Antonio/Tavares, Gema/Gómez, Marcos/Hernández, Ana: „Easy-to-read Texts for Students with Intellectual Disability. Linguistic Factors Affecting Comprehension". In: *Journal of Applied Research in Intellectual DisabilitOies* 27 (2), 2014, S. 212–225.

Foucault, Michel: *Mikrophysik der Macht. Über Strafjustiz, Psychiatrie und Medizin.* Merve: Berlin, 1976.

Foucault, Michel: *Dispositive der Macht. Über Sexualität, Wissen und Wahrheit.* Merve: Berlin, 1978.

Foucault, Michel: *Der Wille zum Wissen. Sexualität und Wahrheit 1.* Suhrkamp: Frankfurt am Main, 2003a.

Foucault, Michel: *Die Ordnung des Diskurses.* Fischer: Frankfurt am Main, 2003b.

Foucault, Michel: „Subjekt und Macht". In: Defert, Daniel/Ewald, François (Hg.): *Schriften in vier Bänden. Dits et Ecrits. Band 4.* Suhrkamp: Frankfurt am Main, 2005, S. 269–294.

Holly, Werner: „Sprache in Massenmedien. Medialität, Intermedialität und kulturelle Praxis". In: Volodina, Maja N. (Hg.): *Mediensprache und Medienkommunikation im interdisziplinären und interkulturellen Vergleich.* Institut für deutsche Sprache: Mannheim, 2013, S. 57–64.

Humboldt, Wilhelm von: „Theorie der Bildung des Menschen". In: Humboldt, Wilhelm von (Hg.): *Schriften zur Bildung. Herausgegeben von Gerhard Lauer.* Reclam: Stuttgart, 2019, S. 5–12.

Jekat, Susanne J./Jüngst, Heike Elisabeth/Schubert, Klaus/Villiger, Claudia: „Barrieren abbauen. Einleitung zum Sammelband Sprache barrierefrei gestalten: Perspektiven aus der angewandten Linguistik". In: Jekat, Susanne J./Jüngst, Heike Elisabeth/Schubert, Klaus/Villiger, Claudia (Hg.): *Sprache barrierefrei gestalten. Perspektiven aus der Angewandten Linguistik.* Frank & Timme: Berlin, 2014, S. 7–15.

Kaczmarzik, Janine: „Prüfen von Leichte-Sprache-Texten: Gewusst wie! Ziele der Textprüfung, Systematisierung der Prüfmethoden und Konzeption von Prüfungsinstrumenten". In: *Teilhabe* 57 (4), 2018, S. 174–180.

Kaczmarzik, Janine: „Prüfung von Leichte-Sprache-Texten: Gewusst wie! Probleme bei der Textprüfung, Grundprinzipien im Prüfungsprozess und erste Lösungsvorschläge". In: *Teilhabe* 58 (1), 2019, S. 10–17.

Kahl, Sylvia/Pöld-Krämer, Silvia: „Haben Menschen mit Behinderung ein Recht auf Schulden? Zur Finanzkompetenz von Menschen mit Lernschwierigkeiten". In: *Teilhabe* 53 (1), 2014, S. 30–35.

Karreman, Joyce/ van der Geest, Thea/ Buursink, Esmee: "Accessible Website Content Guidelines for Users with Intellectual Disabilities". In: *Journal of Applied Research in Intellectual Disabilities* 20 (6), 2007, S. 510–518.

Kellermann, Gudrun: „Leichte und Einfache Sprache – Versuch einer Definition". In: *Aus Politik und Zeitgeschichte* 64 (9–11), 2014, S. 7–10.

Köhler, Tanja: „Barrierefreie Sprache – Nachrichten für alle". In: *Gemeinsam leben* (3), 2016, S. 132–141.

Krasmann, Susanne: „Simultaneität von Körper und Sprache bei Michel Foucault". In: *Leviathan* 23 (2), 1995, S. 240–262.

Kupke, Charlotte/Schlummer, Werner: „Kommunikationsbarrieren und ihre Überwindung. Leichte Sprache und Verständlichkeit in Texten für Menschen mit Lernschwierigkeiten". In: *Teilhabe* 49 (2), 2010, S. 67–73.

Kurzenberger, Stephan/Niehoff, Ulrich/Walther, Helmut/Sack, Rudi: „Barrierefreiheit für Menschen mit kognitiver Beeinträchtigung – Ergebnisse einer Befragung". In: *Teilhabe* 51 (3), 2012, S. 121–126.

Lange, Daisy/Bock, Bettina M.: „Was heißt „Leichte" und „einfache Sprache"? Empirische Untersuchungen zu Begriffssemantik und tatsächlicher Gebrauchspraxis". In: Mälzer, Nathalie (Hg.): *Barrierefreie Kommunikation – Perspektiven aus Theorie und Praxis.* Frank & Timme: Berlin, 2016, S. 117–134.

Ledergerber, Bettina: „Leichte Sprache. Ein Praxiskonzept verbreitet sich in der Schweiz". In: *Schweizerische Zeitschrift für Heilpädagogik* 25 (2), 2019, S. 26–32.

Leitner, Gerhard: *Weltsprache Englisch. Vom angelsächsischen Dialekt zur globalen Lingua franca.* Verlag C. H. Beck: München, 2009.

Linz, Erika: „„Leichte Sprache ist nicht Kindersprache". Zur sozialen und pragmatischen Relevanz stilistischer Aspekte in Leichte-Sprache-Texten". In: Bock, Bettina M./Fix, Ulla/Lange, Daisy (Hg.): *„Leichte Sprache" im*

Spiegel theoretischer und angewandter Forschung. Frank & Timme: Berlin, 2017, S. 147–162.

Maaß, Christiane: *Easy Language – Plain Language – Easy Language Plus. Balancing Comprehensibility and Acceptability*. Frank & Timme: Berlin, 2020.

Maaß, Christiane/ Rink, Isabel/Zehrer, Christiane: „Leichte Sprache in der Sprach- und Übersetzungswissenschaft". In: Jekat, Susanne J./Jüngst, Heike Elisabeth/Schubert, Klaus/Villiger, Claudia (Hg.): *Sprache barrierefrei gestalten. Perspektiven aus der Angewandten Linguistik*. Frank & Timme: Berlin, 2014, S. 53–85.

Poncelas, Angela/Murphy, Glynis: „Accessible Information for People with Intellectual Disabilities: Do Symbols Really Help?" In: *Journal of Applied Research in Intellectual Disabilities* 20 (5), 2007, S. 466–474.

Przybyla-Wilkin, Agnieszka: "Easy-to-read in English, German and Polish". In: Mälzer, Nathalie (Hg.): *Barrierefreie Kommunikation – Perspektiven aus Theorie und Praxis*. Frank & Timme: Berlin, 2016, S. 135–150.

Reckwitz, Andreas: „Grundelemente einer Theorie sozialer Praktiken. Eine sozialtheoretische Perspektive". In: *Zeitschrift für Soziologie* 32 (4), 2003, S. 282–301.

Reichstein, Martin F.: „Teilhabe an der digitalen Gesellschaft? Über (vorgelagerte) Barrieren bei/in der Nutzung digitaler Medien durch Menschen mit einer sogenannten geistigen Behinderung". In: *Teilhabe* 55 (2), 2016, S. 80–85.

Rink, Isabel: „Zur Übersetzung juristischer Fachtexte in Leichte Sprache am Beispiel des Pilotprojekts „Leichte Sprache in der Niedersächsischen Justiz"". In: Mälzer, Nathalie (Hg.): *Barrierefreie Kommunikation – Perspektiven aus Theorie und Praxis*. Frank & Timme: Berlin, 2016, S. 257–273.

Rocktäschel, Lucia Clara: *Gendern in Leichter Sprache – eine Anleitung* (19.11.2020). https://www.genderleicht.de/gendern-in-leichter-sprache-anleitung/ [30.06.2022].

Rüstow, Nadine/Volkmann, Tobias: „Bildung durch Leichte Sprache – Barrierefreie Gestaltung kultureller und geschichtlicher Bildungsangebote im Museum". In: *Teilhabe* 52 (4), 2013, S. 186–190.

Schiewe, Jürgen: „„Leichte Sprache" aus der Perspektive von Sprachkritik und Sprachkultur. Überlegungen zur Anwendbarkeit der Kategorie „Angemessenheit"". In: Bock, Bettina M./Fix, Ulla/Lange, Daisy (Hg.): *„Leichte Sprache" im Spiegel theoretischer und angewandter Forschung*. Frank & Timme: Berlin, 2017, S. 71–85.

Schubert, Klaus/Klein, Martina: *Das Politiklexikon*. 7., aktual. u. erw. Aufl. Bundeszentrale für politische Bildung: Bonn, 2020. https://www.bpb.de/kurz-knapp/lexika/politiklexikon/ [30.06.2022].

Schuppener, Saskia/Goldbach, Anne/Bock, Bettina M.: „LEICHTE SPRACHE – ein inklusionssensibles Konzept zur Förderung beruflicher Teilhabe?" In: Feyerer, Ewald (Hg.): *System – Wandel – Entwicklung. Akteurinnen und Akteure inklusiver Prozesse im Spannungsfeld von Institution, Profession und Person*. Klinkhardt: Bad Heilbrunn, 2018, S. 361–367.

Seitz, Simone: „Leichte Sprache? Keine einfache Sache". In: *Aus Politik und Zeitgeschichte* 64 (9–11), 2014, S. 3–6.

Stefanowitsch, Anatol: „Leichte Sprache, komplexe Wirklichkeit". In: *Aus Politik und Zeitgeschichte* 64 (9–11), 2014, S. 11–18.

Stertkamp, Wolf: *Sprache und Kommunikation in Online-Computerspielen. Untersuchungen zu multimodaler Kommunikation am Beispiel von World of Warcraft*. Dissertation: Gießen, 2017.

Sutherland, Rebekah Joy/Isherwood, Tom: "The Evidence for Easy-Read for People With Intellectual Disabilities: A Systematic Literature Review". In: *Journal of Policy and Practice in Intellectual Disabilities* 13 (4), 2016, S. 297–310.

Trescher, Hendrik: *Inklusion. Zur Dekonstruktion von Diskursteilhabebarrieren im Kontext von Freizeit und Behinderung*. VS: Wiesbaden, 2015.

Trescher, Hendrik: *Ambivalenzen pädagogischen Handelns. Reflexionen der Betreuung von Menschen mit ‚geistiger Behinderung'*. Transcript: Bielefeld, 2018a.

Trescher, Hendrik: *Kognitive Beeinträchtigung und Barrierefreiheit. Eine Pilot-Studie*. Klinkhardt: Bad Heilbrunn, 2018b.

Trescher, Hendrik: „Selbstbestimmung. Ambivalenzen pädagogischen Handelns". In: *Schweizerische Zeitschrift für Heilpädagogik* 24 (7/8), 2018c, S. 6–12.

Trescher, Hendrik: „Leichte Sprache und Barrierefreiheit". In: *Schweizerische Zeitschrift für Heilpädagogik* 26 (10), 2020, S. 48–54.

Trescher, Hendrik: „Ambivalenzen Leichter Sprache". In: *Zeitschrift für Inklusion* 15 (1), 2021, online.

Trescher, Hendrik/Hauck, Teresa: „Zwischen Teilhabe und Ausschluss. Eltern und ihre erwachsenen Kinder mit geistiger Behinderung". In: *Schweizerische Zeitschrift für Heilpädagogik* 26 (1), 2020, S. 37–43.

Trescher, Hendrik/Klocke, Janos: „Kognitive Beeinträchtigungen mit Butler verstehen – Butler im Kontext kognitiver Beeinträchtigung verstehen". In: *Behindertenpädagogik* 53 (3), 2014, S. 285–308.

Villa, Paula-Irene: *Judith Butler. Eine Einführung*. Campus: Frankfurt am Main, 2012.

Zurstrassen, Bettina: „Inklusion durch Leichte Sprache? Eine kritische Einschätzung". In: Dönges, Christoph/Hilpert, Wolfram/Zurstrassen, Bettina (Hg.): *Didaktik der inklusiven politischen Bildung*. Bundeszentrale für politische Bildung: Bonn, 2015, S. 126–138.

Zurstrassen, Bettina: „Leichte Sprache – eine Sprache der Chancengleichheit?" In: Bock, Bettina M./Fix, Ulla/Lange, Daisy (Hg.): *„Leichte Sprache" im Spiegel theoretischer und angewandter Forschung*. Frank & Timme: Berlin, 2017, S. 53–69.

Renate Delucchi Danhier

Diversitätsembleme als individualisierte Visualisierungsform persönlicher Daten im Sinne des Datenhumanismus

Abstract: Data emblems are personalized graphic representations of personal information. These have gained popularity in recent years, especially on the Internet. This paper presents digital emblems specifically designed to represent individuals working in the field of diversity studies. The paper explains what information has been pictorially encoded in the emblems, the variables operationalized, the design decisions, and possible uses of the emblems. The personalized emblems are designed according to a predefined visual system that depicts the personal background as well as information about the academic career of the individual. The contribution of the paper is not the analysis of the data but rather a discussion of the design process of the visualization. The overall goal of the project is not to rank or quantify scientists or their work, like a publimetric project would do, but to design identity. Readers are invited to reflect on how personal characteristics may affect research in the field of diversity studies.

Keywords: data visualization, digital space, data humanism, diversity, personalized emblems

1. Einleitung

Ein Emblem ist eine abstrakte oder gegenständliche Darstellung, die ein Konzept oder eine Person repräsentiert. Embleme stehen zum Beispiel für Könige, Adelshäuser, Heilige oder sogar moralische Wahrheiten oder Allegorien. Beispiele für Embleme werden in Abbildung 1 gezeigt. Historisch gesehen, ist die Funktion von Emblemen für eine einflussreiche Person, Familie oder Institution zu stehen. Adelsgeschlechter, beispielsweise, haben Gegenstände wie Urkunden oder Gebäude mit ihren Emblemen versehen, um sie als ihnen zugehörig zu kennzeichnen. Somit stehen Embleme – im Unterschied zu einem Porträtfoto – nicht direkt für eine Person, sondern symbolisieren eher die Macht und den Einfluss einer Person oder einer ganzen Gruppe. Demnach können verschiedene Personen über Generationen hinweg dasselbe Emblem tragen, wie zum Beispiel im Fall des Emblems des britischen Königshauses Windsor oder des Emblems des Vereinigten Königreichs von Großbritannien und Nordirland. Letzteres ist gleichzeitig auch das Emblem von König Charles III und wird als Symbol der königlichen Herrschaft benutzt. Die Person, die das Amt übernimmt, wird durch die Weiterführung des schon bekannten und sich längst im Umlauf befindlichen Emblems legitimiert. Nur Könige und Mitglieder der königlichen Familien hatten ursprünglich das Recht, ein Emblem zu tragen, dieses Recht wurde später auf den Adel erweitert.

Die visuellen Elemente eines Emblems, wie Farbe oder Symbole, tragen eine Bedeutung und werden entsprechend als Attribute benutzt. Beispielsweise ist das Cavallino Rampante das Logo des italienischen Sportwagenherstellers Ferrari. Auf Rennwagen wird als Hintergrund des Logos die Form eines heraldischen Schildes verwendet. Bei Straßenfahrzeugen hat das Logo stattdessen eine rechteckige Form. Das Emblem selbst bildet ein schwarzes Pferd ab, das sich auf einem gelben Hintergrund aufbäumt, wobei die Farben der italienischen Flagge waagerecht darüber liegen. Die italienische Flagge bezieht sich darauf, dass Ferrari ein italienischer Hersteller ist. Der gelbe Hintergrund ist eine Hommage an die Stadt Modena, aus der der Gründer Enzo Ferrari stammt, und die schwarze Farbe steht für die Trauer um den verstorbenen legendären Jagdflieger und italienischen Nationalheld Francesco Baracca. Die Buchstaben „S F" stehen für Scuderia Ferrari, wörtlich „Rennstall Ferrari", als Ort, an dem Rennpferde gezüchtet werden. Das Pferd selbst wurde von dem Familienwappen der Familie Baracca übernommen. Das sich aufbäumende Pferd vermittelt als persönliches Emblem Dynamik, Kraft und ungezügeltes Temperament. Dies ist ein Beispiel für ein Symbol, welches im Laufe der Zeit vom Familienwappen zum Logo übergegangen ist. Embleme bleiben in vielen Fällen lange im Umlauf, weil sie an veränderte Anforderungen angepasst werden können.

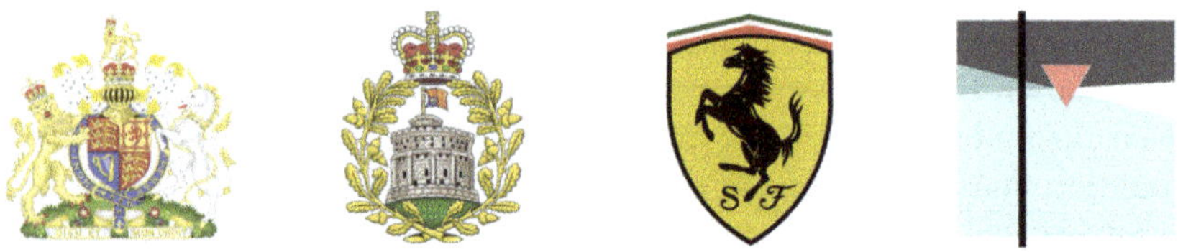

Das Wappen des Vereinigten Königreichs | Emblem des Hauses Windsor | Logo der Scuderia Ferrari | Diversitäts-Emblem

Abbildung 1: Auswahl von Emblemen, die für Personen oder Institutionen stehen. Ein Beispiel für die in diesem Beitrag vorgeschlagenen Embleme befindet sich ganz rechts

In den letzten Jahren haben Embleme in Form von Datenemblemen den Sprung in die digitale Welt geschafft. Genau wie die heraldischen Embleme werden diese digitalen Auffassungen des Emblemkonzepts verwendet, um Personen oder Institutionen digital und online zu repräsentieren. Digitale Datenembleme sind aber formell etwas anderes als ihre heraldischen Vorgänger, denn sie haben die Form von maßgeschneiderten Visualisierungen, die auf der Basis von persönlichen Daten von Menschen erstellt werden. Anstatt Symbole und Attribute werden hier Informationen durch abstrakte Formen, Farben und Winkel zum Ausdruck gebracht. Die zugrundeliegenden Daten, die zur Herstellung der Datenembleme herangezogen werden, können aus allen möglichen Bereichen des Lebens einer Person stammen. So können zum Beispiel die Anamnese eines*r Patienten*in (Plaisant et al. 1998) oder die unternommenen Reisen einer Person (Rekimoto, Miyaki & Ishizawa 2007) emblematisch dargestellt werden.

Spezialisierte Software, die es ermöglicht, anhand solcher vielfältigen Daten Datenvisualisierungen zu erstellen, wird zunehmend finanzierbar und benutzerfreundlicher. Gleichzeitig wird die Datenkompetenz der Nutzer*innen, d. h. die Fähigkeit, Datenpunkte als Informationen zu lesen, zu verstehen, zu erstellen und zu kommunizieren, immer früher und intensiver als Teil der Fertigkeiten der Digital Natives trainiert (Carlson & Johnston 2015, Tygel & Kirsch 2015). Dieser technische Fortschritt in der Visualisierungssoftware in Kombination mit der allgemeinen Verbesserung der Data Literacy von nicht speziell ausgebildeten Nutzer*innen, hat zu einer erhöhten Popularität solcher Embleme im Internet geführt. Datenembleme, die virtuell im Internet Gebrauch finden, stehen in derselben Traditionslinie der Heraldik, da sie abstrakte Informationen über eine Person, Familie oder Gruppe visuell kodieren und eher repräsentativ als erklärend zu interpretieren sind. Die Datenporträts, die im Internet Verwendung finden, entsprechen weder wissenschaftlichen Ansprüchen an die Qualität der genutzten Datengrundlage noch verfügen sie über eine systematische Methodik der Darstellung. In diesem Beitrag soll daher deren Potential als wissenschaftliche Methodik einer humanistisch orientierten Datenanalyse exploriert werden.

Ziel dieses Beitrags ist es, eine Visualisierung ausgewählter Wissenschaftler*innen im Bereich der Diversitätsstudien zu erstellen, um anhand dieser Visualisierung Diversität selbst im Denken der Nutzer*innen anzuregen: Kognitive Vielfalt ist Vielfalt im Denken. Diversitätswissenschaftler*innen weisen eine Menge persönlicher und beruflicher Diversitätsmerkmale auf, die oft nicht von diesen Wissenschaftler*innen selbst wahrgenommen und wertgeschätzt werden. Die vorgeschlagenen Embleme sollen diese diversen Profile sichtbar machen. Dabei steht nicht die Datenanalyse im Vordergrund, sondern die Datenvisualisierung, um die hinter den Emblemen stehenden Daten im Sinne eines Storytellings greifbar zu machen. Um aber ein ausdrucksstarkes Design zu erzielen, das dem Datenhumanismus zugeordnet werden kann, ist es unabwendbar, Daten von echten Menschen zu nutzen. Denn das ist genau, worum es im *Data Humanism* geht: „Daten nutzen, um die menschliche Geschichte hinter den Zahlen und Statistiken zu entdecken und die Vorstellung von Daten als etwas Unpersönliches und Einschüchterndes in Frage zu stellen" (Lupi 2017). Datenembleme können dabei eine Methodik darstellen, Daten und deren Interpretation in der Wissenschaft kritisch zu hinterfragen und implizite Machtstrukturen aufzudecken. Ziel des Beitrages ist es daher anhand des o.g. Beispiels ausgewählter Wissenschaftler*innen das Datenemblem als Methode der Kontextualisierung und Visualisierung von Daten in einem wissenschaftlichen Kontext zu explorieren.

Der Bereich der Diversitätsstudien ist aufgrund seiner Auseinandersetzung mit verschiedenen Ausprägungen von Identität, seiner inter- und transdisziplinären Orientierung und seiner damit verbundenen Offenheit für neue Methoden und Perspektiven der ideale Kontext für diese Bestrebungen. Die Diversitätsforschung untersucht Konstruktionsprozesse von Zugehörigkeiten und Zuschreibungen von sozialer Identität. Dieser Beitrag ist ein Versuch, die soziale Identität der Diversitätsforscher*innen selbst zu visualisieren, um zu zeigen wie durch Embleme Daten personalisiert und kontextualisiert werden können. Aspekte von Identität und Intersektionalität werden dabei in Form eines Emblems auf einen Blick sichtbar und für Dritte nachvollziehbar. Wenn ein Forschungsbereich von Diversität profitieren kann, dann sind dies die Diversitätsstudien selbst. Dabei ist die Diversität gemeint, die potentiell die wissenschaftliche Tätigkeit beeinflussen könnte: Diversität im Selbstbild, Diversität sozialen Ursprunges, aber auch in erster Linie Diversität in der Kognition: Wie denken diese Forscher*innen, wie sehen sie die Welt, auf welcher Sprache denken sie? Mit Hilfe dieser Visualisierung soll eine Übersicht über die Vielfalt der in diesem Bereich tätigen Kolleg*innen gewonnen werden. Außerdem soll ausprobiert werden, inwieweit diese Embleme zu Repräsentationszwecken von den Wissenschaftler*innen selbst in verschiedenen Kontexten benutzt werden könnten. Es soll exploriert werden, inwiefern sich Embleme für die Untersuchung und Darstellung verschiedener Diversitätsdimensionen und deren Intersektionalität als Einfluss auf Identität eignen.

Die in diesem Artikel vorgestellten Datenembleme sollen Personen repräsentieren und gleichzeitig Eigenschaften und Informationen über Diversitätseigenschaften dieser Akademiker*innen integrieren. Diese Visualisierungen werden Diversitätsembleme genannt, um deren Repräsentationswert in den Vordergrund zu stellen. Die Visualisierung wird die Form eines personalisierten

Datenemblems einnehmen, welche biographische Informationen verschlüsselt. Da es sich um personenbezogene Daten handelt, die unter die Datenschutzgrundverordnung (DSGVO) fallen, werden die Informationen bei der Visualisierung absichtlich teilweise undurchsichtig dargestellt, um die Privatsphäre der Personen zu schützen. Dies hat jedoch gleichzeitig zur Konsequenz, dass die Embleme nicht für das Lesen optimiert sein werden, weil keine Rückschlüsse über die hinter den Emblemen liegenden Daten möglich sind. Somit sind die Embleme für eine formale Analyse ungeeignet, dennoch können sie die Vielfalt und verschiedene Identitäten innerhalb der Gemeinschaft der Menschen aufzeigen, die im Bereich Diversitätsstudien arbeiten und forschen. Somit ist das Ziel dieser Darstellungsform nicht Genauigkeit; diese Art von Darstellung ist kein reines Werkzeug für wissenschaftliche oder soziologische Analysen, sondern ein Stück funktionale Kunst (Cairo 2012), welche zu Repräsentationszwecken, als ein Introspektionsintrumentarium oder als Impuls für Gespräche zwischen den Diversitätswissenschaftler*innen dienen kann.

Der Beitrag ist wie folgt strukturiert: Nach einer kurzen Einführung in die Thematik folgt ein kurzer Exkurs in den historischen Ursprung der Embleme und deren Nutzung in Literatur und Film. Es wird hier gezeigt, wie Embleme in unterschiedlichen Kulturen und zu verschiedenen Zeiten als ein symbolischer Gegenstand zu Zwecken der Repräsentation und der Wiedererkennung benutzt worden sind. Nachfolgend wird auf andere, ähnliche Visualisierungsprojekte eingegangen, um Kontext für die hier vorgeschlagene Visualisierung zu geben. Im nächsten Kapitel geht es um die Erörterung der designspezifischen Prinzipien, die das Visualisierungsprojekt leiten. Anschließend wird das Konzept der Visualisierung zusammen mit den Rahmenbedingungen und Parametern welche das Design inspiriert bzw. eingeschränkt haben, vorgestellt. Diese umfassen den Internetauftritt der Konferenz „Diversity in Cognition" (5. bis 7. Februar 2020, TU-Dortmund), auf der dieses Projekt erstmalig präsentiert wurde, sowie die unternehmenskommunikativen Auftrittselemente der Universität, auf denen die Konferenz stattgefunden hat. Daraufhin wird der Schlüssel zum Lesen der Visualisierung erklärt. Es folgen die Erklärung der Methode der Datenerhebung und kurze Einsichten in den Datensatz, die aus der Verwendung der Embleme bis jetzt gewonnen werden konnten. Danach werden Möglichkeiten zur Anwendung der Embleme vorgestellt. Der Beitrag wird mit einem Fazit abgeschlossen.

2. Beispiele für die historische Relevanz und Funktion von Emblemen und ihre Nutzung in Literatur und Film

Ein Emblem ist ein abstraktes oder gegenständliches Bild, das für ein Konzept oder eine Person steht. Die Tradition von Emblemen, Logos und anderen Symbolen ist in einer langen Reihe von repräsentativen ikonographischen Darstellungen einzuordnen, die schon seit der Antike zu Repräsentationszwecken genutzt worden sind. Auch in Literatur und Film werden Embleme bis heute zu Zwecken des Wordbuilding, der Konstruktion in sich schlüssiger fiktiver Welten, verwendet. Ziel des folgenden Abschnittes ist es, zum besseren Verständnis des Emblemkonzepts, einen Überblick über die historische Entwicklung der Nutzung und der Typen von Emblemen zu geben und darzustellen, welche Funktion Embleme in Literatur und Film einnehmen.

2.1 Die historische Nutzung von Emblemen

Manche der frühesten historischen Beispiele für den sozialen und politischen Gebrauch von Emblemen finden wir im Alten Ägypten. Als bekanntes Beispiel können an dieser Stelle die königlichen Kartuschen genannt werden, denn die Kartuschen haben ikonographisch den königlichen Namen hervorgehoben. Es gab aber eine noch frühere ikonographische Konvention, welche den Kartuschen vier Dynastien vorausgeht (ca. 700 Jahre): Das Serekh (Hieroglyphen-Transkription srḫl). Es besteht aus einem rechteckigen Rahmen, der die mit Nischen oder Toren versehene Fassade eines Palastes darstellt und (üblicherweise) vom Horus-Falken gekrönt wird. Wie bei den Kartuschen steht der königliche Name in Serekh eingeschlossen. Eines der frühesten erhaltenen Beispiele für den Gebrauch eines Serekh als Emblem ist in der sogenannten Prunkpalette des Narmer (Abbildung 2) zu sehen, die auf ca. 3100 v. Chr. datiert wird. Narmer war ein Pharao der Frühzeit bzw. der sogenannten 0. Dynastie. Die Prunkpalette zeigt das Serekh von Pharao Narmer auf beiden Seiten im obersten Bereich. Narmers Serekh ist insoweit als ein Emblem zu deuten, als es im Inneren der Fassadendarstellung die Hieroglyphen *nʿr* (Wels) und *mr* (Meißel) trägt. Diese geben die phonetische Darstellung des Königsnamens Nar+mer, übersetzt „Schlagwels", wieder und folgen dabei dem Rebus-Prinzip: Die Hieroglyphen werden hier als Phonogramme verwendet, ohne Rücksicht auf die ursprüngliche Bedeutung der Zeichen. Somit wird im Emblem der Name des Pharaos durch die Hieroglyphen und dessen Stellung durch die einrahmende Palastfassade repräsentiert. Der Gebrauch der Serekh als Emblem war damals auf den Pharao beschränkt, als Teil der Repräsentationsmöglichkeiten des Königs.

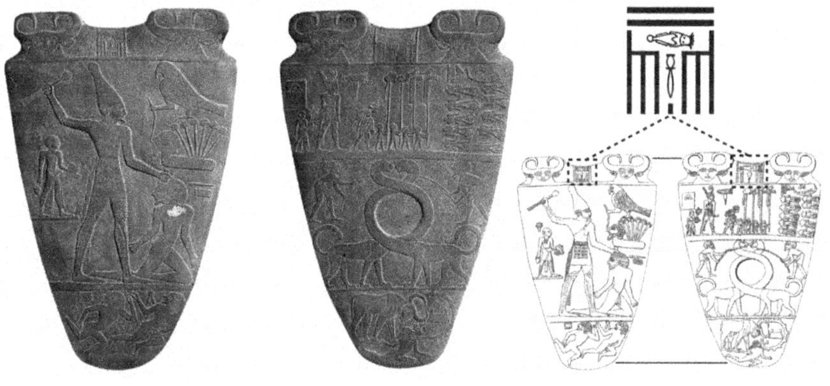

Abbildung 2: Prunkpalette des Narmer mit Serekh des Pharaos

Im Laufe der Zeit wurde der Gebrauch solcher Embleme verbreitet und auch allmählich weiteren Bevölkerungsgruppen zugänglich gemacht, was in der Archäologie als Demokratisierungsprozess bezeichnet wird (Willens 2008). Ein Beispiel hierfür findet sich im Mittelalter: Im 11. und 12. Jahrhundert n. Chr. hat sich in Zusammenhang mit der mittelalterlichen Heraldik der Gebrauch von Emblemen verbreitet: Ritter in Westeuropa begannen die freie Fläche der Schilder als Erkennungszeichen mit geometrischen Figuren, Tieren oder anderen Ausschmückungen zu verzieren. Solche geschmückten Schilderflächen sind beispielsweise in einer der Abbildungen in der Bamberger Motettenhandschrift (Suckale-Redlefsen 1984), auch Codex Bamberg genannt (ca. 1170 n. Chr.), zu sehen. Abbildung 3 zeigt zwei Illustrationen in kolorierter Federzeichnung vom sogenannten Davidmeister, die den Kommentar zu den 150 Psalmen des Alten Testaments von Petrus Lombardus schmücken. Die Illustrationen zeigen kämpfende Ritter mit Rüstungen sowie mit Emblemen versehene Schilder. Es ist in der Forschung noch umstritten, ob der Gebrauch von Emblemen auf den Schildflächen mit Rüstungsentwicklungen (Pastoureau 2003:27) oder mit sozialen Entwicklungen des ritterlichen Status (Jones 2008) in Verbindung zu bringen ist: Diese frühen Wappen können entweder als Ausdruck eines ritterlichen und individuellen Selbstverständnisses angesehen werden oder als eine eher praktische Notwendigkeit, im Turnier oder Kampf erkannt zu werden. Es ist aber wahrscheinlich, dass der Gebrauch der Embleme zeigt, dass der Ritter um diese Zeit nicht mehr nur als Kämpfer angesehen wurde, sondern als Teil der exklusiven Klasse des höfischen Rittertums. Der Gebrauch solcher piktographischer und farbiger Wappenschilder bzw. Fahnen war sehr nützlich in Zeiten, in denen nur ein kleiner Anteil der Bevölkerung lesen und schreiben konnte (Wendehorst 1986). Die meisten Ritter selbst waren Analphabeten. Über bildliche Zeichen und Farben konnten semantische Inhalte auch für Analphabeten zugänglich gemacht werden, oder zumindest als Wiedererkennungsfaktor genutzt werden.

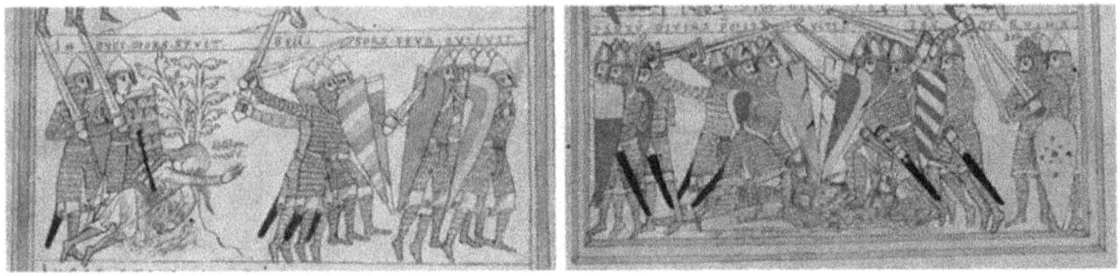

Abbildung 3: Kämpfende Ritter des Codex Bamberg

Der Gebrauch von Emblemen als repräsentative Darstellungsform ist nicht nur in der westlichen Tradition zu finden. Auch in östlichen Kulturen wurden Embleme genutzt. Ein Beispiel für asiatische Embleme sind die japanischen Hausmarken, auf Japanisch 紋(*mon*) genannt. Mon sind beim Kriegeradel schon im 12. Jahrhundert belegt, bis heute als Familienzeichen (*kamon* 家紋) in Gebrauch (Hawley & Chappelear 1976) und manchmal in Firmenlogos integriert (Abbildung 4). Das Mon des japanischen Kaisers, die sechzehnblättrige Chrysantheme, dient zugleich als Staatswappen Japans und steht u.a. auf dem japanischen Pass.

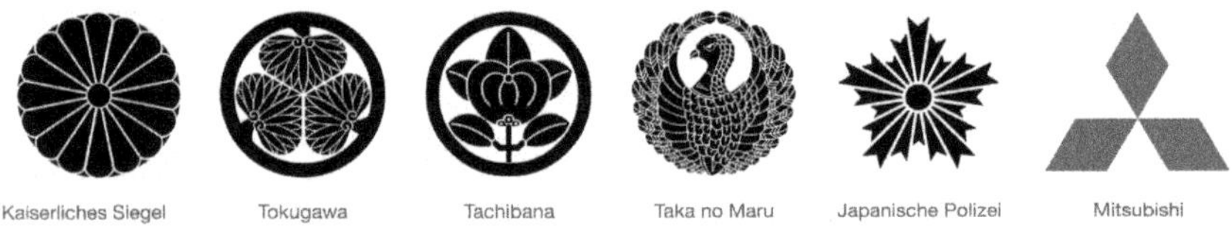

Abbildung 4: Beispiele für japanische Mons. Das Mon der Mitsubishi ist gleichzeitig die Marke des Unternehmens

Mons sind, anders als europäische Embleme, typischerweise kreisförmig und monochrom, d. h. dass die Farbe nicht Teil des Designs ist. Entsprechend kann ein Mon in jeder Farbe gezeichnet werden, weil keine symbolische Bedeutung an die Farbe gekoppelt ist. Grund für die vorherrschende Kreisform der Mons ist, dass sie zuerst als Aufnäher für Kleidung und Fahnen sowie als Emblem auf Laternen dienten (Hartmann 2016). Die runde Form zusammen mit der

Umrandung vereinfacht das Aufnähen von vorgefertigten Emblemen. Somit ist die runde Form der Embleme für Asien typisch, die Schildform hingegen für (Nordwest)-Europa charakteristisch. Diese Unterschiede in Ausprägung und Form der Embleme sind, wie oben beschrieben, auf die unterschiedliche Nutzung zurück zu führen. Die unterschiedlichen Designentscheidungen sind in diesen Beispielen von Anforderungen an den Gebrauch geprägt, auch wenn beide Arten von Emblemen mit der ikonographischen Repräsentation primär dieselbe Funktion erfüllen.

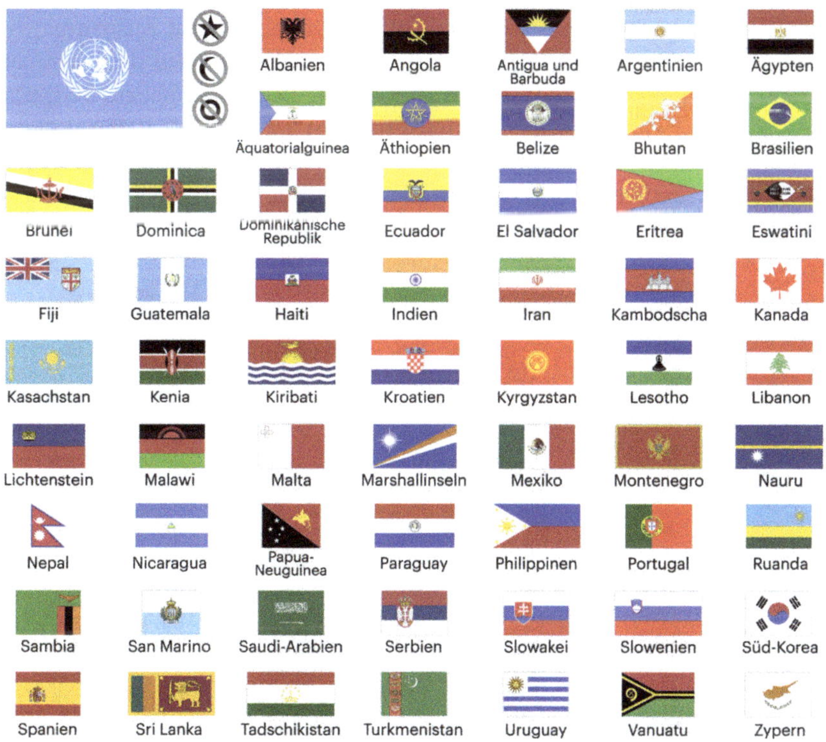

Abbildung 5: Flaggen der Welt, welche ein Emblem im Design tragen

Ab dem 13. Jh. haben auch Länder in Europa angefangen, Flaggen als Symbole zu nutzen. Manche Flaggen nutzen auch Embleme, die, wie wir gesehen haben, bis dahin nur mit einzelnen Rittern oder Familien in Verbindung gebracht wurden, und jetzt auch zur Repräsentation von geopolitischen Einheiten verwendet werden. Die früheste Flagge, die ein Emblem trägt und noch heute in Gebrauch ist, ist die von Albanien, die zum ersten Mal 1443 als Skanderbeg gebraucht wurde, als der albanische Nationalheld die Flagge hisste, um den eindringenden Türken zu trotzen. Das Design des doppelköpfigen Adlers wurde dem byzantinischen Reich entlehnt, die Flagge wurde 1912 nach der endgültigen Unabhängigkeit vom Osmanischen Reich offiziell von der neuen albanischen Republik angenommen. So wie im Fall Albaniens, tragen viele moderne Flaggen Embleme, z. B. Spanien oder Ecuador. Von 193 Nationalflaggen der Mitglieder der Vereinten Nationen tragen 59 heute ein Emblem, was 30,6 % aller Flaggen der Mitglieder der Vereinten Nationen entspricht. Dabei wurde jedes symbolische Zeichen als Emblem betrachtet, mit Ausnahme von fünfzackigen Sternen, der Halbmondsichel oder Kreisen, weil diese sehr oft vorkommen und eine standarisierte symbolische Bedeutung haben. Beispielsweise gilt die Halbmondsichel mit fünfzackigem Stern (*Hilal*) als Symbol des Islams und ist in vielen Flaggen der islamischen Welt verbreitet. Alle Flaggen, die diesen Kriterien entsprechen, sind in Abbildung 5 dargestellt. Die Flagge der Vereinten Nationen trägt selbst auch ein Emblem.

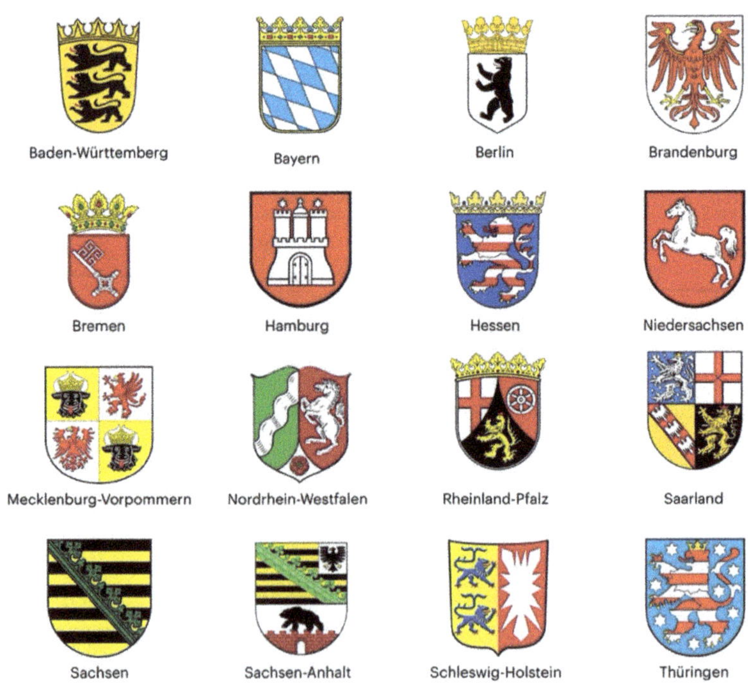

Abbildung 6: Wappen der deutschen Bundesländer

Embleme sind, auch unabhängig von Flaggen, noch heute im Gebrauch, je nach Form werden sie auch Wappen genannt: Das Wort Wappen selbst offenbart den militärischen Ursprung dieser Tradition. Das Wort kommt aus dem Mittelniederländischen *wāpen*, was „Zeichen auf der Waffe" bedeutete. Es wurde erst im 16. Jahrhundert im Sprachgebrauch zwischen dem Schild als Verteidigungsgerät und dem ikonographischen Zeichen auf dem Schild unterschieden. Der Ursprung kann bis heute an der schildartigen Form der Wappen als Untergruppe der Embleme erkannt werden. Beispielsweise haben alle sechszehn deutschen Bundesländer ein eigenes schildförmiges Wappen (Abbildung 6). Dabei funktionieren solche modernen Wappen ikonographisch oft genauso wie die ältesten Embleme, indem sie auf dem Gebrauch von Symbolen, Metaphern und des Rebus-Prinzips, der Verwendung von Emblemen als Phonogramme, basieren. Beispielsweise trägt das Wappen von Berlin seit ungefähr 1280 einen Bären. Die Stadt Berlin ist mit dem Bären über dasselbe Rebus-Prinzip verbunden, das schon beim Serekh des Pharao Narmer in Gebrauch war: Der Ortsname Berlin ist slawischen Ursprungs, abgeleitet von *Berl*, was „Sumpf" bedeutet und phonetisch dem deutschen Wort *„Bärlein"* ähnlich ist (Fischer 2005).

2.2 Embleme in Literatur und Film

Auch in der literarischen Darstellung fiktiver Königreiche und Länder werden Embleme benutzt, um kriegerische oder politische Fraktionen auseinander zu halten und allgemein zu Zwecken des *Worldbuilding,* also der Konstruktion einer in sich nachvollziehbaren Welt. Embleme finden sich besonders im Bereich der Fantasy-Literatur, wie zum Beispiel bei *The Lord of the Rings* oder *A Song of Ice and Fire (Game of Thrones)*. Die Embleme werden in mittelalterlicher Tradition in diesen Texten bei Festzügen oder vor einer Schlacht beschrieben. Die Wichtigkeit der Embleme wird oft in solchen Fantasy-Werken *in-world* diskutiert, d. h. im Werk selbst. Ein Beispiel dafür ist in „A Clash of Kings" (*A Song of Ice and Fire*) zu finden. Jon Snow erklärt dem Wildlingsmädchen Ygritte die Bedeutung der Heraldik in den Sieben Königslanden:

Ygritte: *„Is that how you lot do your fighting? You march down the road banging drums and waving banners?"*
Jon Snow: *„Most of the time, yes."*
Ygritte: *„How do the men holding the banners fight?"*
Jon Snow: *„They don't, really. It's a great honor to carry your House sigil."*

Ebenfalls bei *Game of Thrones* hat jedes Adelshauses eine eigene Heraldik, die aus einem Wappen mit festen Symbolen und Farben sowie einem Motto besteht. Das Familienwappen wird oft auf der Kleidung der Charaktere abgebildet (Abbildung 7). Familienmottos haben in der Regel die Form von Schlachtrufen oder Prahlereien. Eine große Ausnahme bildet das Haus Stark, dessen Ruf die unheilvolle Warnung „Der Winter naht“ lautet.

Auch in den Filmen der „Herr der Ringe“ erscheinen Embleme hauptsächlich auf Kleidung und Fahnen, gelegentlich auch auf Schilden. Im zweiten „Herr der Ringe“ Film, „Die zwei Türme“, kommt es zu einer Schlacht zwischen Rohan und Isengard. Hierbei werden die Rohirrim als die Guten und Isengard als die Bösen dargestellt. Auf beiden Seiten sind die Krieger mit Emblemen dargestellt, die sie als Gruppe ausweisen. Die Bösewichte tragen eine weiße Hand, eine Anspielung auf Saruman den Weißen, den Herrscher von Isengard. Die Bewohner von Rohan tragen ein weißes Pferd auf grünem Grund, weil Rohan gelegentlich das *Reiterland* genannt wird und die Armee Rohans überwiegend aus Kavallerieeinheiten besteht. Lediglich die Anbringung dieser Symbole auf einem Schild macht sie nicht automatisch zu heraldischen Emblemen. Ein Wappen würde auf eine bestimmte Person referieren, wie z. B. Saruman, den Herrn von Isengard, oder Théoden, den König von Rohan. Es dient der Identifizierung seines Trägers im Kampf, in dieser Schlacht jedoch tragen alle das gleiche Emblem. Diese beiden Embleme identifizieren die gesamte Gruppe, aber nicht einzelne Personen, anders als die historischen heraldischen Wappen. Damit sind sie den modernen Flaggen ähnlicher. Solche Embleme spielen eine wichtige Rolle bei der Film-Ausstattung und dem *Merchandising* literarischer Fantasie-Werke.

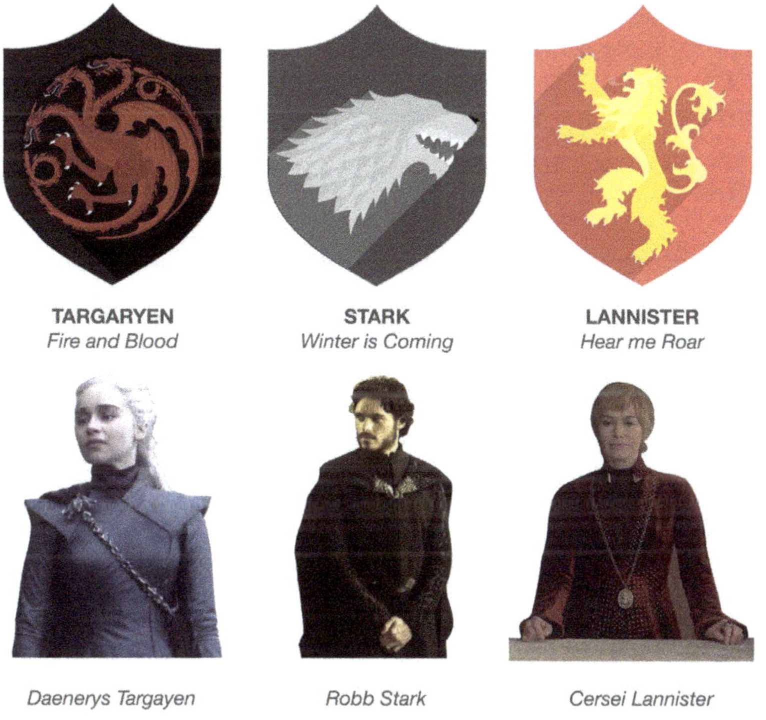

Abbildung 7: Familienembleme bei *Game of Thrones* (rechts), die von den Charakteren an ihren Kostümen z. B. als Broschen oder Schmuck getragen werden

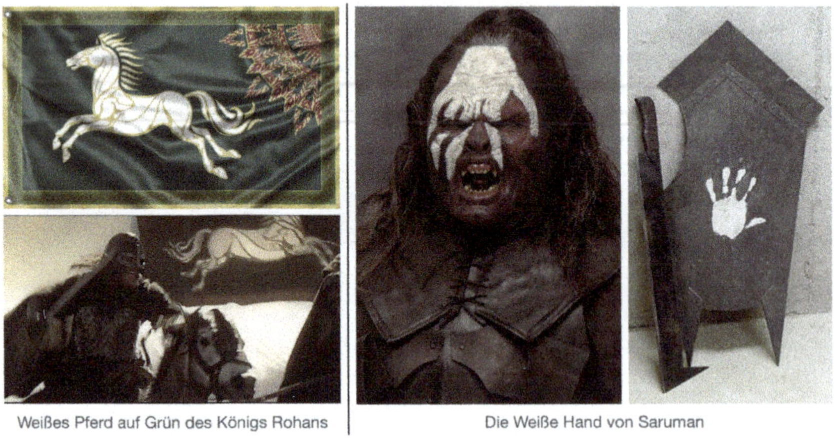
Weißes Pferd auf Grün des Königs Rohans
Die Weiße Hand von Saruman

Abbildung 8: Embleme aus dem Film *The Two Towers* von *The Lord of the Rings*: Die guten Rohirrim und die Bösen Uruk-Hai werden zusätzlich durch Embleme identifiziert

In Tolkiens Legendarium findet sich die Idee einer komplexen elbischen Heraldik bereits in frühen Texten wie "The Fall of Gondolin". Sein schöpferischer Eifer hat Tolkien zu der Erfindung eines ausgedachten Systems von regelgeleiteten Emblemen motiviert, was zur Illustration der von ihm geschaffenen Geschlechter, Helden und mythischen Reiche verwendet werden konnte. Es handelt sich um eine Gruppe von einfachen Zeichnungen, gezeichnet mit Zirkel und Lineal von Tolkiens Hand, die auf das letzte Jahrzehnt von Tolkiens Leben datiert sind (Hammond & Scull 1995). Die Embleme, die Tolkien für die Elbenvölker mit Lineal und Zirkel entworfen hat, sind farbige, abstrakte geometrische Zeichnungen: Tolkien schuf ein persönliches System gegenständlicher, und genealogischer, Bilder, das von Regeln bestimmt war. Die Embleme für das Haus des Finwës, das Königshaus der Ñoldor, wird in Abbildung 9 gezeigt. Die Elbenembleme sind sowohl horizontal als auch vertikal symmetrisch. Die Form bestimmt, für wen das Emblem steht: Die Embleme der Frauen haben die Form eines Kreises, die der Männer die Form einer Raute und die Wahrzeichen von Familien, Häusern oder Reichen haben die Form eines Quadrats. Der Rang wird durch die Anzahl der Berührungspunkte des Musters mit dem äußeren Rand bestimmt: Vier Berührungspunkte stehen für einen Fürsten, sechs bis acht Berührungspunkte für einen König. Die großen Urväter haben manchmal sechzehn Berührungspunkte, wie der Hochkönig Finwë.

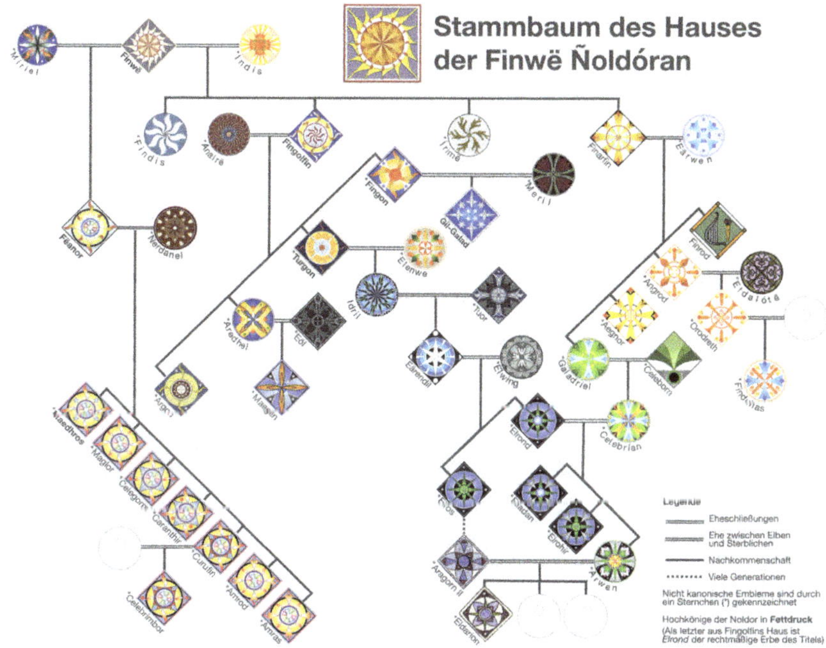

Abbildung 9: Elbenembleme von J.R.R.Tolkien integriert im Stammbaum der Finwë, erster Hochkönig der Ñoldor

Zusätzlich werden familiäre Beziehungen oft durch Ähnlichkeiten im Muster gekennzeichnet: Das lässt sich zum Beispiel bei den Motiven für das Haus von Finwë, für Finwë selbst, seinen ältesten Sohn Fëanor und seinen zweiten Sohn Fingolfin erkennen. Die Darstellung erfolgt immer sehr gründlich, bei Tolkien sollen „die heraldischen Regeln und der visuelle Kanon mit der gleichen philologischen Sorgfalt behandelt werden wie die Vokabular- und Grammatikregeln seiner geschaffenen Sprachen“ (Hriban 2011). Die Verwendung von regelbasiertem Verhalten für die Embleme hat den Vorteil, dass – auch wenn Tolkien selbst kein persönliches Emblem für alle Ñoldor entworfen hat – die fehlenden Embleme von anderen Tolkien-Gelehrten und engagierten Tolkiendili (Tolkien-Fans) unter Anwendung dieser Regeln re- bzw. nachkonstruiert werden können, wie in Abbildung 9 gezeigt wird.

2.3 Moderne Nutzung von Emblemen

Die Tradition, Bilder, Wappentiere und Farben zur Repräsentation und zu Wiedererkennungszwecken zu nutzen, bleibt bis heute bestehen. Die Wappenkunde als Teil der mittelalterlichen Rezeption hat zudem immer noch eine besondere Stellung in der kollektiven Vorstellungskraft sowie Pop-Kultur (Petersen 2009) und kann auf Spielzeugen, als Markenzeichen von Unternehmen auf der Ausrüstung von Sportmannschaften oder in Fernsehserien gefunden werden. In Abbildung 10 werden drei moderne Emblembeispiele gezeigt: Ein Detail eines Trikots des Ballspielverein Borussia mit den assoziierten Anfangsbuchstaben BVB und den Vereinsfarben schwarz-gelb (links); eine Playmobilfigur eines Ritters (mittig) und das Wappen des Hauses Targaryen mit dessen Familienmotto aus G.R.R. Martins *A Song of Ice and Fire* bzw. der Fernsehadaptation *Game of Thrones* des Senders HBO (rechts). Der Gebrauch von Emblemen ist also nach wie vor aktuell und weltweit verbreitet.

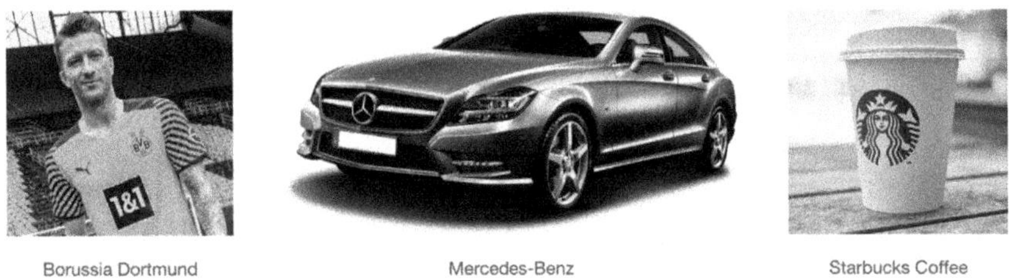

Abbildung 10: Moderne Beispiele für den Gebrauch von Emblemen in der Sportausrüstung und als Marke

Es wurde in diesem Abschnitt gezeigt, dass Embleme kontinuierlich von der Vorgeschichte bis heute in verschiedenen Kontexten genutzt worden sind. Datenembleme, die im virtuellen Raum Verwendung finden, stehen in derselben Traditionslinie der Heraldik, da Datenembleme thematische Eigenschaften einer Person, Familie oder Gruppe visuell kodieren und eher repräsentativ als erklärend zu interpretieren sind. Die weiter unten vorgestellten Visualisierungen werden als Emblem bezeichnet, da sie hauptsächlich als symbolische Erkennungszeichen dienen sollen. Zusätzlich enkodieren diese Datenembleme durch Formen und Farben zusätzliche Informationen über die dargestellten Personen, Gruppen und Institutionen, so dass sie über eine rein symbolische Anspielung hinausgehen.

3. Graphiken und Best Practices bei der Datenvisualisierung

Wie oben gezeigt, wurden seit Jahrtausenden Embleme benutzt, um Menschen und Gruppen hinsichtlich ihrer sozio-ökonomischen oder politischen Eigenschaften zu repräsentieren. Es wurden die Kontexte und die formellen Mittel (Form, Farben und Symbole) erklärt, mit denen Embleme ihre Botschaften visuell kommunizieren. In der Forschung wurde aber bisher nicht versucht, diese Darstellungsmittel auf Akademiker*innen anzuwenden. In diesem Beitrag werden Diversitätsembleme vorgestellt, die wie traditionelle Embleme funktionieren, jedoch zugleich maßgeschneiderte Visualisierungen sind. Sie orientieren sich hierbei entsprechend an den Best Practices der Datenvisualisierung. Aus einer Datenvisualiserungsperspektive verleiht die Einhaltung dieser formellen Kriterien den Emblemen Validität und macht diese somit zu graphischen Datenrepräsentationen.

Im Folgenden sollen Best Practices für die Visualisierung von Daten beleuchtet werden, die eine Orientierung geben sollen, worauf es bei einer aussagekräftigen und nachvollziehbaren Darstellung ankommt. Für die Darstellung quantitativer Daten in wissenschaftlichen Kontexten findet die Nutzung von Emblemen bisher noch keine verbreitete Anwendung, es wird vielmehr mit verschiedenen Formen graphischer Diagramme gearbeitet. Ein graphisches Diagramm ist eine Form der Datendarstellung quantitativer Art, in der visuelle Mittel (Linien, Vektoren, Flächen oder Symbole) verwendet werden, um die mathematische Beziehung oder statistische Korrelation zwischen den Variablen sichtbar zu machen. Es gibt eine große Anzahl verschiedener Diagramme bzw. Visualisierungsformen. Die besser bekannten und meist gebrauchten, wie Streudiagramme, Säulendiagramme oder Tortendiagramme werden standarisierte Visualisierungsformen genannt. Jede Visualisierungsform hat ihre Vor- und Nachteile. Im Bereich der Wahrnehmungsforschung und Psychologie sind in den letzten Jahrzenten Untersuchungen durchgeführt worden, um besser nachvollziehen zu können, wie visuelles Denken und visuelle Kommunikation funktionieren (Arnheim 1969). Auf dieser Basis kann begründet entschieden werden, welche graphischen Enkodierungen von Informationen beim Designen von Visualisierungen bevorzugt werden sollten (Franconeri 2021; Heer et al. 2010; Cairo 2019), weil sie besser von den Leser*innen verstanden werden und nachhaltiger in der Erinnerung der Nutzer*innen bleiben. Aus diesen Untersuchungen entstehen *Best-Practices-Prinzipien* für den Bereich des Visualisierungsdesigns (Munzner 2014, Meirelles 2013). Beispielsweise sind Länge und Position leichter visuell zu vergleichen als Winkel, sodass, wenn die genauen Werte von Bedeutung sind, allgemeine (gestapelte) Säulendiagramme vor Tortendiagrammen zu bevorzugen sind. Neben diesen grundlegenden und sehr breit verbreiteten Formen der Graphiken finden sich andere, die, wenn auch ebenfalls standardisiert und lange im Umlauf, weniger bekannt sind. Boxplots zum Beispiel wurden 1970 vom Mathematiker John Tukey (Tukey 1970) eingeführt.

Seine Kolleg*innen und Studierenden haben die Graphikform stark beworben (Kleiner & Graedel 1980, Cox & Jones 1981) und die Boxplots verbreiteten sich über die Statistik hinaus in mehreren quantitativen Wissenschaften. Der Bekanntheitsgrad ist so groß geworden, dass das Boxplot heute als Standarddiagramm der Statistik gilt. Wenn eine Graphikform ein solch hohen Bekanntheitsgrad erlangt, muss beim Gebrauch nicht mehr erklärt werden, welche Daten genau dargestellt werden oder wie die Graphiken zu lesen sind. Die Diagramme werden durch diese Art Lexikalisierungsprozess zu standardisierten Graphiken. Radardiagramme, auch Spinnendiagramme genannt, wurden fast gleichzeitig mit den Boxplots 1973 eingeführt (Kolence 1973), haben aber nicht denselben Lexikalisierungsprozess durchlaufen, und finden heute vornehmlich im Sportjournalismus Anwendung. Der Grund dafür ist, dass die Radardiagramme sich am besten für Situationen eignen, in denen mehrere Messgrößen in Daten mit unterschiedlichen quantitativen Skalen zusammen dargestellt werden und in denen das Ziel darin besteht, die Symmetrie der Werte zu bewerten, und nicht ihre Größenordnungen direkt zu vergleichen. Eine solche Situation wird z. B. in Abbildung 11 dargestellt. Außerhalb des Kontextes der Wissenschaft oder des Sportjournalismus sind Radardiagramme nicht ohne weitere Erklärung anzuwenden, da sie sich nicht ohne Weiteres durch Laien alleine erschließen lassen. Radardiagramme stellen ein Beispiel für eine Visualisierungsform dar, die heutzutage relativ verbreitet ist, obwohl man als Informationsvisualisierer*in vor einigen Jahren noch nicht davon ausgehen konnte, dass das allgemeine Publikum sie lesen kann, was auf eine Verbesserung der allgemeinen Datenkompetenz hindeutet (Friel, Curcio & Bright 2001, D'Ignazio 2017).

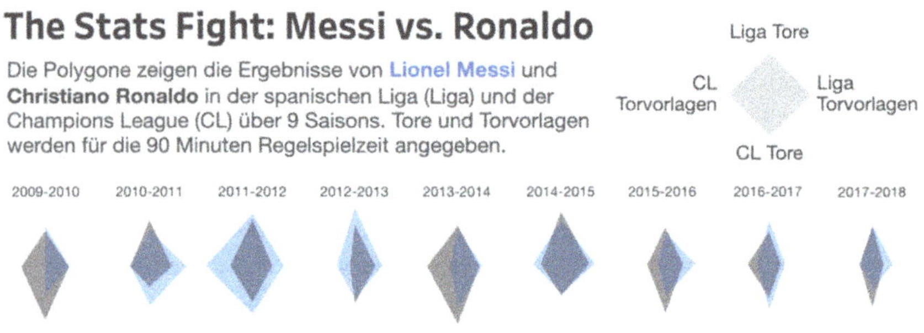

Abbildung 11: *Small multiples* von geordneten Radar-Charts für die wichtigsten Statistiken von zwei legendären Fußballspielern – Lionel Messi und Cristiano Ronaldo – über neun Saisons hinweg. Die Daten stammen von Transfermarkt.com

Abbildung 10 zeigt eine Visualisierung von Evelina Judeikyte, in der eine Reihe von Radardiagrammen jeweils für die Leistung der Fußballspieler Christiano Ronaldo und Lionel Messi stehen. Sinn der Darstellung war es, die Leistungen beider Spieler vor dem Hintergrund der damaligen Diskussion um den weltbesten Fußballspieler zu vergleichen. Mittlerweile wird Messi als der beste Fußballspieler aller Zeiten angesehen. Jedes Radardiagramm steht für eine Saison und alle Radardiagramme teilen dieselbe Skala. Wenn eine Visualisierung aus mehreren Einheiten besteht, wird auf Grundlage der *Best Practices* empfohlen, die Einheiten in einer Form anzuordnen, welche die visuelle Erschließung der Daten unterstützt. In diesem Fall wird ein Raster dafür benutzt. Diese Visualisierungsform wird *Small Multiples, Grid* oder *Panel Charts* genannt.

Die erforderlichen Daten für *Small Multiples* werden in der Regel aus einer Tabelle entnommen, deren Zeilen oder Spalten die Daten für jede der einzelnen darzustellenden Reihen enthalten. *Small Multiples* sind besonders in Situationen effektiv, in denen die visuelle Gegenüberstellung der Daten erschwert ist, beispielsweise, wenn viele unterschiedliche Variablen enkodiert werden oder wenn sich die Daten oder Beschriftungen in einer Datenvisualisierung überschneiden. Wenn wir dagegen nur eine Variable vergleichen wollen, sind *Small Multiples* möglicherweise nicht die passende Visualisierungsform.

Diese Bemühungen hin zu *Best Practises* im Bereich der Visualisierungen kommen nicht nur bei Standarddiagrammen wie Säulendiagrammen oder Tortendiagrammen zum Einsatz, sondern auch bei so genannten maßgeschneiderten Visualisierungen. Diese sind Visualisierungsformen, die speziell für den zu visualisierenden Datensatz kreiert worden sind. Beispiele werden im nächsten Abschnitt präsentiert. Solange die Prinzipien des Visualisierungsdesigns befolgt werden, bleiben sie trotzdem verständlich, obwohl die Leser*innen einer Visualisierung dieser Art nie zuvor gesehen haben. Maßgeschneiderte Visualisierungen können herangezogen werden, um entweder sehr komplexe Datensätze zu explorieren, oder um Visualisierungen mehr emotionalen Gehalt zu verleihen, indem sie persönlicher und als weniger objektiv dargestellt werden, wie beispielsweise die außergewöhnlichen Arbeiten von Informationsdesigner*innen Giorgia Lupi oder Stefanie Posavec (Lupi & Posavec 2016). Maßgeschneiderte Visualisierungen finden immer häufiger Anwendung und Akzeptanz, allmählich sogar in eher methodologisch strengen akademischen Kontexten (Delucchi Danhier 2017).

4. Beispiele für emblemähnliche maßgeschneiderte Visualisierungen

Die in diesem Artikel vorgestellten Embleme sind keineswegs die ersten ihrer Art. In diesem Kapitel werden einige relevanten Beispiele für Vorarbeiten in diesem Bereich präsentiert. Die vorgestellten Projekte umfassen datenbasierte Logos, Infographiken, Poster und Ansteckbuttons.

Ein Beispiel für die Anwendung einer maßgeschneiderten Visualisierung für Branding-Zwecke stellt das neue Logo für die *Open Knowledge Foundation* dar, das von Johnson Banks entwickelt wurde. Das Logo samt einer Erklärung des Entwurfsprozesses wird in Abbildung 12 gezeigt. Die *Open Knowledge Foundation* ist eine technologische Pionierstiftung, die sich für eine offene Welt einsetzt, in der alle nicht-personenbezogenen Informationen offen und frei für alle nutzbar sind – Regierungen, Unternehmen und Personen. Beispielsweise werden Finanzdaten des öffentlichen Bereichs gesammelt und bereitgestellt.

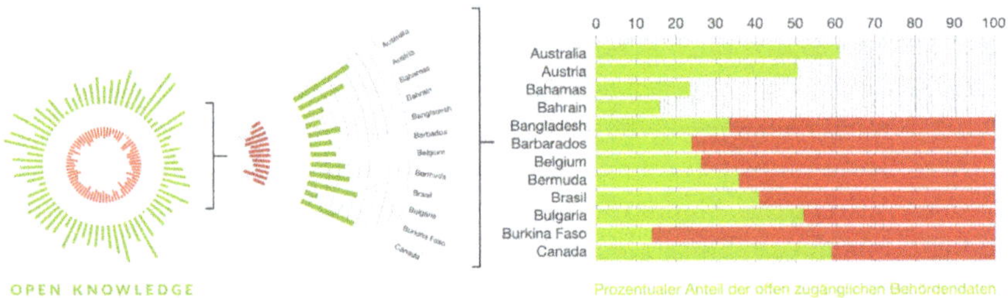

Abbildung 12: *Open Knowledge* Logo (rechts) mit Erklärung des Entwurfsprozesses

Das Logo ist so gestaltet, dass es auf mehreren Ebenen funktioniert: Es stellt die Welt dar, sieht wie ein Auge aus und erinnert an den Anfangsbuchstaben des englischen Wortes „*open*". An diesem Logo ist besonders interessant, dass es auf echten Daten basiert: Das Logo wurde direkt aus den Datensätzen der damals 72 Länder, die für das Projekt des *Global Open Data Index* – die umfassendste Aufnahme zum Stand der Veröffentlichung offener Behördendaten in der Welt – gesammelt worden waren, zusammengestellt. Es zeigt, wie offen (grün) oder geschlossen (rot) die Daten der teilnehmenden Länder sind. Insgesamt sind nur 11 % der Datensatzeinträge im Index offen. Die Werte für die Offenheit bzw. Geschlossenheit der Behördendaten für jedes Land sind in einem kreisförmigen Muster alphabetisch im Uhrzeigesinn angeordnet, wobei offene Daten in einem äußeren grünen Ring und geschlossene Daten in einem kleineren roten Ring eine Art Datenerde bilden. Das Logo ist dahingehend interessant, da es aufzeigt, wie individuelle Darstellungsformen für echte Daten in speziellen Kontexten aussehen können. Darüber hinaus kombiniert es die Darstellung von Daten anhand eines graphischen Diagramms mit emblematischen Darstellungsformen.

Die meisten Ansätze für Datenembleme sind informativ und reflektierend und basieren auf vorab gesammelten Daten, die auf eine vordefinierte Weise visualisiert werden. *Small Multiples* werden oft benutzt, um datengesteuerte emblemähnliche Visualisierungen zu präsentieren. Im Folgenden werden ausgewählte Beispiele vorgestellt, um die in diesen Beitrag präsentierten Diversitätsembleme in einen Kontext stellen zu können. Viele dieser Beispiele für maßgeschneiderte Visualisierungen ordnen die Diagramme in einem *Small-Multiples*-Raster an, um sie besser miteinander vergleichen zu können.

Das erste Beispiel kommt aus dem Einzelhandel. Mymuesli bietet auf ihrer Webseite sowie auf den Verpackungen ihrer Müslisorten eine Visualisierung von fünf Merkmalen ihrer Müsli-Geschmacksrichtungen, basierend auf den Variablen süß, sauer, fruchtig, knusprig und breiig, an. Jede Variable wird durch ein Blütenblatt in einer 5-blättrigen Blume, Geschmacksblume genannt (Abbildung 13), dargestellt.

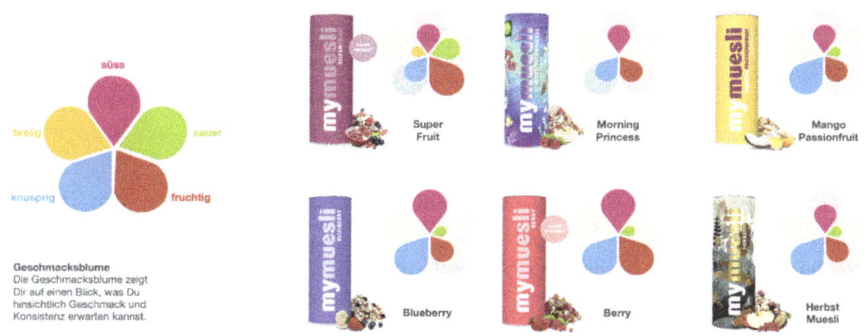

Abbildung 13: Geschmacksblumen für Müslisorten von Mymuesli

Ein weiteres Beispiel für emblemähnliche maßgeschneiderte Visualisierungen stellen die Sonnenblumen von Shirley Wu dar (Abbildung 14), die vor allem für ihre 3D-Visualisierungen bekannt ist. Bei dieser Visualisierung zeigt sie die *Top-Sommer-Blockbuster* aus unterschiedlichen Jahren als Sonnenblumen. Hierbei steht die Form der Blütenblätter für das Genre des Films, die Farbe für die im Film behandelten Themen, die Anzahl der Blütenblätter für die Anzahl der *imdb*-Stimmen, die der Film online erhalten hat, und die Größe der Blume für die Bewertung des Films durch Kritiker*innen. Dieses Beispiel zeigt emblemartige Visualisierungen, die eine Mischung aus kategorischen und skalierten Daten darstellen.

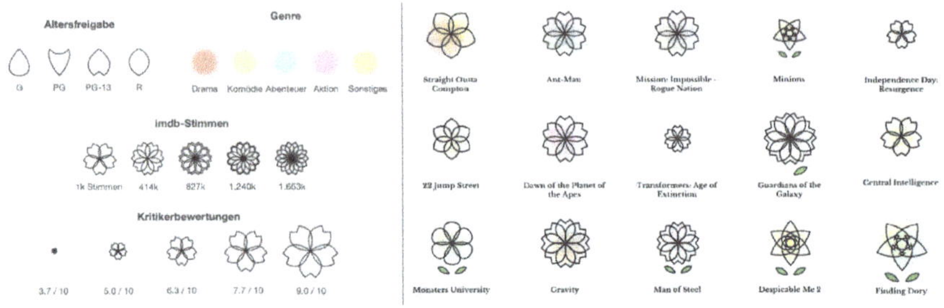

Abbildung 14: Sonnenblumen für Filme von Shirley Wu

In seinem Poster „*Weather Portraits*" hat Nicholas Rougeux Wetterdaten für jeweils eine Stadt in jedem der 50 US-Bundesstaaten für das Jahr 2014 visualisiert (Abbildung 15). Das Poster zeigt Diagramme der täglichen Temperaturen und Windkonditionen während eines Jahres für die bevölkerungsreichste Stadt jedes Bundesstaates. Jedes der einzelnen Diagramme, die jeweils für eine Stadt stehen, enthält 365 lollipopförmige Elemente, welche die fünf täglichen Messungen (Windrichtung, Windgeschwindigkeit, höchste und niedrigste Temperatur und Variationsbreite der Temperaturen) darstellen. Die Wetterdaten wurden aus den von der *National Oceanic and Atmospheric Association* (NOAA) frei zur Verfügung gestellten *Quality Controlled Local Climatological Data* (QCLCD) gewonnen. Die Daten für jede Stadt wurden vom Hauptflughafen der jeweiligen Stadt ermittelt (z. B. LAX für Los Angeles usw.). Die Windrichtung wird durch den Winkel und die Windgeschwindigkeit durch die Länge der Verankerungslinie abgebildet. Die Tageshöchsttemperatur wird durch einen höheren Halbkreis, der die höchste Temperatur angibt, und einen niedrigeren Halbkreis, der die niedrigste Temperatur angibt, dargestellt. Die Temperatur wird durch eine Farbe kodiert, und die Größe des Konstrukts steht für die Temperaturvariation (je größer der Lollipop, desto größer die Variation der Temperaturen). Die Lollipops, die für jeden Tag stehen, sind um ein zentrales Etikett angeordnet, das den Namen der jeweiligen Stadt zeigt. Jedes Stadt-Diagramm sieht aus wie eine Paintball-Uniform nach einer Spielrunde. Es ist eine äußerst kreative Art, Daten zu präsentieren, die sonst langweilig aussehen würden.

Ein anderer Bereich, in dem der Gebrauch von datengesteuerten Graphiken in den letzten Jahren populär geworden ist, ist der der Darstellung von

Personen, die Mitglieder von Organisationen oder Teilnehmende von Veranstaltungen sind. Bei diesen Vorschlägen geht es darum, auf subtile Weise durch personalisierte und auf der Kleidung tragbare Visualisierungen persönliche Merkmale dieser Personen visuell darzustellen, damit verschiedene Personen ihre personalisierten Embleme vergleichen können und auf diese Art Gleichgesinnte erkennen können. In diesen Bereich fallen auch die Diversitätsembleme, die der Fokus dieses Artikels sind.

Ein populäres Beispiel sind die Datenporträts von Accurat Studio für TED (Abbildung 16), die einen humanistischen Ansatz der Datenverarbeitung und -visualisierung verfolgen. Basierend auf den Antworten einfacher Fragen entwarf und produzierte Lupis Team 2017 für die TED-Konferenz in Vancouver Datenporträts. Die Fragen zielten darauf ab, qualitative und „weiche" Daten zu kodieren, welche Mehrdeutigkeit und Personalisierung jenseits absoluter Zahlenwerte begünstigen: z. B. „Welcher TED-Buchstabe sind Sie? (Technologie, Unterhaltung oder Design)", „Wie unordentlich ist Ihr Schreibtisch?" „Glauben Sie, dass die Zukunft rosig oder trübe ist?". Es handelt sich dabei um nicht-invasive Fragen, die lustige Fakten über die Teilnehmer*innen enthüllten. Die Antworten wurden in Formen, Farben und Symbolen umgesetzt, um die Ansichten und die Persönlichkeiten der Teilnehmer*innen darzustellen. Die Farbe, die Position und die Drehung jedes Elements zeigten eine andere Antwort an und machten aus den Daten, die jeden Menschen einzigartig machen, ein Kunstwerk. In den Vortragspausen auf der Hauptbühne war Lupi selbst anwesend und verwandelte die Antworten der Teilnehmer*innen auf die Fragen mit ihrem iPad unmittelbar in handgezeichnete Datenvisualisierungen. Diese wurden anschließend umgehend auf einen Druckserver übertragen, sodass ein Ansteckbutton gedruckt und dem/der Teilnehmer*in ausgehändigt werden konnte. Durch die Präsenz der Künstlerin bzw. der Designerin wurde das Ganze zu einer Art künstlerischem *Happening*.

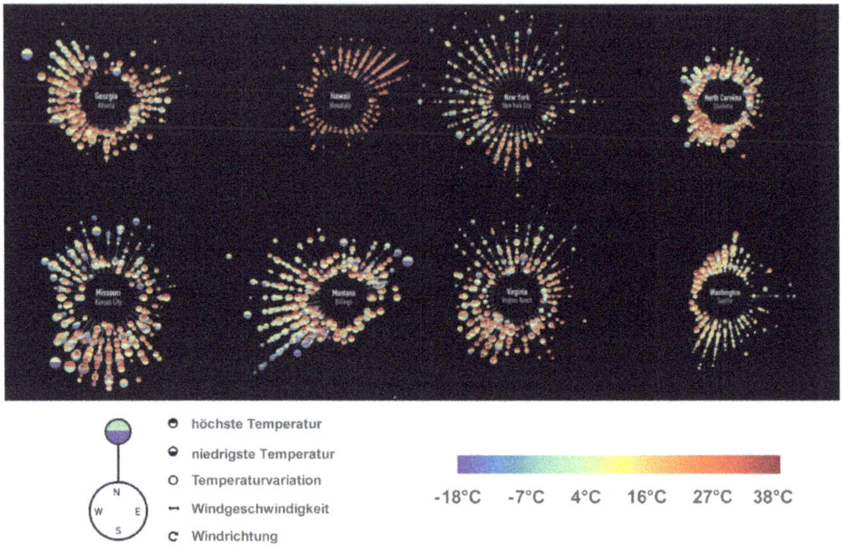

Abbildung 15: Wetterporträts von Nicholas Rougeux

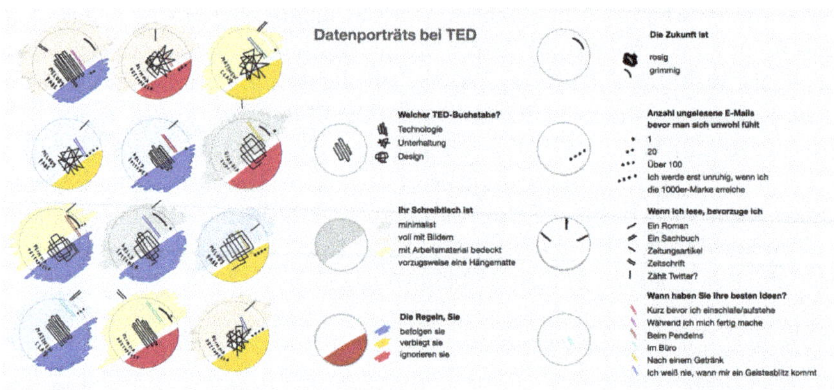

Abbildung 16: Ansteckbuttons für TED-Teilnehmer*innen von Giorgia Lupi

Ein weiteres Beispiel für datenbasierte Embleme sind das Logo und die einzelnen Mitgliederembleme der *Data Visualization Society* (Abbildung 17). Das Design stammt von Amy Cesal, einer Datenvisualisierungsdesignerin und einer der Mitbegründer*innen der Gesellschaft. Die Embleme basieren auf der Selbsteinstufung der Mitglieder in neun Kategorien, die sich auf ihre

Fähigkeiten in den Bereichen Daten, Visualisierung und Gesellschaft beziehen: Zu jedem der Wörter im Namen der *Data Visualization Society* wurden drei Fähigkeiten in einer Umfrage erfragt, drei Fähigkeiten pro Wort im Namen der Organisation: Unter der Kategorie „*Data*" (in grün) wurden die Fähigkeiten des Sammelns, Bereinigens und Analysierens von Daten erfragt. Unter „*Visualization*" wurden das Entwerfen, Erstellen und Storytelling erfragt. Und in der Kategorie „*Society*" Projektmanagement, *Community Building* und Führung. Für jede Fähigkeit wurden die Teilnehmer*innen gebeten, sich selbst in eine von fünf Stufen einzuordnen: Neuling, Lernende, Anfänger*in, Mittelstufe, Fortgeschrittene oder Expert*in. Die Ränge wurden visuell in drei sich überschneidende Dreiecke übersetzt, wobei jede Ecke eines Dreiecks für eine Kategorie steht. Je höher der Rang für die Kategorie ist, desto größer die Fläche der jeweiligen Ecke. Auf den drei sich überlappenden Dreiecken steht eine vertikale Linie für die jeweilige Zeitzone, in der sich die Person befindet, da die *Data Visualization Society* Mitglieder auf der ganzen Welt zählt. Für das Logo der Gesellschaft werden alle Einzelerhebungen gemittelt. Auf diese Weise repräsentiert das Logo die Summe aller ihrer Mitglieder (oben links in Abbildung 17). Das aktuelle Logo spiegelt wider, dass die Fähigkeiten der Mitglieder recht ausgewogen sind, wenn man alle Mitglieder als Gruppe betrachtet. Das Logo ist dynamisch und kann sich weiter verändern, wenn mehr Menschen der Organisation beitreten.

Die Datenausweise (Abbildung 18) für ein Seminar über *Data Physicalization* (Panagiotidou et al. 2020) sind ein weiteres Beispiel für personalisierte Designs. In diesem Ansatz wurde – sehr naheliegend – eine Datenphysikalisierung angewendet, sodass die Teilnehmer*innen selbst die Zusammenstellung der Ausweise vor Ort übernommen haben. Die enkodierten Informationen umfassen den beruflichen Hintergrund, die Forschungsinteressen, die Reisestunden für die Teilnahme am Workshop, die Anzahl der Veröffentlichungen und der besuchten *Sessions* auf der Konferenz. Unterhalb des Ausweises ist zusätzlich der Name des*r Teilnehmer*in zu sehen. Die Zusammensetzung der Elemente, die für diese Informationen stehen, ist so konzipiert, dass sie modular, ineinandergreifend und einfach zu befestigen ist. Da die Nutzer*innen selbst für die Erstellung der Datenausweise zuständig sind, ist diese emblemähnliche Visualisierung weniger standarisiert und nicht so stark vordefiniert wie die vorherigen Beispiele. Die Auseinandersetzung mit den eigenen Daten, die durch die Erstellung der Embleme vorausgesetzt wird, und die Freiheit des Zusammensetzens fördern die Selbstreflektion der Teilnehmer*innen und ermutigen sie außerdem, sich ihre Datenausweise zu eigen zu machen, was den beabsichtigten Repräsentationsraum der Datenembleme von der reinen Repräsentation zu mehr Provokation erweitert.

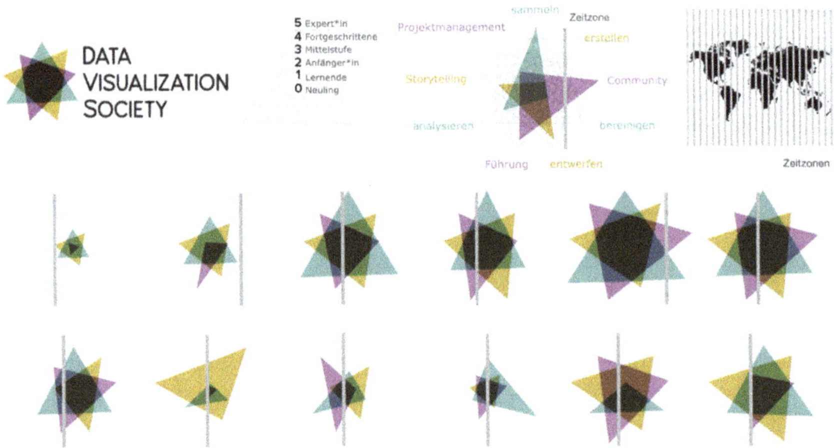

Abbildung 17: Embleme für die Mitglieder der *Data Visualization Society*

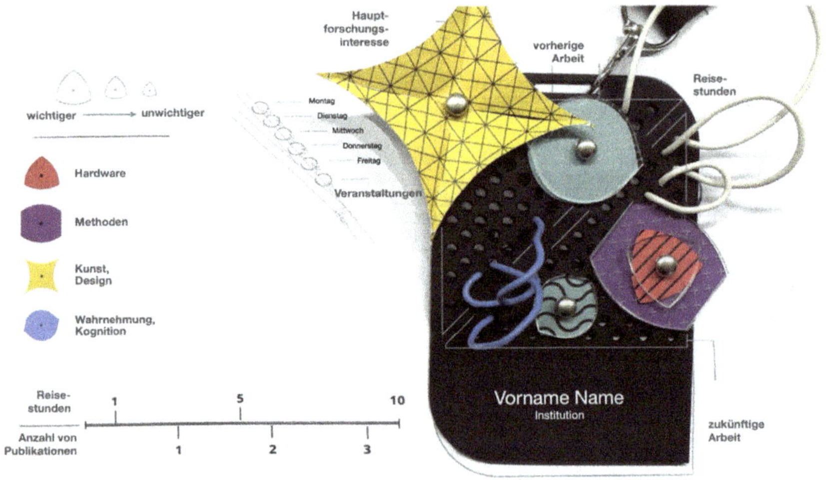

Abbildung 18: Selbstgemachte Datenausweise für die Teilnehmer*innen einer Konferenz über *Data-Physicalization* von Panagiotidou, Görücü und Moere

Die hier vorgestellten Beispiele zeigen, wie spannend und dynamisch sich der Bereich der maßgeschneiderten emblemähnlichen Visualisierungsdesigns in den letzten Jahren entwickelt hat. Diese Beispiele dienen als Inspiration für das Design der hier vorgesellten Diversitätsembleme. Im Folgenden wird der Designprozess der Diversitätsembleme näher diskutiert.

5. Design-Grundsatzerklärung

Nachdem in den vorangegangenen Abschnitten die historische Entwicklung der Embleme und ihre Funktion in Literatur und Film behandelt wurde und gezeigt wurde, was diese in modernen Kontexten alles leisten können, wird im Folgenden aufgezeigt, welche Designprinzipien das vorliegende Projekt leiten und den hier entwickelten Emblemen zugrunde liegen. Sie bilden jenseits des hier dargestellten konkreten Projektes die Grundlage für die Ziele, die ich allgemein bei der Erstellung von maßgefertigten Visualisierungen verfolge: Die Visualisierung soll es ermöglichen, Komplexität abzubilden, sich nicht auf standarisierte Lösungen verlassen und nach Ästhetik streben. Im Folgenden wird auf diese drei Designkriterien einzeln eingegangen.

Komplexität ist ein inhärentes Merkmal der menschlichen Welt. Sie sollte daher nicht vermieden werden, indem Sachverhalte vereinfacht werden, die von Natur aus vielseitig und vielschichtig sind. Bei der Darstellung von komplexen Zusammenhängen wird oft ein Kompromiss zwischen der Lesbarkeit der Visualisierung und der Integration eines möglichst hohen Grades an Komplexität eingegangen. Ein zu hoher Grad an Komplexität in einer Visualisierung kann in diesem Zusammenhang dazu führen, dass die*er Nutzer*in unter einer Informationsüberflutung leidet und die Aussage der Abbildung verwässert wird. Dieser Kompromiss kann jedoch bei der Darstellungsform der Embleme in Kauf genommen werden. Anders als bei üblichen Visualisierungen besteht das Ziel hier nicht darin, die Informationen so klar und lesbar wie möglich darzustellen, sondern einen Mittelweg zu finden zwischen Lesbarkeit, Schutz von privaten Informationen – durch absichtliche Intransparenz der dargestellten Informationen – und ästhetischem Erscheinungsbild (Benoit 2016). Das Ziel der Visualisierung ist daher nicht eine Vereinfachung der Multidimensionalität der Kolleg*innen, sondern die Ermöglichung eines mehrdimensionalen und menschlichen Blicks auf diese Personen. Hierfür ist es essenziell, quantitative Daten nicht als kontextlose Zahlen zu verstehen, sondern als ein messbares Konstrukt, das auf operationalisierten Variablen beruht, aber für Ideen und konkrete Menschen steht. Jedoch geht eine Reduktion auch immer mit einer gewissen Unschärfe und Verzerrung in der Visualisierung einher. Die

Visualisierung soll den zugrundeliegenden Datensatz akkurat abbilden jedoch gleichzeitig gefühlsreich und ästhetisch sein. Anstatt auf eine schon bekannte Lösung zurückzugreifen, wie es standarisierte Visualisierungsformen sind, soll im Projekt eine originelle, maßgeschneiderte und projektspezifische Visualisierung entwickelt werden, die zugleich den oben beschriebenen *best practises* der Datenvisualisierung folgt.

Hierbei geht es nicht darum, Standardlösungen zu entwickeln, sondern eine Mindestqualität der Darstellung sicher zu stellen. In der Regel versuche ich, mir visuelle Metaphern für die Darstellung eines Datensatzes vorzustellen und damit zu arbeiten. Mit anderen Worten, ist es der Anspruch, ein Gleichgewicht zwischen vertrauten visuellen Motiven und unerwarteter, schöner Ästhetik zu finden – auch wenn diese Schönheit notwendigerweise subjektiv sein wird. Erfahrungsgemäß weckt diese Kombination Neugier und Interesse und schafft erinnerungswürdige Bilder für die Nutzer*innen.

Das vorliegende Projekt hat zum Ziel, die vielseitigen Profile von Akademiker*innen abzubilden, anstatt diese im Sinne eines Wettbewerbs einzustufen (Crameri 2022). Hierdurch soll zu einem gesunderen akademischen Arbeitsumfeld beigetragen werden. Eine Art abstrakter Daten-Avatar soll entstehen, der das Aufzeigen von Mustern der Vielfalt innerhalb der Gruppe darstellt. Ziel der Visualisierung ist, die Akademiker*innen in einer Art und Weise darstellen zu können, in der sowohl die Gemeinsamkeiten zwischen den Kolleg*innen als auch die Eigenschaften, die sie unterscheiden, wertgeschätzt werden. Dabei soll bewusst eine Einstufung der Kolleg*innen, wie es so oft bei *publication metrics* der Fall ist, vermieden werden. Viel mehr kann das Projekt unter dem Konzept des *Data Humanism* eingeordnet werden, da dem Grundsatz gefolgt wird, dass „Daten uns menschlicher machen“ (Koblin 2011). Ziel der Diversitätsembleme ist es also, einen Blick auf die Kolleg*innen als Menschen zu werfen, so dass sie als solche von anderen Menschen gesehen werden können, ohne zu sehr in die Privatsphäre dieser Personen einzugreifen. Dafür muss differenziert ausgewählt werden, welche persönlichen Daten mit welchem Grad an Transparenz in den Emblemen enkodiert werden. Trotzdem sollten die Embleme aktualisierbare Erkundungen von Identitätsaspekten der Kolleg*innen ermöglichen. Dafür werden der persönliche Hintergrund, die akademischen Interessen und die Berufserfahrung miteinbezogen. Zusammenfassend verfolgt das Projekt das Ziel der Erstellung einer maßgeschneiderten, explorativen und optisch ansprechenden Darstellung von Daten. Der ästhetische Aspekt wird als ebenso wichtig erachtet, wie die Daten selbst, in der Hoffnung, dass die angenehme Ästhetik Nutzer*innen motivieren wird, die Feinheiten der Visualisierung zu erkunden.

6. Kontextbezogene Einschränkungen im Designprozess

Bei der Erstellung der Embleme musste ich als Informationsdesignerin folgende Fragen beantworten:

1. Welche Variablen soll die Darstellung beinhalten?,
2. Welche Art von Diagramm ist für den Datentyp und für die Zwecke der Visualisierung geeignet?
3. Welcher visuellen Inspiration soll das Aussehen der Embleme folgen?

In diesem Abschnitt werden die zweite und dritte Frage beantwortet und es erfolgt eine Darstellung des Design-Prozesses.

Da die Datenembleme hauptsächlich im digitalen Raum Anwendung finden sollen, wurde eine quadratische Form gewählt, da es die übliche Form der Bilder im Internet ist. Hier folgt die Form der Funktion, wie bei den schildförmigen europäischen Wappen und den runden angenähten japanischen Mons. Das Design, das die Fragebogenantworten in einzigartige Kombinationen aus gezeichneten Formen, Farben und Symbolen umsetzt, wurde in einem ersten Schritt per Hand auf Papier entworfen. Künstlichere Beispiele mit ausgedachten Daten wurden ausprobiert, um zu überprüfen, ob das Design eine Taxonomie der Akademiker*innen ermöglicht. Erst in einem zweiten Schritt wurde dieses Schema als ein programmierter Code in R übersetzt, um eine schnelle und automatisierte Umsetzung der Fragebogenantworten in die Embleme zu ermöglichen. Die Visualisierung hat letztendlich die Form einer Reihe von datengesteuerten Emblemen. Diese Embleme unterscheiden sich formal von Graphiken, da Embleme eher dekorativ sind und ein einzelnes abgegrenztes Thema darstellen. Eine große Anzahl von Emblemen kann wie *Small Multiples* in einer Reihe nebeneinander dargestellt werden.

KSLM Kognition ∩ Literatur ∩ Medien ∩ Sprache
diversitätsstudien

Abbildung 19: Logo des Instituts für Diversitätsstudien mit Bildmarke

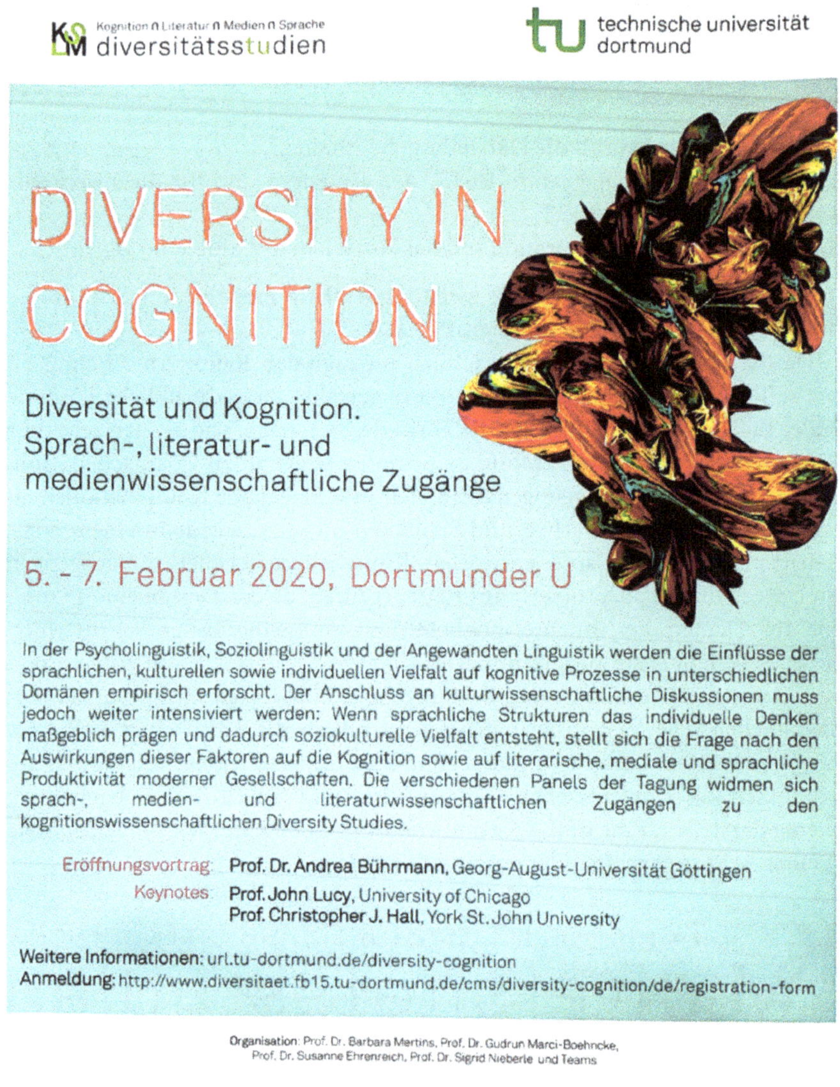
Kognition ∩ Literatur ∩ Medien ∩ Sprache
diversitätsstudien
technische universität
dortmund
DIVERSITY IN COGNITION
Diversität und Kognition.
Sprach-, literatur- und medienwissenschaftliche Zugänge
5. - 7. Februar 2020, Dortmunder U
In der Psycholinguistik, Soziolinguistik und der Angewandten Linguistik werden die Einflüsse der sprachlichen, kulturellen sowie individuellen Vielfalt auf kognitive Prozesse in unterschiedlichen Domänen empirisch erforscht. Der Anschluss an kulturwissenschaftliche Diskussionen muss jedoch weiter intensiviert werden: Wenn sprachliche Strukturen das individuelle Denken maßgeblich prägen und dadurch soziokulturelle Vielfalt entsteht, stellt sich die Frage nach den Auswirkungen dieser Faktoren auf die Kognition sowie auf literarische, mediale und sprachliche Produktivität moderner Gesellschaften. Die verschiedenen Panels der Tagung widmen sich sprach-, medien- und literaturwissenschaftlichen Zugängen zu den kognitionswissenschaftlichen Diversity Studies.
Eröffnungsvortrag: Prof. Dr. Andrea Bührmann, Georg-August-Universität Göttingen
Keynotes: Prof. John Lucy, University of Chicago
Prof. Christopher J. Hall, York St. John University
Weitere Informationen: url.tu-dortmund.de/diversity-cognition
Anmeldung: http://www.diversitaet.fb15.tu-dortmund.de/cms/diversity-cognition/de/registration-form
Organisation: Prof. Dr. Barbara Mertins, Prof. Dr. Gudrun Marci-Boehncke, Prof. Dr. Susanne Ehrenreich, Prof. Dr. Sigrid Nieberle und Teams

Abbildung 20: Poster der Konferenz „*Diversity in Cognition*“

Da die intendierten Nutzer*innen ursprünglich die Kolleg*innen am Institut für Diversitätsstudien der TU Dortmund waren, orientiert sich das Emblemdesign an der Bildmarke des Instituts. Erst später wurde die Nutzung auf die Konferenzteilnehmer*innen ausgeweitet. Das Logo des Instituts, das von der Autorin dieses Artikels entwickelt wurde, besteht aus einer Kombination aus einer Wortmarke und einer Bildmarke und steht mit der neuen *Corporate Identity* der Universität (TU Dortmund 2017) im Einklang. Die Bildmarke repräsentiert die vier thematischen Schwerpunkte, die inhaltlich am Institut in der Lehre und Forschung behandelt werden: Kognition, Sprache, Literatur und Medien, jeweils widergespiegelt durch ihren Anfangsbuchstaben. Abbildung 19 gibt das offizielle Logo der damaligen Arbeitsgruppe wieder. Die Farben des Emblemdesigns, sowohl das Cyanblau als Hauptfarbe als auch die die lachsfarbenen Akzente, wurden vom Poster der durch das Institut organisierten Konferenz „Diversity in Cognition" übernommen, das in Abbildung 20 abgebildet ist. Bei der Konferenz lag der Schwerpunkt auf den Schnittstellen der sprachlichen, kulturellen und sozialen Vielfalt in einem Dialog zwischen Sprach-, Literatur-, Medien- und Kognitionswissenschaft. Die vier Themen, die auch an der Bildmarke des Logos des organisierenden Instituts wiederzufinden sind, wurden als Ankerpunkte für die Positionierung der Forschungsinteressen gewählt.

Die Visualisierung hat die Form einer Reihe von datengesteuerten Emblemen. Alle Embleme teilen eine gemeinsame Skala und es wurden stets dieselben Farben für alle Embleme genutzt. Zudem wurden die Embleme nach den Werten einer Kategorie in einem Raster angeordnet, um den Vergleich zu erleichtern. Dafür wurde die Kategorie „Expertise" gewählt, operationalisiert als Erfahrungsjahre. Abbildung 21 gibt die geordnete Auswahl der Datenportraits der Kolleg*innen als *Small Multiples,* geordnet von oben nach unten und von links nach rechts, nach Laufbahnabschnitt und Erfahrungsjahren, wieder. Die Auswahl zeigt die große Vielfalt innerhalb der Gruppe.

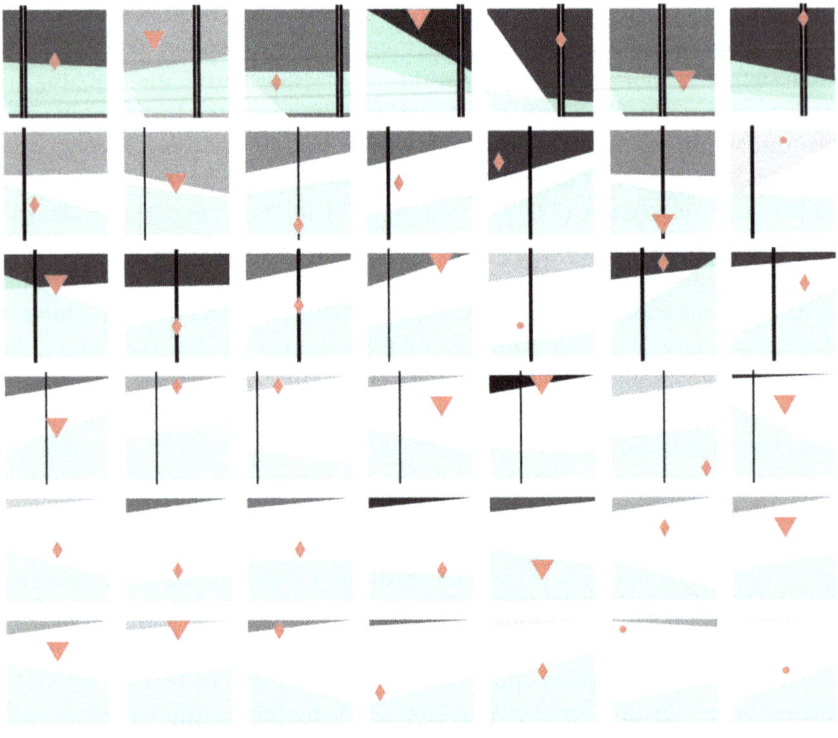

Abbildung 21: Auswahl der Datenembleme der Teilnehmer*innen an der Konferenz „Diversity in Cognition“

7. Regeln zur Erstellung der Embleme

Bei der Visualisierung werden die über einen Fragebogen erfassten Informationen in Formen und Farben umgewandelt, um die Daten visuell zu untersuchen. Die Visualisierung funktioniert nach dem Prinzip eines Codes, bzw. wie eine visuelle Sprache mit einer eigenen Grammatik: In der Linguistik ist die Grammatik einer natürlichen Sprache die Gesamtheit der Regeln für die Zusammensetzung von Sätzen, Phrasen oder Wörtern durch die Sprecher*innen. Die Embleme werden auch auf der Grundlage von Regeln, die einer Grammatik ähneln, erschaffen. Man kann lernen, sie zu lesen, so wie man auch lernen kann, das geschriebene Wort zu lesen. In diesem Abschnitt wird das Vorgehen zur Erstellung bzw. Entschlüsselung der Embleme erklärt. Diese grammatischen Regeln werden in Abbildung 22 bildlich zusammengefasst.

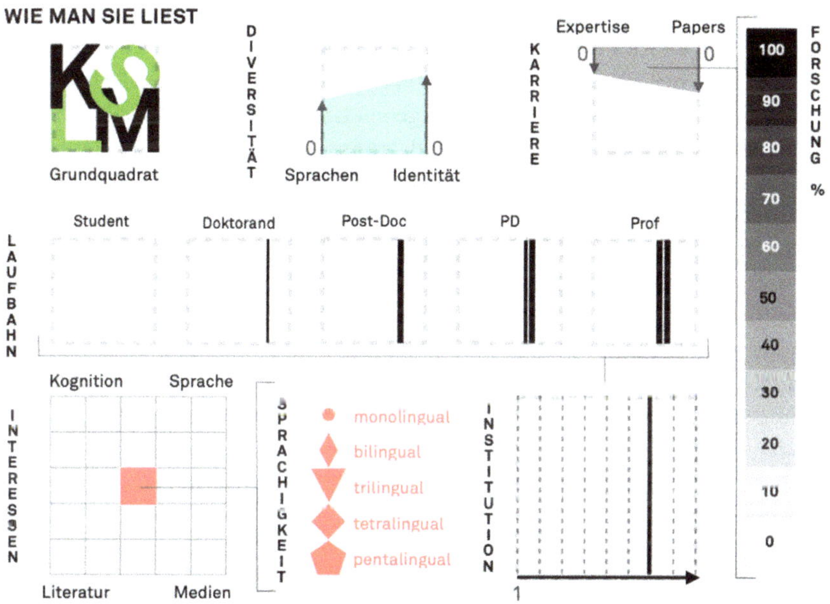

Abbildung 22: Entschlüsselung der Embleme

Das Wort Grammatik leitet sich vom Griechischen γραμματική τέχνη (grammatikḕ téchnē) ab, was „Kunst der Buchstaben" bedeutet, von γράμμα (grámma), „Buchstabe", was wiederum von γράφειν (gráphein), „zeichnen, schreiben" abgeleitet ist. Somit teilen die Begriffe Grammatik und Graphik im Griechischen dieselbe Wurzel, was für dieses Projekt sehr passend ist.

Das Design des Emblems basiert auf einem Grundquadrat, das für das organisierende Institut steht. Dieses Quadrat wird durch zwei geometrische Figuren (meistens Trapeze) überlagert: Die erste geometrische Figur ist in grau schattiert und ist am oberen Rand des Quadrats verankert. Sie steht symbolisch für die berufliche Seite der dargestellten Menschen. Die zweite geometrische Figur ist in Cyan farblich markiert und am unteren Rand des Quadrats verankert. Die cyanblaue Figur steht für die private und sprachliche Seite der Kolleg*innen. Die genaue Form dieser geometrischen Figuren ist von den Werten von jeweils zwei Variablen anhängig, welche die Position der Ecken der Figuren an den vertikalen Seiten des Grundquadrats bestimmen. Je größer die Werte sind, desto weiter wandern die Ecken der Figuren in Richtung des gegenüberliegenden Rands des Quadrats und die entstehenden geometrischen Figuren werden entsprechend großflächiger (d. h. die Figur in Graustufen wächst nach unten, und die cyanblaue Figur nach oben). Die geometrischen Figuren verlassen jedoch nie die Ränder des Grundquadrats. Wenn die Werte dieser vier Variablen groß genug sind, kann es sein, dass sich die beiden geometrischen Figuren überlagern.

Die geometrischen Figuren sind halb transparent, damit immer die genaue Platzierung ihrer Ecken sichtbar ist, unabhängig von den Werten der Variablen. Die genaue Graustufenschattierung der obersten Figur ist von dem Verhältnis zwischen Lehre und Forschung abhängig. Die Farbe der unteren cyanfarbigen Figur bleibt unverändert und vergibt allen Emblemen eine Einheitsnote. Über dieser beschriebenen ersten Schicht, welche das Basisquadrat darstellt, werden zwei Verzierungen platziert: ein schwarzes vertikales Band und ein kleines regelmäßiges Polygon in Lachsfarbe. Platzierung und Form der zwei Ornamente enkodieren jeweils zwei weitere Informationen. Die schwarzen Bänder stehen für den spezifischen akademischen Karriereschritt, in der sich die Person befindet, operationalisiert als berufliche Stellenbezeichnung, und die Anzahl der Bildungseinrichtungen, an welchen die Person tätig gewesen ist. Die kleine geometrische Figur repräsentiert hingegen die kognitiven Fähigkeiten der Person, operationalisiert als ihre Forschungsinteressen und die Anzahl der Sprachen, die sie spricht. Die Anzahl der Sprachen wird an der Form der orangenen Figur erkannt und die Forschungsinteressen an der Platzierung der lachsfarbenen Figur in Bezug auf die vier Ecken des Basisquadrats, die jeweils für eine der Hauptthemen der Konferenz stehen. Das quadratische Feld ist in ein Raster von 5 x 5 gleichgroßen kleineren Feldern unterteilt, sodass es 25 unterschiedliche Möglichkeiten gibt, die eigenen Forschungsinteressen in Bezug auf die vier Ankerthemen zu platzieren. Beispielsweise würde jemand, der ausschließlich literaturwissenschaftliche Forschung betreibt, sich in dem untersten linken Feld verorten, während eine andere Person, die an den vier Themen gleichermaßen interessiert ist, sich im mittleren Feld positionieren würde, in gleicher Entfernung zu den vier Ecken.

8. Methodik

Die Daten für die Embleme wurden mittels eines online Fragebogens erhoben. Dieser Fragebogen wird vollständig übersetzt unter Tabelle 1 wiedergegeben. Der Originalfragebogen war auf englischer Sprache, da die Konferenz international war. Mit dem Ziel, den Zeitaufwand für die Kolleg*innen möglichst gering zu halten und gleichzeitig die graphische Komplexität des Emblems zu begrenzen, wurden die Fragen auf zehn in der Anzahl beschränkt. Die Fragen beziehen sich entweder auf quantifizierbare Informationen (Verhältnisskala) oder es musste eine Auswahl zwischen verschiedenen Optionen getroffen werden (nominale Variable). Zudem wurde die Frage nach den erlernten Sprachen (Frage 9) absichtlich offen formuliert, um erkunden zu können, was genau die Teilnehmer*innen unter Sprache verstehen (natürliche Sprachen, Programmiersprachen, oder etwas anderes). Auch wie hoch das Beherrschungsniveau der Sprache sein muss, um als erlernte Sprache zu gelten, wurde den Teilnehmer*innen überlassen.

Table 1: Fragebogen für die Datenerhebung (deutsche Übersetzung)

1	Name
2	Akademische Stelle: ▢ Student*in ▢ Doktorand*in ▢ Post-Doc, Akademische (Ober-)Rät*in ▢ Privatdozent*in ▢ (emeritierte/r) Professor*in
3	In welchem Jahr haben Sie Ihr Studium in diesem Fachbereich begonnen? (z. B. Linguistik, Literaturwissenschaft, usw.)
4	An wie vielen Universitäten (oder Forschungseinrichtungen) haben Sie studiert oder gearbeitet?
5	Wie viel Prozent Ihrer Arbeitszeit widmen Sie der Lehre im Verhältnis zur Forschung? 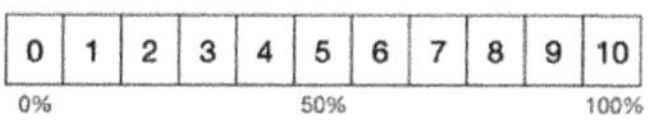
6	Wie positionieren Sie Ihre Arbeit (Lehre und/oder Forschung) in Bezug auf die vier Pole, die im Bild dargestellt sind? (Nennen Sie Koordinaten wie bei einer Seeschlacht oder beim Schach) 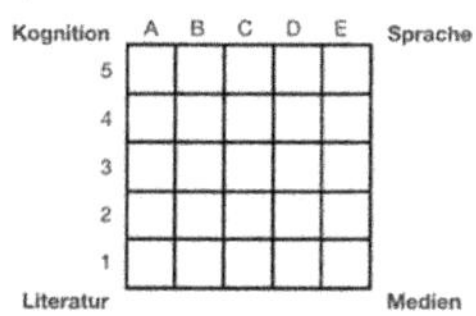
7	Wie viel haben Sie veröffentlicht? (Wenn Sie die genaue Zahl nicht kennen ist eine ungefähre Zahl der Publikationen in Ordnung)
8	Im Folgenden finden Sie zwei Listen mit sich gegenseitig ausschließenden Merkmalen. Bitte zählen Sie, wie oft die Kategorie auf der linken Seite auf Sie zutrifft. (Sie müssen sie nur zählen, es wird nicht nach Einzelheiten gefragt)
9	Wie viele Sprachen können Sie oder haben sie erlernt?
10	Wie viele dieser Sprachen verwenden Sie täglich (entweder sprechen/hören/schreiben oder lesen?)

Die Fragen zu den Diversitätseigenschaften sind ein besonders sensibles Thema, weil es sich um personenbezogene Daten handelt, die möglicherweise zu Diskriminierung führen können. Gleichzeitig ist es eine besonders interessante Frage, da sich die Teilnehmer*innen professionell diesen Themen widmen. Um dieses Thema taktvoll einzubinden, wurden die Diversitätsmerkmale, die auf eine Person zutreffen, anhand einer Liste (siehe unten) gewertet, und nicht als getrennte Fragen. Somit werden die Eigenschaften lediglich zusammengezählt und dementsprechend keine potentiell sensiblen Informationen wie z. B. Religion oder sexuelle Orientierung durch die Visualisierung offenbart. Die in diesem Projekt berücksichtigten Diversitätskategorien sind lose an die *Power Flower* (Burke et al. 1991) angelehnt. Die *Power Flower* (siehe Abbildung 23, oben) ist ein Instrument, das von kanadischen Pädagog*innen für sozialen Wandel entwickelt wurde. Diese arbeiteten mit Gruppen, um herauszufinden, wie verschiedene Identitäten einer bestimmten Person mit denjenigen interagieren, die in der Gesellschaft Macht ausüben. Das Zentrum des gänseblümchenartigen Diagramms ist in Segmente unterteilt, die jeweils eine Facette oder Kategorie unserer sozialen Identität darstellen. Dieses Zentrum ist von einem doppelten Satz von Blütenblättern umgeben. Die äußeren Blütenblätter beschreiben die dominanten oder mächtigen Identitäten in der Gesellschaft. Die inneren Blütenblätter stehen für die vergleichsweise weniger mächtigen Identitäten. Das ursprüngliche Ziel der Übung ist es, herauszufinden, wie nahe oder wie weit entfernt jede Person von der dominanten Identität ihrer Gesellschaft ist, denn als pädagogisches Instrument sollte die *Power Flower* ihnen helfen, die eigenen sich überschneidenden Identitäten intersektionell zu erforschen.

Im Rahmen dieses Projektes, und um die möglicherweise sensiblen Eigenschaftsmerkmale der Teilnehmer*innen zu schützen, wurden die 16 Kategorien, die bei der *Power Flower* berücksichtigt werden, auf 20 erweitert. Für die Erstellung des persönlicheren Emblems werden also die Kategorien Geschlecht, Ethnie, Nationalität, sozialer Status, Altersgruppe, Beeinträchtigung, Geistlichkeit/Konfession, Familienstand, Wohnsituation, geographische Herkunft, soziale Schicht, sexuelle Orientierung, sexuelle Identität, Bildungstand, finanzielle Lage, Schuldenstand, Fremdsprachkenntnisse, Arbeitssprache, Essgewohnheiten, familiäre Situation und Beförderungsmittel zur Arbeit berücksichtigt. Die komplette Liste der Identitätsmerkmale und Lebensstilentscheidungen, die für die Operationalisierung des Diversitätsgrades berücksichtigt wurden, wird in der Tabelle in Abbildung 23 unten wiedergegeben. Dabei werden Eigenschaften, die in der heutigen deutschen Gesellschaft als privilegiert angesehen werden (links in der Tabelle) mit vergleichbaren entmachteten Eigenschaften gepaart (Tabelle 1, rechts).

Hier wird das Geschlecht der Teilnehmer*innen bewusst mit anderen persönlichen Identitätsmerkmalen aggregiert, um das Geschlecht lediglich als ein weiteres Diversitätsmerkmal in einer Reihe von vielen verschiedenen Eigenschaften zu betrachten. Dennoch scheint der Bereich der Diversitätsstudien, so wie andere Geisteswissenschaften, weiblich dominiert zu sein: Autorinnen spezialisieren sich unter anderem auf Themen wie Feminismus, Politik und Gewalt, während männliche Autoren keine Vorliebe für bestimmte Themen aufzeigen (Sokil & Osorio 2022). Deshalb soll der Fokus hier bewusst nicht auf das Geschlecht gelenkt werden, viel mehr sollen in diesem Projekt alle berücksichtigen Diversitätsmerkmale gleich gewertet werden. Oft wird für eine Analyse, sei es eine wissenschaftliche Untersuchung oder *Market Research*, wenn Informationen über eine Gruppe von Menschen graphisch wiedergeben werden sollen, nach Geschlechtern aufgeschlüsselt. Dies passiert oft ohne zunächst zu diskutieren, ob für den zu behandelnden Sachverhalt eine Unterscheidung nach Geschlechtern sinnvoll ist oder nicht. Dies führt zu einer statistischen Überrepräsentierung der Kategorie Geschlecht in *Market Research* oder als Erklärungsgröße von gesellschaftlichen Entwicklungen. Die Tatsache, dass in den Emblemen nicht erkennbar ist, was für ein Geschlecht die Person hat, ist intendiert. Das Geschlecht wird somit als nicht wichtiger als andere Differenzmerkmale angesehen.

Es wurde darauf geachtet, dass die Fragen aussagekräftige Antworten liefern, ohne konfrontativ zu wirken. Die Fragen wurden so formuliert, dass die Teilnehmer*innen zu ehrlichen Antworten ermuntert wurden und die soziale Erwünschtheit so niedrig wie möglich gehalten wurde: Bei Frage 8 wurde z. B. absichtlich nicht danach gefragt, in wie vielen Kategorien man zu einer benachteiligten Gruppe gehört, sondern es wurde indirekt nach der Zugehörigkeit zu privilegierteren Gruppen gefragt. Bei anderen Fragen, wie z. B. Frage 3, wurde nach dem spezifischen Jahr des Studienbeginns gefragt, anstatt zu fragen, seit wie vielen Jahren man schon im akademischen Bereich tätig ist, um unmissverständlich auch die Ausbildungsjahre miteinzubeziehen. Diese Jahre tragen zweifellos zur Expertise der Wissenschaftler*innen bei und dies erlaubt somit auch die Inklusion von jungen Studierenden in der Umfrage. Da es in erster Linie darum geht, Wissenschaftler*innen zu quantifizieren, schien eine Frage zur akademischen Produktivität unvermeidlich. Diese wird üblicherweise anhand von Publikationsmetriken festgehalten. Unter Publikationsmetriken versteht man die Zählung der Anzahl wissenschaftlicher Veröffentlichungen akademischer Autor*innen und andere Metriken, die von dieser grundlegenden Zählung abgeleitet werden.

In der Bibliometrie scheint es üblich geworden zu sein, die Forschungsproduktivität (*Productivity*) als die Anzahl der Veröffentlichungen pro Forscher*in zu definieren und sie von dem *Impact* zu unterscheiden, der durch Zitationen gemessen wird: Produktivität wird direkt an der Zahl der Veröffentlichungen gemessen; Qualität anhand der Anzahl der Zitate, die auf der Grundlage des Artikels getätigt worden sind. Denn ein Artikel, der häufiger zitiert wird, hat mehr Einfluss in der wissenschaftlichen Gemeinschaft und spiegelt somit eine höhere Qualität wider. Manche Metriken, wie der bekannte h-Index kombinieren beide Parameter: Die Anzahl der Publikationen (n) die mindestens n-Mal zitiert worden sind. Für das Konferenzemblem wollte ich die Publikationsmetriken einfach halten, um der Überoptimierung der akademischen Metriken entgegenzuwirken, und mich auf die Darstellung der vollständigen Profile anstatt des wertenden Einstufens der Akademiker*innen zu konzentrieren. Daher entschied ich mich für eine einfache Aufzählung der Gesamtanzahl der Publikationen. Obwohl dies eine sehr einfache Metrik ist, findet sie sehr breite Anwendung, z. B. bei den drei bekanntesten Hochschulrankings – *Academic Ranking of World Universities* (ARWU), *QS World University Rankings* und *THE World University Rankings* – als Operationalisierung für die Qualität der Forschung (die Anzahl von Publikationen pro Professor*in).

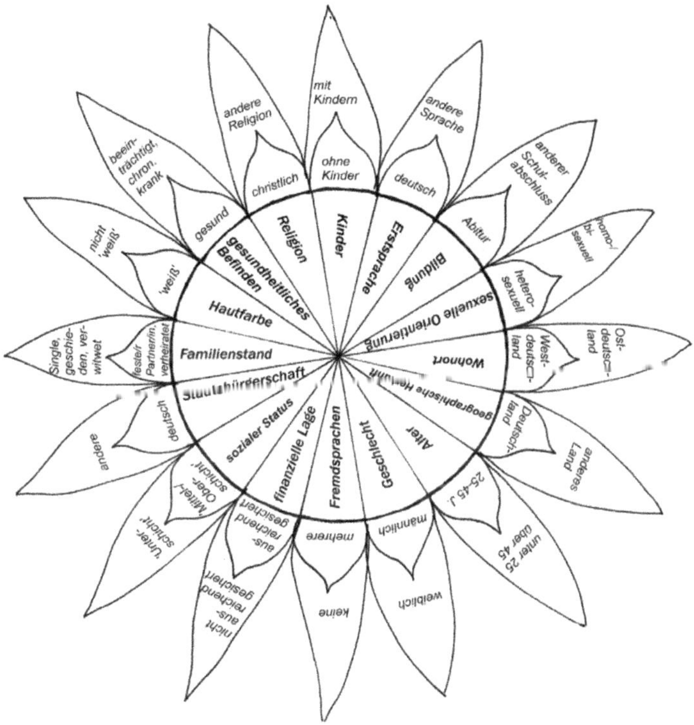

privilegiert	vergleichsweise entmachtet
männlich	weiblich; nicht-binär
"weiß"	*person of color*
zwischen 25-45 Jahre alt	unter 25 Jahre; über 45 Jahre
verheiratet, verpartnert	ledig; getrennt lebend; geschieden;
heterosexuell	homosexuell; *queer*; asexuell; bisexuell;
gleichgeschlechtlich; *cisgender*	transgender; nicht-binär
körperlich gesund; keine chronischen	Menschen mit Behinderung; chronisch krank
christlich	andere Religion, Atheist, Agnostiker
keine diätetischen Einschränkungen	Veganer; Vegetarier
Staatsbürger des Landes, in dem Sie	Staatsbürger eines anderen Staates;
Oberschicht, Mittelschicht	Arbeiterklasse; Unterschicht
aufgewachsen in der ersten Welt	aufgewachsen in einem anderen Land
akademischer Familienhintergrund	Akademiker der ersten Generation
Zugang zu Sprachunterricht gehabt	keine Fremdsprachenausbildung
Arbeitssprache ist auch erste Sprache	Arbeitssprache ist eine andere Sprache
Hauseigentümer	Wohnt zur Miete, andere Wohnformen
keine Kinder oder abhängige ältere Eltern	Kinder oder/und andere abhängige Personen
finanziell abgesichert	nicht finanziell abgesichert
keine Studiendarlehen	zahlt Studiendarlehen ab
fährt mit dem Auto zur Arbeit	benutzt öffentliche Verkehrsmittel, Fahrrad

Abbildung 23: *Power Flower* (oben) und Identitäten für den Fragebögen (unten)

Wenn die Umfrage nur zum Teil beantwortet worden wäre, wäre aufgrund der Lücken im Datensatz die Erstellung der Embleme nicht mehr möglich gewesen. Deswegen war es von großer Wichtigkeit bei der Planung der Umfrage alle möglichen Hürden, vom durch die Befragten zu erbringenden Aufwand über das Verständnis des Fragebogens bis zu möglichen technischen Schwierigkeiten, so niedrig wie möglich zu halten. Die Tatsache, dass die meisten Konferenzteilnehmer*innen den Fragebogen vollständig beantwortet haben, zeigt, dass der Aufwand für die befragten Personen akzeptabel war.

9. Auswertung des Datensatzes

In diesem Abschnitt wird über Einblicke in den Datensatz berichtet. Die Einsichten basieren auf der Konferenz-Stichprobe, an der insgesamt 44 Kolleg*innen teilgenommen haben, einschließlich der Autorin selbst. Erste interessante Befunde werden direkt aus dem Fragebogen gewonnen. In Bezug auf Frage 9, „Wie viele Sprachen können Sie oder haben sie erlernt?", wurden 20 verschiedene moderne Sprachen von den Teilnehmer*innen genannt: Albanisch, Arabisch, Deutsch, Englisch, Französisch, Griechisch, Italienisch, Japanisch, Mazedonisch, Niederländisch, Norwegisch, Persisch, Polnisch, Portugiesisch, Russisch, Serbo-Kroatisch, Slowakisch, Spanisch, Tschechisch und Türkisch. Keine der Befragten hat Dialekte miteinbezogen (auch ich nicht, obwohl ich selbst einen Dialekt als Muttersprache spreche). Dialekte sind jedoch, psycholinguistisch gesehen, komplett ausgebildete Sprachsysteme. Dabei *switchen* Sprecher*innen genauso zwischen Dialekt und der Hochsprache wie es auch bilinguale Sprecherinnen zwischen zwei Sprachen tun (Delucchi Danhier & Mertins 2018). Unter den sogenannten toten Sprachen wurden Latein (relativ oft), Altgriechisch (einmal) und Mittelägyptisch (einmal) angegeben. Bisher wurden keine konstruierten Sprachen (*Conlangs)* oder Programmiersprachen genannt. Auch „Musik" wurde von einer Teilnehmer*in als eigenständige Sprache angeführt, was umstritten, jedoch nicht ausgeschlossen ist (Patel 2003), denn es handelt sich um eine hochgradig entwickelte Expertise, in der Syntax eine erhebliche Rolle spielt und Gefühle kommuniziert werden. Inwieweit diese Kriterien jedoch für die Klassifizierung als Sprache ausreichen, ist derzeit noch umstritten, weshalb Musik hier nicht berücksichtigt wurde.

Eine weitere Erkenntnis aus dem Datensatz ist, dass die große Mehrheit der Kolleg*innen multilingual ist. Es können auch Zusammenhänge zwischen mehrere Variablen festgestellt werden: Personen, die akademische Titel tragen (Prof., PD, Dr.) verfügen zugleich über eine sehr weitreichende Erfahrung (beurteilt nach Expertise und Publikationen) und waren im Laufe Ihrer akademischen Karriere bei vielen Universitäten tätig, was auf eine höhere Karrieremobilität hindeutet. Dies kann anhand der Kombination aus großflächigen grauen geometrischen Formen im obersten Bereich des Emblems mit schwarzen Doppellinien im rechten Bereich des Emblems erkannt werden. Es zeigt sich darüber hinaus eine klare Korrelation von vielen Publikationen mit einem hohen Anteil der Gesamtarbeitszeit, die für Forschung aufgewandt wird. Auch wenn diese Zusammenhänge nicht überraschen, liefern sie wertvolle Beispiele, um das Potential der Diversitätsembleme aufzuzeigen und Erkenntnisse aus komplexen Daten sichtbar zu machen.

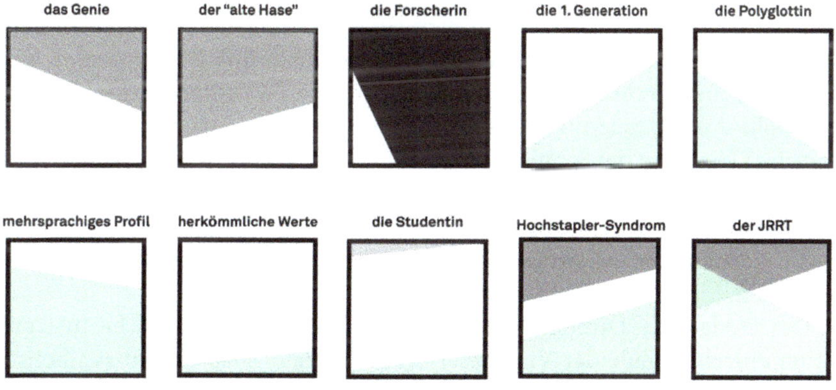

Abbildung 24: Prototypische Muster, die sich bei den Emblemen identifizieren lassen

Gute Visualisierungen sollten unsichtbare Muster sichtbar machen. Die in Abbildung 24 gezeigten Diversitätsembleme bilden mit einer Prise Humor eine Reihe unterschiedlicher archetypischer Muster der akademischen Tätigkeit ab. Große graue Vierecke im oberen Bereich weisen auf lange Expertise in der akademischen Laufbahn hin. Ein graues Viereck, das rechts viel weiter unten als links verortet ist, deutet auf ein Genie oder Wunderkind hin, das innerhalb weniger Jahren viel publiziert hat. Dunklere Vierecke, die im oberen Bereich platziert sind, deuten darauf hin, dass der Schwerpunkt auf der Forschung liegt. Student*innen lassen sich durch eine breite weiße Fläche in der Mitte erkennen, die auf ihre relative Unerfahrenheit zurückzuführen ist. Kolleg*innen mit schmalen weißen Streifen in der Mitte des Emblems, die aber keine Studierende mehr sind, könnten u.U. am Hochstapler-Syndrom leiden, was dem Stereotyp für den Mittelbau entsprechen würde. Wenn sich das oberste und unterste Viereck überkreuzen, signalisiert dies ein*e erfahrene*r Linguist*in, die/der viele Sprachen spricht. Ich bezeichne dieses Muster als John Ronald Reuel Tolkien

(JRRT), nach dem Professor für englische Sprachwissenschaft, der konstruierte Sprachen zum ersten Mal für literarische Zwecke verwendete.

Ein großes cyanblaues rechtwinkliges Dreieck mit dem rechten Winkel unten links steht für jemanden, der oder die viele Sprachen spricht. Kleinere Formen hingegen deuten darauf hin, dass jemand vielleicht neu in der Wissenschaft ist und gerade erst anfängt. Auf dem anderen Ende der Skala stehen Professor*innen, die so viel publiziert haben, dass sie die Skala sprengen und die oberste geometrische Figur zu einem unregelmäßigen Pentagon wird. Angehörige der ersten Generation würde man typischerweise an einem großen farbigen rechtwinkligen Dreieck mit dem rechten Winkel unten rechts erkennen. Menschen mit „Migrationshintergrund" werden eher ein großflächiges farbiges Viereck im unteren Bereich aufweisen, denn ihre Profile werden häufig durch überdurchschnittlich zahlreiche soziale Diversitätsmerkmale sowie eine hohe Anzahl gelernter Sprachen charakterisiert, da sie zusätzlich zu den Sprachen, die sie in der Schule gelernt haben, weitere von zu Hause mitbringen. Das Gegenbild davon sind Menschen mit einem bürgerlichen Hintergrund, deren Profile häufig durch eine geringere Anzahl an sozialen Diversitätsmerkmalen geprägt sind, weswegen sie eher kleinere Vierecke im unteren Bereich aufweisen.

Das Design der Diversitätsembleme erlaubt eine metaphorische Interpretation einzelner Teile der Visualisierung: Das graue Trapez steht symbolisch für die berufliche Seite der dargestellten Menschen. Die cyanblaue Figur steht für die private und sprachliche Seite der Kolleg*innen. Dieses Zusammenspiel und ggf. die Überlagerung der grauen und cyan-farbigen Polygone kann metaphorisch für den *Work-Life-Ausgleich* im akademischen Leben stehen: Denn es interagieren die beiden traditionellen Messgrößen der akademischen Tätigkeit, des Dienstalters und der Publikationen, mit zwei Messgrößen des alltäglichen Lebens – Identitätsmerkmale und Sprachen, die man erworben hat.

10. Anwendungsmöglichkeiten

In diesem Abschnitt wird auf eine Auswahl von Möglichkeiten der Anwendung der Diversitätsembleme eingegangen. Diese sind hauptsächlich dafür entwickelt worden, um für sich alleine stehend für die betreffende Person verwendet zu werden. Dennoch können sie auch gruppenweise eingesetzt werden, denn die Bildsprache der Diversitätsembleme kann weiter ausgebaut werden, um z. B. ganze Arbeitsgruppen darzustellen. Die folgenden Ideen werden in aufsteigender Reihenfolge von vollkommen seriös bis hin zu erfinderisch vorgestellt.

10.1 Persönliche Embleme als Repräsentation einer Person

Die einfachste Verwendung der Diversitätsembleme ist die Darstellung einer bestimmten Person. Es bestehen verschiedene Möglichkeiten, die Embleme in diesem Kontext zu verwenden. Die erste und einfachste Möglichkeit ist die stationäre Verwendung des Emblems, z. B. auf einer Webseite oder Visitenkarte oder als Bild für ein Namenschild. Diese letzte Option wurde auf der hier beschriebenen Konferenz verwendet.

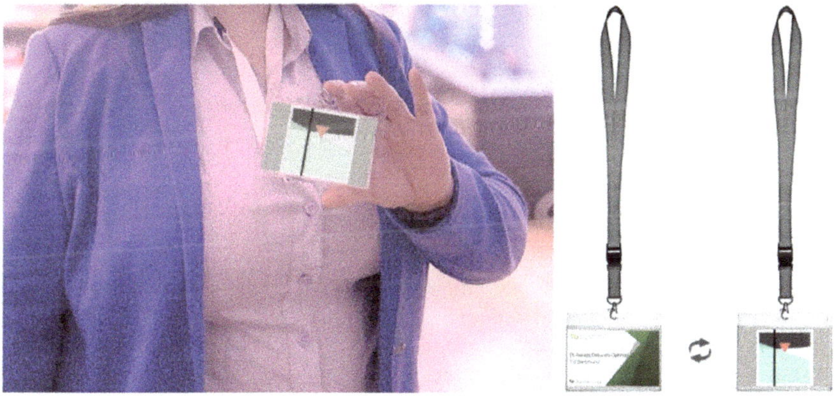

Abbildung 25: Beispiel für den Einsatz der Embleme auf dem Namensschild. Auf der Vorderseite sind, wie auf einem Namensschild üblich, Namen und Universitätszugehörigkeit abgebildet. Auf der Rückseite ist das Datenemblem zu sehen

Abbildung 25 zeigt ein Beispiel eines Namenschildes mit Emblem, welches die Konferenzteilnehmer*innen bekommen haben. Die mit Emblemen verzeichneten Namenschilder führten zu einer Art datengesteuerten Aktivierung zu Konferenzanfang, die zu interessanten neuen Begegnungen der Teilnehmer*innen bei Tagungseröffnung geführt hat. Denn die Datenportraits auf der Rückseite des Namenschildes fungierten als Gesprächsanreger, sodass zunächst fremde Konferenzteilnehmer*innen zu Gesprächen angeregt wurden. Schon zu Anfang der Konferenz konnte beobachtet werden, wie neugierige Kolleg*innen ihre Embleme miteinander verglichen und Hypothesen zur Bedeutung und Symbolik der Embleme aufgestellt haben. Die Semantik der Embleme bzw. wie genau diese zu lesen sind, wurde in einem der Vorträge im ersten Panel der Konferenz zum Zusammenhang von Kognition und Psycholinguistik enthüllt. In der Präsentation wurde der Schlüssel der Visualisierung vorgestellt und die Frage beantwortet, wie divers das Feld der Konferenzteilnehmer*innen ist und wie sich intra- und interpersonelle Diversitätsaspekte in Graphiken visualisieren lassen. Die personalisierten Embleme wurden von den Teilnehmer*innen während der gesamten Dauer der Konferenz getragen. Die Aktivierungsaktivität sorgte für Aufregung und Neugier weit über das Konferenzfoyer und sogar über die Dauer der dreitägigen Konferenz hinaus, sodass die Datenporträts zu bedeutungsvollen Souvenirs bzw. Andenken an die Veranstaltung wurden. Manche Konferenzteilnehmer*innen, die im Vorfeld nicht an der Umfrage teilgenommen hatten, kontaktierten mich anschließend per E-Mail, um ihre personalisierten Embleme nachträglich zu erhalten.

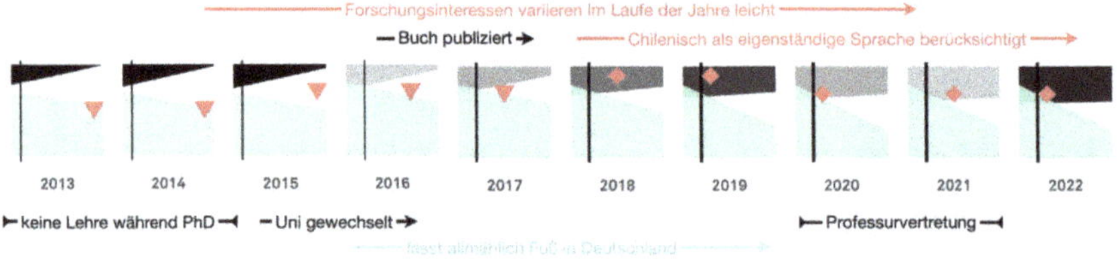

Abbildung 26: Darstellung meines Emblems über ein Jahrzehnt. Änderungen in den Metriken verändern das allgemeine Bild

Die Embleme können zudem auch zeitliche Veränderungen anzeigen, indem die dargestellten Informationen in regelmäßigen Abständen aktualisiert werden. Ein Beispiel dafür wird in Abbildung 26 mit der Entwicklung des Emblems der Autorin über die letzten Jahre gegeben. Die Abbildung zeigt ein Jahrzehnt zusammengefasst in zehn Embleme geordnet von links nach rechts, die jeweils für ein Jahr stehen. Es werden Muster sichtbar, beispielsweise kann anhand der Farbe des obersten grauen Poligons nachverfolgt werden, wie sich die Verteilung der Arbeitszeit im Laufe der Jahre von einer forschungsintensiven Promotion zu einer durch eine von einer intensiven Lehrtätigkeit geprägten Professurvertretung verändert. Es kann auch beobachtet werden, wie nach der Publikation der Dissertation im Jahr 2017 der Doktortitel erworben wurde, was sich in den Emblemen als eine breitere Laufbahnlinie widerspiegelt.

10.2 Arbeitsgruppen

Für die Visualisierung von Gruppen bieten sich zwei Optionen an: Die Mitglieder der Gruppe entweder als nebeneinander aufgereihte Fliesen darzustellen (Abbildung 27, links) oder die gesamte Gruppe als eine Summe von sich überlappenden und transparenten Kacheln zu repräsentieren (Abbildung 27, rechts). Die erste Option bietet erheblich mehr Lesbarkeit, während die zweite

Option visuell ästhetischere Ergebnisse liefert. Auf diese Weise könnte jedes Team durch ein komplexes, eigenes Emblem dargestellt werden, das gleichzeitig die Teammitglieder und ihre thematischen Schwerpunkte visualisiert.

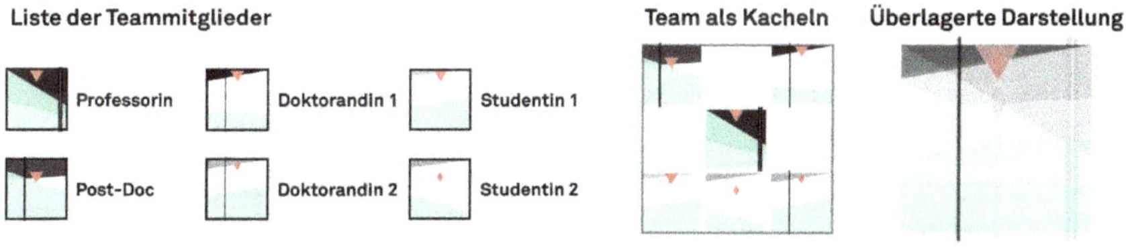

Abbildung 27: Alternativdarstellungen für dieselbe Forschungsgruppe. Hier beispielhaft mit sechs Teammitgliedern

Diese Darstellung kann auch verwendet werden, um gruppenübergreifende Teams zu repräsentieren oder sogar Gruppen von Kolleg*innen unterschiedlicher Institutionen, die gemeinsam an einem Projekt arbeiten. Mitglieder anderer Institutionen könnten z. B. dadurch gekennzeichnet werden, dass im Emblem die beiden Hauptfarben der anderen Einrichtung anstelle der institutionellen Farben der TU Dortmund verwendet werden. Obwohl große wissenschaftliche Errungenschaften oft als Einzelleistungen angesehen werden, handelt es sich meist um kollektive Leistungen, und dies sollte auch so anerkannt und dargestellt werden.

10.3 Visualisierung von Kolleg*innen in einem geteilten Forschungsfeld

Alternativ zu der Darstellung einzelner Personen könnte eine weitere Visualisierung alle Personen an einer Forschungseinrichtung aufgreifen: Bei dieser Darstellung wird das Institut als ein quadratisches Feld repräsentiert, in der die vier Ecken für die Forschungsprofile Kognition, Literatur, Medien und Sprache stehen. Die am Institut tätigen Personen werden innerhalb dieses Feldes als Kacheln dargestellt, die Position der Kacheln in Bezug auf die vier thematischen Schwerpunkte spiegelt die Gewichtung der Forschungsinteressen seitens der Kolleg*innen wider. Auf diese Weise stellt diese Visualisierung des Instituts, die ich „Forschungsfeld" genannt habe, jede Forscher*in als ein komplexes Konstrukt im breiteren Institutssystem dar, hebt die Ähnlichkeiten zwischen den Individuen innerhalb des Netzwerks hervor und zeigt, wie sich die einzelnen Individuen zueinander verhalten. Abbildung 27 gibt das Forschungsfeld wieder.

Diese Visualisierung kann auch hervorheben, wer an ähnlichen Themen arbeitet und so Möglichkeiten für neue Kooperationen schaffen. Als Beispiel werden in Abbildung 28 die Teilnehmer*innen der Konferenz im Forschungsfeld platziert. Eine klare Erkenntnis dieser Visualisierung ist, dass sich fast jede*r Wissenschaftler*in als interdisziplinär (bzw. interthematisch) ansieht.

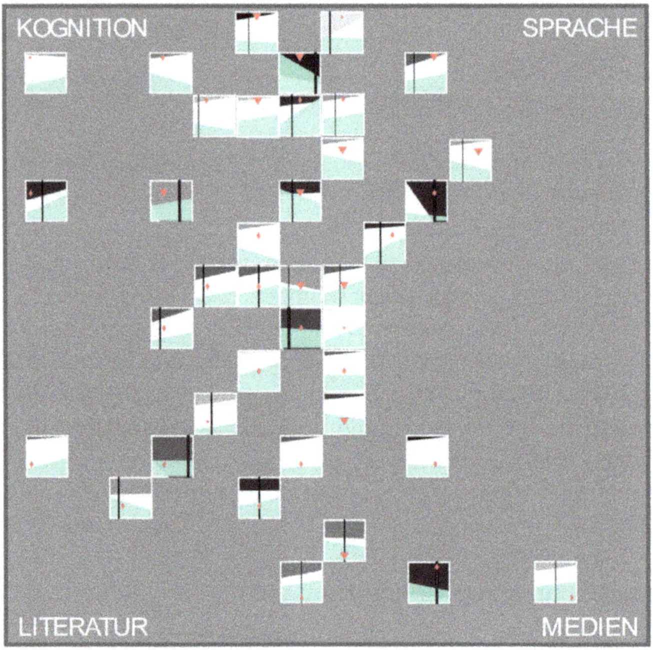

Abbildung 28: *Die Forschungsfeld-Visualisierung.* Mehrere Wissenschaftler*innen werden auf dem Feld positioniert, sodass die Mitarbeiter*innen, welche dieselbe Gewichtung von Interessen haben, in einem Cluster angeordnet werden

10.4 Research-Scooper (das „akademische Minesweeper")

Embleme können sogar auf spielerische Art und Weise verwendet oder in Spiele integriert werden. Im Journalismus ist ein *Scoop* (englisch *to scoop*, „ausschöpfen, abräumen") eine Nachricht, über die eine Journalist*in oder eine Nachrichtenorganisation vor anderen berichtet, und die von außergewöhnlicher Originalität, Bedeutung, Überraschung, Aufregung oder Geheimhaltung geprägt ist. In der Wissenschaft bedeutet ein *Scoop,* dass eine Erkenntnis von einer anderen Forschungsgruppe geklaut und im Anschluss daran als die eigene Idee veröffentlicht wird, wodurch die anderen die wissenschaftliche Priorität und Anerkennung erhalten. Entsprechend möchten Wissenschaftler*innen vermeiden, *gescooped* zu werden. Diese Situationen sollen mittels eines Computer-Spiels, welches die Embleme integriert, inszeniert werden. Das Spiel ist in Anlehnung an *Minesweeper* („Minenräumer") aufgebaut. Ziel des Spiels ist es, ein rechteckiges Spielfeld mit versteckten „Wissenschaftler*innen" zu räumen, ohne auf die Felder zu kommen, die schon von Kolleg*innen besetzt sind, wobei Hinweise auf die Anzahl der benachbarten Wissenschaftler*innen in jedem Feld helfen. Bei *Research-Scooper* werden die Wissenschaftler*innen, die von ihren Emblemen repräsentiert werden, über ein in Zellen unterteiltes Spielfeld nach dem Prinzip der Forschungsfeld-Visualisierung verstreut.

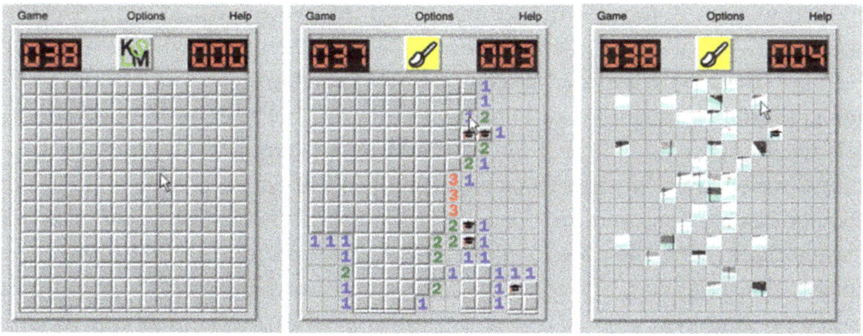

Abbildung 29: Drei Beispiele für das Interface des Spiels *Research-Scooper* basierend auf Windows' *Minesweeper*

Um ein neues Spiel zu beginnen, klickt man auf die Schaufel oben in der Mitte. Das Spielfeld ist zu Spielbeginn komplett bedeckt. Man klickt mit der linken Maustaste auf ein zufälliges Feld, um ein Feld freizulegen. Ein nummeriertes Feld zeigt an, wie viele durch Kolleg*innen besetzte Felder an dieses Feld angrenzen (entweder oben, unten, rechts, links oder diagonal). Man klickt mit der rechten Maustaste auf ein Feld, um eine Stelle zu markieren, an der man eine tätige Kolleg*in vermutet. Dann wird dieses Feld mittels einer Zipfelmütze gekennzeichnet. Mit Hilfe von Verstand und Deduktion findet der/die Spieler*in anhand der bekannten Informationen aus den aufgedeckten Zahlen heraus, wo genau die Kolleg*innen schon tätig sind und kann so in der akademischen *Terra Ignota* in Ruhe weiterforschen. Das Spiel wird gewonnen, wenn alle anderen Kolleg*innen richtig markiert wurden und keine weiteren bedeckten Felder vorhanden sind. Abbildung 29 zeigt, wie eine Partie zu Anfang, in der Mitte und am Ende des Spiels aussehen würde. Dies wäre eine tatsächlich umsetzbare und spielbare Version von „*Research-Scooper*".

11. Fazit

In diesem Beitrag wurden neue Datenembleme präsentiert, die individuelle Informationen aus den persönlichen und beruflichen Sphären von Diversitätsforscher*innen enkodieren. Diese Embleme lassen sich in einer Taxonomie von ähnlichen maßgeschneiderten Visualisierungen einordnen. Es wurde gezeigt, dass solche Visualisierungen eine große Bandbreite aufweisen: An einem Ende des Spektrums stehen die Visualisierungen zwischen klassischen Graphiken und dekorativen Plaketten, wie die Visualisierung von MyMuesli, die letztendlich wie ein Radarplot funktioniert oder die Wetterporträts von Nicholas Rougeux. Am anderen Ende befinden sich Visualisierungen wie die von Giorgia Lupi, die zugunsten der Betonung von Gefühlen, wie z. B. Verspieltheit, auf Lesbarkeit verzichten. Abbildung 30 gibt die behandelten Visualisierungen wieder, geordnet nach ihrer Ähnlichkeit zu standardisierten Visualisierungsformen. Standardisierte Visualisierungen können sich die Nutzer*innen leichter erschließen, weil ihre visuelle Grammatik schon bekannt ist. Von den dargestellten Beispielen sind die Mitgliederembleme der *Data Visualization Society* den hier vorgestellten Datenemblemen am ähnlichsten. Gemeinsam haben die Embleme auch, dass ihr Design es ermöglicht, sie nicht nur für eine Einzeldarstellung zu nutzen, sondern auch zur Darstellung von Gruppen.

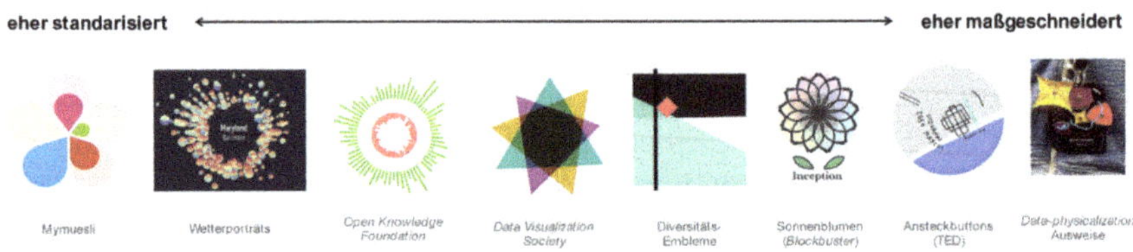

Abbildung 30: Die behandelten maßgeschneiderten Visualisierungen geordnet nach ihrem Standardisierungsgrad. Die Diversitätsembleme befinden sich etwa in der Mitte

Ziel dieses Projektes war es, eine Visualisierung der persönlichen und beruflichen Eigenschaften von Diversitätsforscher*innen zu erstellen, die zu Zwecken der Reflektion und Selbstdarstellung verwendet werden kann. Es wurde durch eine Kombination aus Datenvisualisierung, mittelalterlicher Heraldik, *the quantified Self* und *Branding* eine maßgeschneiderte Selbstdarstellungsmöglichkeit für Diversitätswissenschaftler*innen erstellt. Die Embleme haben eine vielfältige Nutzbarkeit: Sie können reale Informationen in verständliche Glyphen umwandeln, sind personalisierbar, verschlüsseln biographische Informationen auf eine undurchsichtige Weise, zeigen die Vielfalt innerhalb des Forschungsbereiches in einer ansprechenden Weise, fördern die Motivation sowie die Selbstreflexion, erlauben die Identifizierung von Mustern in der beschriebenen Zielgruppe und könnten Kolleg*innen helfen, zukünftige Kooperationspartner*innen zu finden. Außerdem wurden mehreren Verwendungsmöglichkeiten für die Embleme vorgeschlagen. Die Datenembleme stellen einen persönlichen und menschenwürdigen Ansatz für die Darstellung von persönlichen Informationen dar. Hiermit leisten sie einen wichtigen Beitrag zur Weiterentwicklung von durch den *Data Humansim* geprägten Formen der Datenvisulisierung.

Ein weiteres übergeordnetes Ziel des Projektes war es, eine identitätsstiftende Visualisierung der Arbeit der Kolleg*innen im Bereich der Diversitätsstudien zu erstellen, welche ein modernes Konzept einer Universitätsgemeinschaft widerspiegelt: Akademische Teams sollten, nach dem Verständnis der Diversitätsstudien, in erster Linie vielfältig sein, anstatt ausschließlich auf eine hohe Produktivität Wert zu legen, um unser Wissen und Verständnis über den Menschen und die Gesellschaft zu erweitern und auch zu relativieren. Multilingualität und Internationalisierung haben im Zeitalter der Europäischen Union mit ihren 24 Amtssprachen sowie des Bologna-Prozesses, der auf die Schaffung eines einheitlichen Europäischen Hochschulraums ausgerichtet ist und mit einer höheren internationalen Mobilität der Studierenden und Wissenschaftler*innen verbunden ist, an Wichtigkeit gewonnen. Entsprechend bin ich persönlich der Überzeugung, dass gute, moderne Wissenschaft anstatt eines wettbewerbsorientierten Arbeitsumfeldes eine kooperative, faire und unterstützende Gemeinschaft braucht, die alle Forscher*innen auf allen Ausbildungsstufen (auch Student*innen) wertschätzt. Diese Werte sind in den Designprozess der Embleme eingeflossen. Gleichzeitig können die Diversitätsembleme und ihre vielseitigen Nutzungsmöglichkeiten zur Herstellung eines kooperativen akademischen Arbeitsumfeldes beitragen, da sie den Fokus auf die persönlichen und beruflichen Fähigkeiten und Erfahrungen der einzelnen Individuen und deren Beitrag zum Team lenken.

Ein Schlüsselkonzept, das aus diesem Beitrag hervorgeht, ist das Potenzial des personalisierten Emblems als ein mächtiges erzählerisches Mittel, was es ermöglicht sehr spezifisch über die Menschen, die hinter diesen Daten stehen, zu berichten. Da wir mit Hilfe von Technologien immer mehr persönliche Daten mit gesellschaftlicher Relevanz sammeln, entsteht hier eine Chance und vielleicht sogar die Pflicht, im Sinne des *Data Humanism* mit diesen Daten umzugehen und mehr Storytelling in die Darstellung der Daten zu integrieren, um sie verständlicher und emotional relevanter zu machen. „Geschichten sind einfach Daten mit einer Seele." (Brown 2010). Die hier vorgestellten Diversitätsembleme liefern ein Beispiel wie eine solche Geschichte anhand der individuellen Daten von Mitarbeiter*innen eines Instituts für Diversitätsforschung erzählt werden kann. Die so gewonnenen Erkenntnisse über die Potentiale von Datenemblemen lassen sich auch auf andere Forschungsbereiche übertragen.

Das Gebiet der Datenvisualisierung entwickelt sich zurzeit rasant und in diesem Prozess sind nicht nur die Datenwissenschaftler*innen einbezogen, sondern auch die Öffentlichkeit und die Subjekte (also potenziell wir alle). Wissenschaftler*innen aus Psychologie, Kognitionswissenschaften und Design haben in den letzten Jahren große Fortschritte errungen, empirisch und experimentell besser zu verstehen, welche Arten von Daten aussagekräftig und verständlich sind. Auch die Nutzer*innen solcher Datenvisualisierungen, sowohl Expert*innen als auch Lai*innen, werden immer datenkompetenter. Solange sich das Verständnis der Betrachter*innen für das visuelle Vokabular zusammen mit dem der (Daten-)Wissenschaftler*innen weiterentwickelt, werden Datenembleme weiterhin genutzt werden und nützlich sein. Allgemein haben datenbasierte Embleme noch nicht weit verbreitete Anwendung gefunden, wahrscheinlich weil die allgemeine Datenkompetenz nicht hoch genug ist, sodass sich nicht genügend Nutzer*innen die Embleme selbstständig schnell erschließen können. Da jedoch Datenkompetenz immer häufiger verlangt und auch gefördert wird, beispielsweise in Form von grundlegenden Statistikkenntnissen und allgemeinen Lesefertigkeiten im Umgang mit Graphen in einer immer breiteren Auswahl von Studiengängen, können wir davon ausgehen, dass diese Art von datenbasierten Emblemen in naher Zukunft häufiger Anwendung finden wird. Ferner finden immer mehr *Data Scientists* neue Wege, um Daten auf nützlichere, intuitivere und verständlichere Weise in Datenemblemen, die den hier vorgestellten Diversitätsemblemen ähneln, zu kodieren.

Datenbasierte Embleme werden immer beliebter, aber sind sie auch gute Visualisierungen? Wenn es um Präzision und Genauigkeit geht, können sie nicht gegen traditionelle Ansätze wie z. B. *Small Multiples* antreten. Sie sind auch nicht besonders geeignet, um Trends sichtbar zu machen oder *Clusterings* zu enthüllen. Auch bei der Kodierung von Topologien, Hierarchien oder geographischen Daten sind ihre Anwendungsmöglichkeiten eher beschränkt. Jedoch können Embleme zu einer Art Signatur mit einem höheren emotionalen Gehalt für Menschen und sogar ganze Gruppen werden, die täglich mit Daten arbeiten und ein natürliches Interesse an dieser Thematik haben. Sie können verwendet werden, um die Marke und Identität der Gruppe zu stärken. Das sind würdige Ziele, auch wenn es dabei nicht um die Kommunikation oder die Gewinnung von Erkenntnissen geht, den eher traditionellen Zwecken der Datenvisualisierung. Datengesteuerte Embleme sind wertvoll und nützlich, da sie einfach Spaß machen und die Menschen begeistern. Es gibt keinen wirkungsvolleren Akt im Design, als sein Publikum zu erreichen und es glücklich zu machen. Dies zieht die Aufmerksamkeit des Publikums an und die Neugier kann auf diese Weise sehr wohl dazu führen, dass Menschen über das hinter den Daten stehende System nachdenken. Hierdurch können Wissenschaftler*innen auf eine unerwartete Art und Weise neue Erkenntnisse und Interesse an neuen Forschungsfragen gewinnen, die sich ohne die Perspektive der Datenembleme nie offenbart hätten.

12. English summary: Diversity emblems: representations of personal data

Diversity emblems as individualized graphic representations of personal data in the context of Data Humanism

Data emblems are personalized graphic representations of personal information. These have gained popularity in recent years, especially on the Internet. They are used as avatars in digital as well as in analog spaces, such as conventions or conferences. Data emblems are part of a millennia old tradition consisting of using heraldic devices or symbolic objects as a distinctive badge of a nation, organization, or family. Archeological and historical remains show that emblems have been used continuously across cultures for purpose of representation and recognition since the beginning of civilization until today. Some of the earlier examples of emblems are old Egyptian Serekh and Cartouches, while modern examples are found integrated in the flags of some nations like Portugal or Kenia or in the branding of sports teams and other brands. In this paper, elements of data visualization, medieval heraldry, the quantified self and branding are combined to propose digital emblems that have been specifically designed to represent individuals working in the field of diversity studies. This paper explains which information has been pictorially encoded in the emblems and which variables have been operationalized. It also discusses the process of designing the emblems and possible uses. The emblems have been created based on personal and academic information including identity markers, work experience, language use, and thematic research interests. The personalized emblems are drawn according to a predefined visual system that reflects the personal background as well as information about the academic career of a person, including but not revealing private or sensitive information that would not be found in a standard academic curriculum vitae.

The contribution of the paper is not the analysis of the data but rather a discussion of the design process of the visualization. Unlike conventional visualizations, the aim here is not to present the information as clearly and legibly as possible, but to find a balance between legibility, protection of private information (which results in illegibility) and aesthetic appearance. When using the emblems to visualize several scholars, some stereotypical patterns may emerge. Some of these stereotypes include figures such as the researcher, the student, an old hand, the genius, the polyglot, the one with traditional family values, the first generation academic, the academic with a migrant background, the one with impostor syndrome, and the conlanger. A general pattern that an analysis of the emblems has shown is that almost every colleague sees themselves as an interdisciplinary, or rather, in this case, interthematic scholar.

The overall goal of the project is not ranking or quantifying scientists or their work, like a publimetric project would do, but rather designing identity. The main intended use of the emblems is to use them as an avatar in virtual or physical spaces in order to represent a researcher, for example instead of a traditional profile picture. The paper presents and discusses some other, less straight-forward and more creative applications of the emblems, such as the representation of individual scholars, whole research groups, or even an entire "research field", including information about which scholars inside a group have the same or similar shared research interest. One very creative application is a retro computer game designed to help scientists avoid research scoops. The emblems have the potential to be used as an analysis tool in the future, but in their conception, they are rather meant to encourage reflection on one's own personal and professional profiles as well as those of other colleagues, and thereby foment connection between colleagues with similar profiles within the diversity studies research community. Readers are invited to reflect on how personal characteristics may impact research in the field of diversity studies.

Literaturverzeichnis

AccuratStudio (2017). Data portraits at ted 2017, abgerufen am 30.01.2023 unter: https://accurat.it/work/ted-target

Arnheim, Rudolf (1969). *Visual Thinking*. Berkeley, CA: University of California Press.

Benoit, G. (2016). The 'beautiful' in Information: Thoughts about Visual Literacy and Aesthetics. *Journal of Visual Literacy*, 35(1), 60–78.

Bremer, N./Wu, S. (2021). *Data Sketches: A Journey of Imagination, Exploration, and Beautiful Data Visualizations.* Boca Raton, FL: CRC Press.

Brown, B. (2010). *The Power of Vulnerability* [TED Talk], abgerufen am 31.01.2023 unter: https://www.ted.com/talks/brene_brown_the_power_of_vulnerability

Burke, B./Thomas, B./Arnold, R./James, C./Marti, D. (1991). *Educating for a Change.* Toronto: Between The Lines.

Cairo, A. (2012). *The Functional Art: An Introduction to Information Graphics and Visualization.* Berkeley, CA: New Riders.

Cairo, A. (2019). *How Charts Lie: Getting Smarter about Visual Information.* New York: W. W. Norton & Company.

Carlson, J./Johnston, L. (2015). *Data Information Literacy: Librarians, Data, and the Education of a New Generation of Researchers.* West Lafayette, IN: Purdue University Press.

Cesal, A. (2019). *The Data Visualization Society Logo*, abgerufen am 30.01.2023 unter: www.datavisualizationsociety.org

Cox, N. J./Jones, K. (1981). Exploratory Data Analysis. In N. Wrigley/R. J. Bennett (Hrsg.), *Quantitative Geography: A British View* (S. 135–143). London: Routledge.

Crameri, F. (2022). Academic profiling, instead of ranking, with ProAc (0.1.0). Zenodo. https://doi.org/10.5281/zenodo.6569100.

Delucchi Danhier, R. (2017). *Weganweisungen im Deutschen und Spanischen. Eine Vergleichsanalyse unter Anwendung von Visualisierungen.* München: Dr. Hut.

Delucchi Danhier, R./Mertins, B. (2018). Psycholinguistische Grundlagen der Inklusion. Schwerpunkt Bilingualismus. In S. Hußmann/B. Welzel (Hrsg.), *Dortmunder Profil für inklusionsorientierte Lehrerinnen-und Lehrerbildung* (S. 161–178). Münster: Waxmann.

D'Ignazio, C. (2017). Creative Data Literacy: Bridging the Gap between the Data-haves and data-have nots. *Information Design Journal* 23(1), 6–18.

Fischer, R. (2005). *Die Ortsnamen der Länder Brandenburg und Berlin. Alter – Herkunft – Bedeutung. brandenburgische historische studien 13* Berlin: be.bra Wissenschaft Verlag.

Franconeri, S. L./Padilla, L. M./Shah, P. D./Zacks, J. M./Hullman, J. (2021). The Science of Visual Data Communication: What Works. *Psychological Science in the Public Interest,* 22 (3), 110–161.

Friel, S. N./Curcio, F. R./Bright, G. W. (2001). Making Sense of Graphs: Critical Factors Influencing Comprehension and Instructional Implications. *Journal for Research in Mathematics Education,* 32 (2), 124–158.

Hammond, W. G./Scull, C. (1995). *J.R.R. Tolkien, Artist and Illustrator.* Boston: Houghton Milin.

Hartmann, J. (2016): The Japanese Mon and the European Coats of Arms – a Comparative Study. *Armas e Troféus* 18 (2016), 87–113.

Hawley, W./Chappelear, K. (1976). *Mon: The Japanese Family Crest.* Hollywood: Hawley.

Heer, J./Bostock, M./Ogievetskey, V. (2010). A Tour through the Visualization Zoo. *Communications of the ACM* 53 (6), 59–67.

Hriban, C. (2011). The Eye and the Tree. The Semantics of Middle-earth Heraldry. *Hither Shore* 8, 198–211.

Jones, R. (2008). Identifying the Warrior on the Pre-Heraldic Battlefield. *Anglo-Norman studies 30: Proceedings of the Battle Conference 2007* (S. 154–167).

Judeikyte, E., abgerufen am 30.01.2023 unter www.evelinajudeikyte.com.

Kleiner, B./Graedel, T. E. (1980). Exploratory Data Analysis in the Geophysical Sciences. *Reviews of Geophysics* 18, 699–717.

Koblin, A. (2011). *Visualizing Ourselves … with Crowd-sourced Data.* [TED Talk].

Kolence, K. W. (1973). The Software Empiricist. *SIGMETRICS Performance Evaluation Review* 2 (2), 31–36.

Lupi, G. (2017). *Data Humanism: The Revolutionary Future of Data Visualization.* PrintMag.

Lupi, G. (2020). My 2020 in data (so far). *At home. The New York Times.* November 22, 2020.

Lupi, G./Posavec, S. (2016). *Dear Data.* London: Princeton Architectural Press.

Meirelles, I. (2013). *Design for Information: An Introduction to the Histories, Theories, and Best Practices Behind Effective Information Visualizations.* Beverly: Rockport Publishers.

Munzner, T. (2014). *Visualization Analysis and Design. AK Peters Visualization Series.* Boca Raton: CRC Press.

Mymuesli, abgerufen am 30.01.2023 unter www.mymuesli.ch.

Panagiotidou, G./Görücü, S./Vande Moere, A. (2020). Data Badges: Making an Academic Profile through a DIY Wearable Physicalization. *IEEE Computer Graphics and Applications* 40 (6), 5160 ff.

Pastoureau, M. (2003). *Traité d'héraldique.* Paris: Picard.

Patel, A. (2003). Language, Music, Syntax and the Brain. *Nature Neuroscience* 6, 674–681.

Petersen, N. H. (2009). Medievalism and Medieval Reception: A Terminological Question. *Studies in Medievalism* 17, 36–37.

Plaisant, C./Shneiderman, B./Mushlin, R. (1998). An Information Architecture to Support the Visualization of Personal Histories. *Information Management and Processing* 34 (5), 581–597.

Rekimoto, J./Miyaki, T./Ishizawa, T. (2007). LifeTag: WiFi-Based Continuous Location Logging for Life Pattern Analysis. In Hightower, J./ Schiele, B./Strang, T. (Hrsg.), *Location- and Context-Awareness. LoCA 2007. Lecture Notes in Computer Science*, vol. 4718 . Berlin, Heidelberg: Springer.

Sokil, J. P./Osorio, L. (2022). Producción científica en el campo de los estudios de género: analisis de revistas seleccionadas de Web Of Science (2008–2018). *Revista Española de Documentación Científica* 45 (1), e320.

Suckale-Redlefsen, G. (1986). *Der Buchschmuck zum Psalmenkommentar des Petrus Lombardus in Bamberg* (Msc. Bibl. 59). Bamberg: Staatsbibliothek.

TU Dortmund (2017). *Corporate Design, Richtlinien zur Gestaltung.* Stand 11/2017.

Tukey, J. W. (1970). *Exploratory Data Analysis.* Boston: Addison–Wesley.

Tygel, A. F./Kirsch, R. (2016). Contributions of Paulo Freire to a Critical Data Literacy: A Popular Education Approach. *The Journal of Community Informatics*, 12 (3), 108–121.

Wendehorst, A. (1986). Wer konnte im Mittelalter lesen und schreiben? In Fried, J. (Hrsg.), *Schulen und Studium im sozialen Wandel des hohen und späten Mittelalters.* Sigmaringen: Jan Thorbecke Verlag. S. 9–33.

Willens, H. (2008). *Les textes des sarcophages et la démocratie: Éléments d'une histoire culturelle du Moyen Empire égyptien.* Paris: Cybele.

Cognitio

Kognitions- und neurowissenschaftliche Beiträge zur natürlichen Sprachverarbeitung

Herausgegeben von Michael Schecker

Die Bände 1–13 sind bei anderen Verlagen erschienen.

Band 14 Günter Kochendörfer (Hrsg.): Sprache – interdisziplinär. Beiträge zur kognitiven Linguistik, Neurolinguistik und Neuropsychologie. 2007.

Band 15 Anna Jaremkiewicz: Aufmerksamkeit und Sprache. Kindliche Entwicklungsstörungen und ihr wechselseitiger Bedingungszusammenhang. 2007.

Band 16 Sung Eun Lee: Bedeutungsbezüge im Rahmen der zentral-auditiven Verarbeitung. Eine EKP-Studie zu Entwicklungsschritten und -störungen bei 6- bis 10-jährigen Kindern. 2010.

Band 17 Séverine Adam (Hrsg.): ‚Informationsstrukturen' im gesteuerten Spracherwerb. Französisch – Deutsch kontrastiv. 2013.

Band 18 Séverine Adam / Daniel Jacob / Michael Schecker (Hrsg.): Informationsstrukturen in Kontrast. Strukturen, Kompositionen und Strategien. 2015.

Band 19 Carsten Kochler / Tanja Rinker / Eberhard Schulz (Hrsg.): Neurolinguistik, Klinische Linguistik, Sprachpathologie. 2017

Herausgegeben von Tanja Rinker, Barbara Mertins und Sung-Eun Lee

Band 20 Barbara Mertins / Renate Delucchi Danhier (eds.): Diversity in Cognition. 2023.

www.peterlang.com